CLINICAL GUIDE

SKIN &
WOUND
CARE

Sixth Edition

CLINICAL GUIDE

SKIN & WOUND CARE

Sixth Edition

Cathy Thomas Hess,
RN, BSN, CWOCN

President
Wound Care Strategies, Inc.
Harrisburg, Pa.

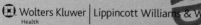

Wolters Kluwer | Lippincott Williams & Wilkins
Health
Philadelphia · Baltimore · New York · London
Buenos Aires · Hong Kong · Sydney · Tokyo

STAFF

Executive Publisher
Judith A. Schilling McCann, RN, MSN

Senior Acquisitions Editor
Margaret Zuccarini

Editorial Director
H. Nancy Holmes

Art Director
Mary Ludwicki

Editorial Project Manager
Ann E. Houska

Editors
Linda Hager,
Elizabeth Jacqueline Mills

Copyeditors
Nicholas J. Bilotta, Laura M. Healy,
Marna Poole

Designer
Joseph John Clark

Digital Composition Services
Diane Paluba (manager),
Joyce Rossi Biletz, Donna S. Morris

Manufacturing
Beth J. Welsh

Editorial Assistants
Megan L. Aldinger, Karen J. Kirk,
Jeri O'Shea, Susan Rainey,
Linda K. Ruhf

Indexer
Barbara E. Hodgson

Library of Congress Cataloging-in-Publication Data
Hess, Cathy Thomas, 1961-
    Skin & wound care / Cathy Thomas Hess. — 6th ed.
        p. ; cm. — (Clinical guide)
    Rev. ed. of: Wound care / Cathy Thomas Hess. 5th ed. c2005
    Includes bibliographical references and index.
    1. Wounds and injuries—Nursing—Handbooks, manuals, etc. 2. Wound healing—Handbooks, manuals, etc. I. Hess, Cathy Thomas, 1961- . Wound care. II. Title. III. Title: Skin & wound care. IV. Series.
    [DNLM: 1. Wounds and Injuries—nursing—Handbooks. 2. Bandages—Handbooks. 3. Skin Care—methods—Handbooks. 4. Skin Ulcer—nursing—Handbooks. 5. Wound Healing—Handbooks. WY 49 H586w 2008]
    RD95.H47 2008
    617.1'4—dc22
    ISBN-13: 978-1-58255-688-8 (alk. paper)
    ISBN-10: 1-58255-688-1 (alk. paper)   2007

CONTENTS

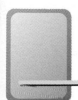

Contributors

David R. Hoffman, Esq.
Private Practice
Philadelphia

N. Blair Hughes, MHS, PT, CWS
Director, Wound and Hyperbaric
Services
Frederick Memorial Healthcare
System
Frederick, Md.

Lucinda J. Rook, RN, CPC
Director, Auditing and
Compliance
Wound Care Strategies, Inc
Harrisburg, Pa.

Susie Seaman, NP, MSN, CWOCN
Sharp Rees-Stealy Medical Group
Wound Clinic
San Diego, Calif.

Jennifer T. Trent, MD
Dermatologist
Private Practice
Sarasota, Fla.

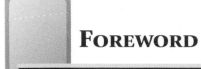

FOREWORD

Chronic wounds exact an emotional toll from the patient and caregivers. Frustration and confusion continue to arise among clinicians when trying to choose which dressing to use on a certain wound type, when to change to another dressing to continue the wound healing process, how to illustrate the wound's progress through appropriate documentation, and how to benchmark outcomes based on care practices. Some of these answers lie within the delicate balance of art and science. *Art* refers to the team member's skill and technique in applying the preferred modality for managing the skin and wound care patient. *Science* refers to the team member's knowledge and understanding of the disease process and its correct treatment. *Art and science*, the fundamental tools of skin and wound healing, have a direct impact on the clinical and financial outcomes of the patient.

The sixth edition of this book has elevated itself in many ways, continuing to support the "delicate balance of art and science." The name of the book has been changed to *Clinical Guide: Skin & Wound Care*, focusing on the importance of caring for the largest organ of the body—the skin—as well as the wound. The reader will welcome the new addition of skin care products that complement and complete the importance of a skin care formulary: skin cleansers, moisture barriers, antifungal and antimicrobial treatments, therapeutic moisturizers, liquid skin protectants, and others. Many new wound care dressings, drugs, and devices added to the book provide cutting-edge choices for formulary development.

Part 1 of the book covers the fundamentals of skin care and wound prevention and treatment modalities. Chapter 1, "Skin care and wound prevention strategies," provides incidence of chronic wounds, anatomy and physiology of the skin, changes that occur in the skin's structure such as xerosis and pruritus, and the ramifications that can occur to the skin due to urinary and fecal incontinence. The chapter instructs the reader on how to establish a skin care formulary and prevention strategies. The chapter also reviews the wound healing principles that occur during the four phases of healing. Local and systemic factors affecting wound healing mechanisms of wound repair, and wound healing complications are reviewed.

Chapter 2, "Assessing and documenting chronic wounds," reviews the importance of assessing the patient, obtaining a history, performing a physical assessment, additional qualifying factors for wound management and nutritional assessment. The chapter stresses the importance of developing documentation guidelines which provide direction for appropriate treatment decisions, evaluation of the healing process, support for reimbursement claims, and a defense for litigation.

Chapter 3, "Types of chronic wounds," provides the pathogenesis, assessment skills, diagnostic testing, and management modalities necessary to oversee patients with the four most common chronic wound types: venous, arterial, diabetic, and pressure ulcers. Useful tools for these wound subsets are incorporated in this chapter to assist the health care professional to create the best care plan for successful outcomes.

Chapter 4, "Laboratory values in chronic wound management," provides the reader with an overview of the common chronic wounds and the laboratory values that can be used to assist in accurately diagnosing those wounds.

Chapter 5, "Developing a skin and wound care formulary," details the need to have a process-driven approach for skin and wound care. In this chapter, the seven skin and wound care processes and their targeted goals are discussed. These important goals include performing a needs assessment, developing an operational formulary, developing a skin and wound care product formulary, developing documentation pathways, developing educational and competency validation pathways, identifying levels of practicing professionals and developing patient educational pathways. This chapter is filled with examples of tools to move these processes forward and assist the reader in understanding the critical elements of formulary development.

Chapter 6, "Tissue load management," focuses solely on the importance of successful pressure ulcer management that includes prevention, relieving pressure, restoring circulation, managing the wound and minimizing related disorders and properly applying support surfaces and off-loading devices to enhance the healing of pressure ulcers and help prevent new ones from developing.

Chapter 7, "Wound care and the regulatory process," details the importance of accurate documentation to support the payment received for the work performed. This chapter specifically reviews the importance of developing and implementing a compliance plan, establishing policies and procedures to support your work, reviewing the importance of internal and external auditing and monitoring and education for providers. The chapter continues by discussing the differences between Medicare, Medicaid, and third-party payers and provides detailed documentation guidelines when caring for individuals with skin and wound care concerns. Many tools are provided to assist the reader in understanding these important concepts.

Part 2 is a practical, quick reference guide to a comprehensive range of the most up-to-date skin and wound care products. Skin care products are well organized for the reader and hundreds of wound care products, primary and secondary dressings, and drugs are arranged alphabetically by category. Each product category begins with a category description, including the action, indication, advantages, and disadvantages of the product category type. Product classification billing codes—the Healthcare Common Procedure Coding System (HCPCS)—are also reviewed with each category and each product, as appropriate.

Each wound care product profile describes the product in detail, including the product's form, available sizes and actions, indications and contraindications, and application and removal instructions. Photographs of the product are displayed on each page, whenever possible. Every attempt has been made to accurately detail the product's information; however, it remains the clinician's responsibility to review each product's insert before use of the product to ensure accurate and timely information.

Part 3 presents additional dressings and products for effective skin and wound management. This section details compression bandage systems, a variety of gauze dressings, tapes, wound cleansers, and pouches. HCPCS codes and sizes are displayed for each of these products when available.

The book concludes with appendices, which serve the health care professional in a number of ways. Tools such as the body mass index, a risk assessment tool, diabetic foot classification scale, laboratory tests to rule out atypical causes of leg ulcers, ankle-brachial index for patients with diabetes, summary of Wound, Ostomy, and Continence Nurses guidelines for pressure ulcer prevention and management and treatment algorithms for pressure, venous, arterial, and diabetic ulcers are illustrated in this section. A comprehensive list of the manufacturers' addresses and websites is included, along with a detailed reference section.

Clinical Guide: Skin & Wound Care, Sixth Edition, continues to prove to be an essential skin and wound care reference for all team members. Coupled with the up-front educational chapters is the skin and wound care product selection guide by category. Use this book as a bedside or desk reference when caring for your patient population.

Robert S. Kirsner, MD, PhD
Professor and Vice Chairman
Department of Dermatology and Cutaneous Surgery
University of Miami (Florida) Miller School of Medicine

PART ONE

WOUND CARE AND PREVENTION

SKIN CARE AND WOUND PREVENTION STRATEGIES

During the past several decades, major advances have been made in the practice of skin and wound care. Clinicians now closely monitor coordinated cellular and biochemical events that occur in skin and wound healing. Manufacturers of skin and wound care products are partnering with clinicians to identify materials that help manage simple and complex skin conditions and wounds. At the same time, standards for describing skin and wounds are being developed to help the clinician document skin and wound assessment. Now more than ever before, a solid foundation of information exists to accelerate skin and wound healing. But despite these advances, the incidence and prevalence of chronic wounds in the United States has risen to epidemic proportions. Consider these statistics:

- About 1% of the general population and 3.5% of people older than age 65 have venous leg ulcers, and the number is rising as the population ages. The recurrence rate of venous ulcers is nearly 70%. It's estimated that the cost of care for venous ulcers exceeds $40,000 *per episode*. At an estimated 2.5 million Americans with venous ulcers, the total cost of treatment may be as high as $3.5 billion annually. As many as 2 million workdays per calendar year are lost because of chronic venous ulcers.
- About 17 million people in the United States have diabetes, with 625,000 new cases diagnosed annually. In addition, another 16 million have a condition known as prediabetes (an elevated blood glucose level that puts them at risk for type 2 diabetes). Some 15% of individuals with diabetes will develop at least one foot ulcer in their lifetimes, and 56% to 83% of the estimated 125,000 lower-extremity amputations performed annually can be directly attributed to diabetes. Moreover, the leading risk factor for ulceration is a previous ulcer—thus, once a person has had an ulcer, he is likely to develop one again.
- It's unclear how many people in the United States have pressure ulcers. A monograph on pressure ulcer incidence and prevalence by the National Pressure Ulcer Advisory Panel found considerable disparity among reported rates, even among the same types of practice. For example, the reported incidence of pressure ulcers is from 0.4% to 38% in general acute-care centers; from 2.2% to 23.9% in long-term care centers; and from 0% to 17% among home health care providers. In general acute

care, the prevalence of pressure ulcers ranges from 10% to 18%; in long-term care, from 2.3% to 28%; and in home health care, from 0% to 29%.

The different types of ulcers are defined and explained in chapter 3, Types of chronic wounds.

One explanation for the dramatic disparities in incidence and prevalence of pressure ulcer data might be the variations in staging definitions and in data sources and methodologies used, making it difficult to compare studies. Other types of wounds, including wounds related to antiphospholipid syndrome, arterial insufficiency, cryofibrinogenemia, cryoglobulinemia, homocystinemia, infection, pyoderma gangrenosum, and sickle cell disease—as well as factitial ulcers, traumatic wounds, surgical wounds, and vasculitic ulcers—may add to the total chronic wound population.

Chronic wounds exact an emotional toll on the patient and his caregivers. Frustration and confusion continue to arise among clinicians when trying to determine which dressing or drug to use on a certain wound type or skin condition, when to change to a different type of dressing or drug, how to document the progress of the wound or skin appropriately, and how to track outcomes based on care practices.

Some solutions to these dilemmas can be found by understanding the delicate balance of art and science. *Art* refers to the team member's skill and application technique in using the preferred management modality for the skin and wound care patient. *Science* refers to the team member's knowledge and understanding of the disease and of the preferred modality used in managing the patient's care. *Art and science* —the fundamental tools of skin and wound healing—directly affect the clinical and financial outcomes of the patient.

Still, after decades of published clinical practice guidelines, research results, and documented best practices for skin and wound care, not to mention the advances in knowledge and available technology, one has to ask. *Why are there so many chronic, nonhealing wounds?*

Reviewing the fundamentals of skin and wound care will help you answer this question. A complete understanding of the anatomy and physiology of the skin, the phases of the healing process, the types of wounds, and the options for wound repair is essential for recognizing factors that may complicate or delay wound healing. Each consideration plays a key role in assessing and managing wounds of all types.

Skin structure

The skin is the body's largest organ, making up about 10% of our total body weight. The skin surface of an average adult covers about 2 square yards. Every day our skin is exposed to physical and mechanical assaults, which may or may not have permanent consequences.

The skin is made up of two major layers—the epidermis and the dermis. Each layer is composed of different types of tissue and has different

Layers of the skin

The skin is composed of two fused layers—the epidermis and dermis. As this illustration shows, the epidermis has five strata—the stratum corneum, stratum lucidum, stratum granulosum, stratum spinosum, and stratum germinativum. Subcutaneous tissue, found beneath the dermis, is a loose connective tissue that attaches the skin to underlying structures.

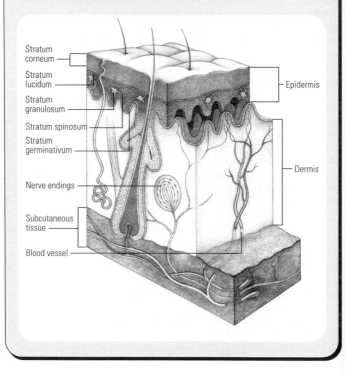

functions. (See *Layers of the skin.*) The dermis provides strength, support, blood, and oxygen to the epidermis.

EPIDERMIS

The epidermis, the outermost layer of the skin layered with epidermal cells, is thin and avascular, normally regenerating every 4 to 6 weeks. Its functions are to maintain skin integrity, to provide a physical barrier against assault by microorganisms and the environment, and to maintain hydration by holding in moisture.

The outer layer of the epidermis, the stratum corneum, plays a key role in hydration. This layer is similar to a brick-and-mortar structure. The keratinocytes (the "bricks") are held together by lipids and proteins (the "mortar"). The epidermis produces the lipids—oily substances that limit the passage of water into or out of the skin—which include cholesterol, ceramide, and fatty acids. If the barrier is deficient in these lipids, moisture can escape. With the loss of water, scales and cracks can develop on the stratum corneum, resulting in dry, flaky, and itchy skin.

If the barrier integrity of the skin is altered, epidermal lipid synthesis increases. Cholesterol and fatty acid synthesis is increased first, followed by ceramide synthesis. This process may be regulated in part by transepidermal water loss (TEWL), which is commonly used to measure the rate of passive diffusion of water from inside the body, through the stratum corneum, and into the external environment.

Healthy skin structure is evident when the epidermis is intact. The substance that helps to maintain an intact epidermis is called natural moisturizing factor (NMF). NMF can absorb water, so it helps to hydrate skin cells. It's found in the cells in the stratum corneum and is made of the breakdown products of proteins. NMF helps prevent individual skin cells from losing water and creates the smooth, nonflaky appearance of healthy, intact skin.

The epidermis also contains melanocytes, which produce pigment, and Langerhans cells, which help the body respond to and process foreign antigens that penetrate the skin surface.

The epidermis may be divided into the following strata, or sublayers:

- *Stratum corneum (horny layer).* This outermost layer of the skin is composed of closely packed, flattened, polyhedral cells. This critical layer serves as the waterproof barrier of the epidermis and protects against infectious microorganisms, harsh chemicals, dirt, and environmental pollutants.
- *Stratum lucidum.* This layer is a translucent line of cells found only on the palms and soles.
- *Stratum granulosum (granular layer).* This layer, two to three cells thick, contains select keratinocytes.
- *Stratum spinosum.* This layer is composed of keratinocytes that become larger, flatter, and contain less water as they travel to the surface of the skin.
- *Stratum germinativum–stratum basale (basal layer).* This innermost layer of the skin contains basal keratinocytes that grow and continually divide, differentiating into the other layers of the epidermis over time. These cells ultimately flatten and lose their nuclei, thereby forming the stratum corneum and eventually replacing select cells that migrate to the skin surface and are lost.

Keratinocytes of the basal layer are anchored to the basement membrane zone (BMZ), which in turn is anchored to the second, thicker layer of the skin, the dermis.

DERMIS

The dermis contains blood vessels, hair follicles, lymphatic vessels, sebaceous glands, and eccrine (sweat) and apocrine (scent) glands. It's composed of fibroblasts, which form collagen, ground substance, elastin, and other extracellular matrix proteins. Ground substance, an amorphous substance composed of water, electrolytes, plasma proteins, and mucopolysaccharides, fills the space between cells and the fibrous components, making the dermis turgid. Collagen fibers, the major structural proteins of the body, give skin its strength. Elastin is responsible for skin recoil or resiliency. Thick bundles of collagen anchor the dermis to the subcutaneous tissue and underlying supporting structures, such as fascia, muscle, and bone.

SUBCUTANEOUS TISSUE

The subcutaneous tissue is composed of adipose and connective tissue, as well as major blood vessels, nerves, and lymphatic vessels. The thickness of the epidermis, dermis, and subcutaneous tissue varies from person to person and from one part of the body to another.

Skin function

The skin has six functions:
- *Protection.* Skin acts as a physical barrier to microorganisms and other foreign matter, protecting the body against infection and excessive loss of fluids. The outer layer (stratum corneum) is slightly acidic, creating a resistance to pathogenic organisms.
- *Sensation.* Nerve endings of the skin allow us to feel pain, pressure, heat, and cold.
- *Thermoregulation.* Skin regulates body temperature through vasoconstriction, vasodilation, sweating, and excretion of certain waste products, such as electrolytes and water.
- *Metabolism.* Synthesis of vitamin D in skin exposed to sunlight activates the metabolism of calcium and phosphate, minerals that play an important role in bone formation.
- *Body image.* The skin performs important body image roles with regard to the skin's appearance (cosmetic), the skin's individual attributes (identification), and skin's ability to convey meaning through expression (communication).
- *Immune processing.* The skin is a portal to the immune system with resident immune cells in both the epidermis (Langerhans cells) and the dermis (dermal dendritic cells).

SKIN PH: ESSENTIAL TO FUNCTION

The skin's pH is acidic, ranging from about 4.2 to 5.6, depending on the area of the body and whether or not the skin is occluded. Skin should be kept in the acidic pH range for several reasons. After an injury to the skin, its barrier function recovers faster when the skin pH is more acidic, rather than more alkaline (less acidic). An acidic environment prevents premature desquamation, or shedding, of dead skin cells. Also, people with an acidic skin pH have less of a tendency toward sensitive skin, which is typically more alkaline.

The pH of the skin helps regulate some of the functions of the stratum corneum, including its permeability, defense against bacteria and fungi, and the integrity and cohesion of skin cells. Skin flora, or the microorganisms that live on or infect the skin, grow differently based on the skin pH. Normal flora grow better at an acidic pH, whereas pathogenic organisms, such as staphylococci, streptococci, and yeast, grow better at a neutral pH. Skin products with a higher pH are thought to promote bacterial growth.

Skin conditions

AGE-RELATED CHANGES

As we age, the overall function of the skin declines or slows. Obvious changes in skin structure and function occur, including the following:

- The epidermal-dermal junction flattens, contributing to the decrease in the overall strength of the skin, leaving us at greater risk for skin tearing or blistering.
- Langerhans cells and melanocyte cells shrink, putting us at greater risk for allergic reactions and increased sensitivity to sunlight, respectively.
- The vascular response is reduced, leading to decreased skin temperature and pallor, or paleness.
- Decreased production of excess sebum and the sweat that moisturizes the skin contribute to skin dryness and flaking.
- Reduced subcutaneous tissue, especially fat, lessens the body's natural insulation or padding and increases the risk of skin breakdown.
- A decline in generalized physical condition, including an altered immune system, puts us at greater risk for a skin or wound infection.
- The reproduction of the stratum corneum slows, which may lead to the skin's inability to absorb topical medications.

XEROSIS AND PRURITUS

A comprehensive assessment of the skin may reveal evidence of skin conditions such as xerosis (dry skin) and pruritus (itching), which are among the most common complaints encountered in nursing homes.

Xerosis affects 59% to 85% of persons older than age 65. More than 70% of hospitalized patients and 90% of nursing home residents over age 65 have dry skin. Many factors contribute to dry skin, including the environment (low humidity, sheets, gowns, elastic stockings or hose), habits (smok-

Skin moisturizing products

Category	Function	Examples
Antimicrobial	Lowers bacteria count	Benzethonium chloride Triclosan
Emollient	Soothes and softens skin; holds and retains moisture	Stearyl alcohol Glyceryl stearate
Humectant	Attracts, holds, and retains moisture	Glycerin Propylene glycol
Preservative	Protects products from spoilage by microorganisms	Methylparaben Propylparaben
Skin protectant	Protects injured or exposed skin from harmful stimuli	Zinc oxide Dimethicone Petrolatum
Surfactant	Cleans	Polysorbate 20 Sodium lauryl sulfate

ing, alcohol, poor diet), diseases (allergies, heart disease, diabetes), medications (diuretics, antibiotics), and skin cleansers (soaps that leave the skin dry, ineffective lotions). (See *Skin moisturizing products*.)

Xerotic skin may appear rough, cracked, fissured, and scaly, and it usually occurs on the lower legs, hands, and forearms. Skin flaking can be seen when a patient removes compression hose; fissuring or cracks can be seen in a patient's heels. Although medications or chronic illnesses can trigger xerosis, it isn't usually associated with a dermatologic condition or systemic disease.

Xerosis is associated with a wide spectrum of clinical findings, from normal-looking skin showing no abnormal dryness to extreme conditions such as ichthyosis, in which the skin becomes dry, thick, and scaly. Xerosis can be classified as acquired, congenital, or inherited.

Pruritus, caused by xerosis in up to 85% of cases, is itchy skin, and it can cause the patient to rub or scratch the affected area. Scratching can cause excoriations, which may progress to secondary eczema or become infected. Pruritus can be caused by many dermatologic and systemic illnesses. It can occur with or without skin lesions.

Low humidity, cold temperatures, frequent bathing, and application of irritants to the skin can worsen pruritus. The condition is most commonly seen in the moisture-depleted skin of elderly people because their sebaceous and sweat gland activity is decreased.

URINARY AND FECAL INCONTINENCE

Loss of skin integrity leaves the patient at greater risk for skin breakdown. Incontinence is the inability of the patient to retain or control urine or feces, or both, until an appropriate time and place for elimination. Urine and stool may contain substances that irritate the epidermis and may make the skin more susceptible to breakdown. Some of the factors that may cause incontinence are:

- delirium
- diabetes
- diuretics
- environmental barriers
- fecal impaction
- high-impact physical activities
- immobility, in chronic degenerative disease
- impaired cognition
- low fluid intake
- morbid obesity
- medications
- neurologic conditions
- pelvic muscle weakness
- psychological conditions such as dementia
- smoking
- stroke
- toileting behaviors.

Incontinence affects patients in all settings. A recent estimate of the direct costs of caring for persons of all ages with incontinence is $11.2 billion annually in the community and $5.2 billion in nursing homes. Given the magnitude of the problem, it is imperative to understand the types of incontinence and the products used to effectively manage this problem.

Fecal incontinence

Fecal incontinence is the loss of normal control of the bowels, leading to stool leaking from the rectum (the last part of the large intestine) at unexpected times. Fecal incontinence is a greater risk factor for pressure ulcer development than urinary incontinence. It affects as many as 1 million Americans and is more common in women and in the elderly of both sexes. The types of fecal incontinence include:

- solid or formed, soft, liquid—the wastes that pass from the rectum in the form of solid, soft, or liquid stool; also called *feces*
- gas—air that comes from the breakdown of food.

Urinary incontinence

The patient with urinary incontinence can't control the passage of urine. This condition may range from an occasional leakage of urine to a complete inability to hold any urine. Urinary incontinence affects about 13 million Americans. Additionally, more than 50% of nursing home residents experience some degree of urinary incontinence. The different types of urinary incontinence include:

- stress incontinence: associated with the impaired urethral closure that allows small amounts of urine leakage when intra-abdominal pressure on the bladder is increased by sneezing, coughing, laughing, lifting, standing from a sitting position, climbing stairs, and so on
- urge incontinence: associated with detrusor muscle overactivity
- overflow incontinence: associated with leakage of small amounts of urine when the bladder has reached its maximum capacity and has become distended
- functional incontinence: occurs in those who can't remain continent because of external factors even though their urinary tract function is intact
- transient incontinence: temporary episodes of urinary incontinence that are reversible once their cause is identified and treated
- mixed incontinence: combination of stress and urge incontinence.

Combined urinary and fecal incontinence

In the presence of both urinary and fecal incontinence, fecal enzymes convert urea to ammonia, raising the alkalinity of the skin pH. Irritation or maceration resulting from prolonged exposure to urine and stool may hasten skin breakdown.

Recently, Centers for Medicare and Medicaid Services (CMS) launched new interpretive guidelines related to incontinence and indwelling catheters, named F Tag 315: Survey Guidance for Incontinence and Catheters (see chapter 7, Wound care and the regulatory process). These guidelines are comprehensive and should be reviewed carefully, as you would with any regulation. In part, the guidelines state:

Skin-related complications

Skin problems associated with incontinence and moisture can range from irritation to increased risk of skin breakdown. Moisture may make the skin more susceptible to damage from friction and shear during repositioning. One form of early skin breakdown is maceration. Lastly, the persistent exposure of perineal skin to urine and/or feces can irritate the epidermis and can cause severe dermatitis or skin erosion. CMS has published clinical tips to include:

1. Keep the perineal skin clean and dry. Research has shown that soap and water regimen alone may be less effective in preventing skin breakdown compared with moisture barriers and no-rinse incontinence cleansers.
2. Because frequent washing with soap and water can dry the skin, the use of a perineal rinse may be indicated.
3. Moisturizers help preserve the moisture in the skin by either sealing in existing moisture or adding moisture to the skin.
4. Moisturizers include lotions or pastes. However, moisturizers should be used sparingly, if at all, on already macerated or excessively moist skin. It's also important to stay abreast of all guidelines for your care setting.

Establishing a skin care formulary

Preserving the barrier function of the skin is imperative. An essential step in preserving—or restoring—the skin's barrier function is choosing the appropriate product which involves establishing a skin care formulary (see chapter 5, Developing a skin and wound care formulary). Be sure to include products in the formulary under such categories as:

- *cleansers,* which effectively remove the urine and/or feces without patient discomfort, provide moisture, and are pH balanced.
- *protectants* or *barrier products,* which protect the skin from urinary and fecal matter during episodes of incontinence. Moisture barriers, sometimes called skin protectants, are ointments, creams, or pastes that shield the skin from exposure to irritants or moisture. Three common protectants are dimethicone, petrolatum, and zinc oxide.
- *moisturizing* or *hydrating products,* such as lotions and creams, which replace lost lipids. (See *Common skin protectants,* page 12.)

Developing prevention strategies

The first step in developing an action plan to prevent the occurrence of pressure ulcers is to identify the at-risk patient population, then base each plan on the patient's needs.

Goals to strive for in each plan include:

- maintaining intact skin
- preventing complications
- identifying and managing complications
- involving the patient and his caregiver in management

ASSESSING PATIENT RISK

The following steps should be included in the action plan:

- Identify patients with high risk for wounds.
- Assess for history of pressure ulcers.
- Inspect bony prominences daily.
- Perform nutritional assessment initially, routinely, and with each change in condition.
- Assess and monitor pressure ulcers with each dressing change.
- Assess for impediments to the healing status (osteomyelitis, fistula formation).
- Assess and evaluate healing.

MINIMIZING ENVIRONMENTAL RISKS

The Agency for Healthcare Research and Quality (AHRQ) provides the following guidelines for prevention of pressure ulcers:

- Minimize environmental factors leading to skin drying such as less than 40% humidity; moisturize skin routinely.

Common skin protectants

Skin protectant	Description
Dimethicone	■ A type of silicone ■ Transparent; doesn't leave residue ■ Allows visual skin inspection ■ Won't wash away ■ Less likely to clog briefs ■ Helps treat and prevent diaper rash
Petrolatum	■ Helps prevent and temporarily protect chafed, chapped, cracked, or wind-burned skin or lips ■ Monograph level 1% to 30% ■ Semitransparent ointment ■ Protects and conditions the skin ■ For treatment and prevention of rash associated with diaper use or continued exposure to urine and feces ■ Monograph level 30% to 100%
Zinc oxide	■ White, nontransparent paste or cream ■ High-level protection ■ Soothing and conditioning properties ■ For treatment and prevention of rash associated with diaper use or continued exposure to urine and feces ■ Monograph level 1% to 40% ■ Cream: may contain lower concentrations of zinc (1% to 25%) ■ Paste: may contain higher concentrations of zinc (25% to 40%)

■ Minimize skin exposure to moisture due to incontinence, perspiration, or wound drainage.
■ Minimize friction and shear forces through proper turning, positioning, and transferring of patient.
■ Document and monitor interventions and outcomes.

POSITIONING AND SUPPORT

Providing the proper mechanical loading and support surfaces (see chapter 6, Tissue load management) is another important step of the action plan for pressure ulcer prevention. The following AHRQ guidelines have been developed to assist the nurse or caregiver when caring for a patient with or at-risk for a pressure ulcer.

- Reposition patients at risk for pressure ulcer development at least every 2 hours if consistent with overall patient goals. Use a written schedule and reevaluate the schedule ongoing.
- For bed-bound patients, use positioning devices such as pillows or foam wedges to keep bony prominences from direct contact with one another based on the care plan.
- Individuals in bed who are completely immobile should have a care plan that includes the use of devices that totally relieve pressure on the heels. Don't use donut-type devices.
- In side-lying positioning, avoid placing the patient directly on the trochanter.
- Maintain the head of the bed at the lowest degree of elevation consistent with medical conditions and other restrictions.
- Use lifting devices such as a trapeze or bed linen to move individuals in bed who can't assist during transfers and position changes.
- Any patient assessed to be at risk for developing pressure ulcer should be placed when lying in bed on a pressure-reducing device, such as foam, static air, alternating air, gel, or water mattresses.
- Any person at risk for developing a pressure ulcer from uninterrupted sitting in a chair or wheelchair should be taught to reposition every hour and reposition body weight by shifting every 15 minutes.

ENSURING NUTRITIONAL SUPPORT

A balanced diet that includes adequate protein and calories is essential to wound healing. Patients with pressure ulcers may need more protein to help ensure a positive nitrogen balance and to replace protein lost through their ulcers. They may also need vitamin and trace element supplementation, especially of vitamin C and zinc. When a patient is unable or unwilling to eat, he may require enteral or parenteral feeding. Expect to individualize the nutritional support plan for each patient, consistent with the overall goals of therapy. (See chapter 2, Assessing and documenting chronic wounds.)

CREATING A PREVENTION
PROGRAM CHECKLIST

In order to create a successful pressure ulcer prevention program, consider these simple steps:

- Assess the types of patients who reside in your facility and determine their skin care needs.
- Implement a pressure ulcer risk assessment tool.
- Determine the support surfaces necessary to manage the patients in your facility (see chapter 6).
- Develop a skin care formulary to maintain or improve the patient's skin integrity (see chapter 5).
- Incorporate a multidisciplinary skin care team to evaluate the patient on admission and periodically thereafter (see chapter 5).

- Assess and reassess the degree of malnutrition associated with the patient's age, weight, intake, and laboratory values (see chapter 2; also see chapter 4, Laboratory values in chronic wound management).
- Develop a laboratory formulary of tests that facilitate managing the patient's nutritional status (see chapter 4).
  - Albumin level is a gross indicator of nutritional status and fluid balance.
  - Prealbumin level reveals acute nutritional status changes.
  - Total lymphocyte count indicates immunosuppression and autoimmunity, which can result from decreased protein intake.
- Include rehabilitation professionals in the skin care team to evaluate the patient for proper off-loading devices to prevent or manage pressure ulcers (see chapter 5).
- Establish a bowel and bladder program for incontinent patients.
- Develop policies, standards, and care procedures to support the facility's practice model (see chapter 5).
- Document care in a progress note or current wound assessment; include the following information:
  - Update the patient's clinical course of treatment.
  - Document and explain the need for diagnostic tests (such as laboratory values).
  - Summarize the patient assessment and care plan.
- Ensure staff's knowledge on documentation standards (see chapter 5).
- Educate the staff at least annually on all aspects of skin and wound care (see chapter 7).
- Maintain head of bed at, or below, 30 degrees or at the lowest degree of elevation consistent with the patient's medical condition (see chapter 6).
- Turn and position patients at least every 2 to 4 hours on a pressure-reducing mattress or at least every 2 hours on a non-pressure-reducing mattress (see chapter 6).
- Reposition chair-bound individuals every hour if they can't perform pressure-relief exercise every 15 minutes (see chapter 6).
- Avoid using foam rings, donuts, and sheepskins as pressure-reducing devices.
- Use pressure-relief devices in the operating room for patients at risk for pressure ulcer development.
- Relieve pressure under heels by using pillows or other devices under the calves.
- Establish a bowel and bladder program for patients with incontinence.
- Use incontinent barriers to protect and maintain skin integrity.
- Consider a pouching system or collection device to contain urine or stool and to protect the skin from the effluent.
- Maintain adequate nutrition that is compatible with the patient's wishes of condition to maximize the potential for healing.
- Educate patients and caregivers about the causes and risk factors for pressure ulcer development and way to minimize risk.

- Develop a plan consistent with the patient's overall plan.

Education is the basis for the development of clinical strategies for skin care.

Providing patient teaching

The final step in developing an action plan for a pressure ulcer prevention program is patient education—which, along with compliance, stands as a cornerstone to successful wound and skin care. The educational needs of the patient should be evaluated on an individual basis beginning with the nonjudgmental assessment of the patient's current knowledge base relevant to the care plan determined.

An educated clinician should direct the educational activities. Principles of adult learning should be used to develop, implement, and evaluate the effectiveness of the educational activity. Validating the impact of the education by measuring retention of the material is paramount for a successful plan.

- The educational activity performed should elicit a change in the patient's actions, comprehension, or competence of the clinician and patient. In order to elicit the change in behavior, the clinician must be educated and her educational skill validated. Once the clinician is educated, she can map the appropriate educational plan for the patient.
- Educational information for the patient and caregiver should include:
  - causes and risk factors for pressure ulcers
  - risk assessment tools and their application
  - skin assessment
  - selection and use of support surfaces
  - development and implementation of the proper program for skin care
  - demonstration of positioning to decrease tissue breakdown
  - instruction on accurate documentation of pertinent data
  - periodic reassessment of patient knowledge.

Wound healing

After skin integrity is altered and a wound results, the healing process begins. This process is generally well orchestrated, leading to repair of the injury. (See *Cascade of wound-healing events,* page 16.) However, chronic wounds don't follow this complex healing model. Because of an impediment to the healing process, these wounds are often thought to be "stuck" in the inflammatory phase. Over time, key cells become senescent. Understanding and correcting the barriers to healing will spark the formation of granulation tissue, leading to the next phase of healing.

Cascade of wound-healing events

This diagram shows the cascade of events that occurs during the wound-healing process.

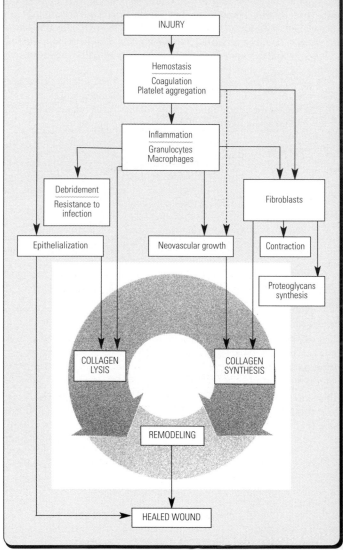

Phases and factors of wound healing

The four phases of wound healing—hemostasis, inflammation, proliferation, and maturation—are described below.

Hemostasis

Hemostasis occurs immediately after the initial injury. The platelet is the key cell responsible for this function, in which the body forms a clot to prevent further bleeding. Platelets also release cytokines, such as platelet-derived growth factor, which gather cells to participate in later phases of healing. After hemostasis, the inflammatory phase begins.

Inflammation

The inflammatory phase, also called the defensive or reaction phase, begins right after injury and typically lasts 4 to 6 days. This phase is characterized by a host of cells infiltrating the wound site. Many of these are inflammatory cells, such as leukocytes and macrophages. Bleeding is controlled by hemostasis, and any bacteria present are destroyed by leukocytes, particularly the polymorphonuclear neutrophils. About 4 days after the injury, macrophages (tissue cells derived from circulating monocytes that migrate to the area) also work to destroy bacteria, cleansing the wound of cellular debris. Macrophages replace the leukocytes (which phagocytize bacteria in the wound, stimulate the inflammatory response, and trigger other biochemical actions) and produce a host of cytokines and growth factors that act as chemoattractants to other cells needed for tissue repair. Macrophages also convert macromolecules into the amino acids and sugars necessary for wound healing.

The cardinal physical characteristics of acute inflammation, first described by Celsus (30 B.C. to 38 A.D.), are still used today. These characteristics are pain, heat, redness, and swelling.

Proliferation

The proliferative phase, also known as the *fibroblastic, regenerative,* or *connective tissue phase,* typically lasts several weeks. In an open wound, granulation tissue forms as red, beefy buds (or granules) of tissue. This tissue consists of macrophages, fibroblasts, immature collagen, blood vessels, and ground substance. With proliferation of granulation tissue, fibroblasts stimulate the production of collagen, which gives the tissue its tensile strength and, ultimately, its structure.

As the wound site fills with granulation tissue, its margins pull together, decreasing the wound's surface. During epithelialization, the final step of this phase, keratinocytes migrate from the wound margins. Subsequently, they divide and, ultimately, become contiguous, closing off the wound. Metalloproteinases (MMPs), such as collagenase 1, are critical in epidermal migration, whereas other MMPs, such as MMP 8 and 9, are important in the normal healing process. The proteins are regulated by a set of inhibitors. Epithelialization can occur only in the presence of viable, vascular tissue. When epithelialization is complete, a scar results.

Maturation

During the maturation or remodeling phase, which can last from 21 days to months or years, collagen fibers reorganize, remodel, and mature, gaining tensile strength. Fibroblasts, MMPs, and their inhibitors play a crucial role in this process, as do certain growth factors, such as transforming growth factor beta. This process continues until the scar tissue has regained about 80% of the skin's original strength. However, because the tensile strength of this tissue is less than that of uninjured skin, it will always be at risk for breakdown.

FACTORS AFFECTING WOUND HEALING

Various factors may delay or impede healing. Local factors occur directly within the wound, whereas systemic factors occur throughout the body.

Local

Wound healing can be delayed by factors local to the wound itself. Such factors include desiccation, infection or abnormal bacterial presence, maceration, necrosis, pressure, and trauma and edema.

- *Desiccation.* A moist environment allows wounds to heal faster and less painfully than a dry environment, in which cells typically dehydrate and die. This causes a scab or crust to form over the wound site, which impedes healing. If the wound is kept hydrated with a moisture-retentive dressing, epidermal cell migration is enhanced, encouraging epithelialization.
- *Infection or abnormal bacterial presence.* A systemic or local infection may delay or impede healing. If an infection is present, as evidenced by purulent drainage or exudate, induration, erythema, or fever, a wound culture should be obtained to identify the offending bacteria and guide antibiotic therapy. When a pressure ulcer or full-thickness wound extending to the bone fails to heal, the patient should be assessed for signs of osteomyelitis. Any abnormal culture or other test results should be reported to the physician so that appropriate antibiotics are prescribed to treat the infection. In addition, an excessive or abnormal bacterial presence may impede healing.
- *Maceration.* Urinary and fecal incontinence can alter the skin's integrity. Educating caregivers about proper skin care is essential for successful skin and wound management.
- *Necrosis.* Dead, devitalized (necrotic) tissue can delay healing. Slough and eschar are the two types of necrotic tissue that may appear in a wound. Slough is moist, loose, stringy necrotic tissue that's typically yellow. Eschar, which appears as dry, thick, leathery tissue, may be black. In most cases, necrotic tissue must be removed before repair and healing can occur.
- *Pressure.* When pressure at the wound site is excessive or sustained, the blood supply to the capillary network may be disrupted. This impedes blood flow to the surrounding tissue and delays healing.

■ *Trauma and edema.* Wounds heal slowly—and may not heal at all—in an environment in which they are repeatedly traumatized or deprived of local blood supply by edema. Edema interferes with the transportation of oxygen and cellular nutrition to the wound.

Systemic

Wound healing can also be delayed by systemic factors that bear little or no direct relation to the location of the wound itself. These include age, body type, chronic disease, immunosuppression, nutritional status, radiation therapy, and vascular insufficiencies.

■ *Age.* Wounds in older patients may heal more slowly than those in younger patients, mainly due to comorbidities that occur as a person ages. Older patients may have inadequate nutritional intake, altered hormonal responses, poor hydration, and compromised immune, circulatory, and respiratory systems, any of which can increase the risk of skin breakdown and delay wound healing.

■ *Body type.* Body type may also affect wound healing. An obese patient, for example, may experience a compromise in wound healing due to poor blood supply to adipose tissue. In addition, some obese patients suffer from protein malnutrition, which further impedes the healing. Conversely, when a patient is emaciated, the lack of oxygen and nutritional stores may interfere with wound healing.

■ *Chronic diseases.* Coronary artery disease, peripheral vascular disease, cancer, and diabetes mellitus are a few of the chronic diseases that can compromise wound healing. Patients with chronic diseases should be followed closely through their course of care to provide the best plan.

■ *Immunosuppression and radiation therapy.* Suppression of the immune system by disease, medication, or age can delay wound healing. Radiation therapy can cause ulceration or changes in the skin, either immediately after a treatment or after all treatment has ended.

■ *Laboratory values.* Nutritional markers aren't the only laboratory values that must be considered when evaluating healing. Measuring the hemoglobin level helps assess the oxygen-carrying capacity of the blood; however, it may also be necessary to assess hepatic, renal, and thyroid functions to determine the patient's healing capacity. (See chapter 4.)

■ *Nutritional status.* Ongoing nutritional assessment is necessary because the visual appearance of the patient or the wound isn't a reliable indicator of whether the patient is receiving the proper amount of nutrients. Albumin and prealbumin levels, total lymphocyte count, and transferrin levels are markers for malnutrition and must be assessed and monitored regularly, as protein is needed for cell growth.

■ *Vascular insufficiency.* Various wounds or ulcers—such as arterial, diabetic, pressure, and venous ulcers—can affect the lower extremities. Decreased blood supply is a common cause of these ulcers. The clinician must identify the type of ulcer to ensure appropriate topical and supportive therapies.

Wound repair mechanisms

Wound repair occurs by primary intention, secondary intention, or tertiary intention. Many acute wounds, such as surgical wounds, are closed by primary intention—that is, the skin edges are brought together manually to facilitate healing. Such wounds have a lower risk of infection, involve little tissue loss, and heal with minimal scarring after 4 to 14 days.

Chronic wounds, such as pressure ulcers, heal by secondary intention. With this type of repair, the skin edges aren't approximated. Because of the delay in healing, chronic wounds are at greater risk for becoming infected.

In healing by tertiary intention, a surgical wound is left open for 3 to 5 days to allow edema or infection to resolve or exudate to drain, after which the wound is closed with sutures, staples, or adhesive skin closures. This type of healing is also called delayed primary closure.

Wound-healing complications

Unfortunately, not all wounds heal. The most common complications of healing include:

- dehiscence—separation of skin and tissue layers that commonly occurs 3 to 11 days after injury
- evisceration—protrusion of visceral organs through a wound opening
- fistula—abnormal passage between two organs or between an organ and the surface of the body
- hemorrhage—internal (hematoma) or external bleeding
- infection—drainage of purulent material and inflamed wound edges that, if uncontrolled, can lead to osteomyelitis, bacteremia, and sepsis.

Accurate assessment skills and diagnosis coupled with the appropriate interventions are the keys to achieving optimal wound-healing results.

ASSESSING AND DOCUMENTING CHRONIC WOUNDS

Stated simply, a chronic wound is an insult or injury to the skin that has failed to heal. The patient with a chronic wound usually has a host of factors that impede the healing process and ultimately lead to generalized patient discomfort. Chronic diseases—such as diabetes, vascular insufficiency, and various autoimmune diseases—can inhibit proper wound healing and affect the overall condition of the patient's skin, including its moisture level and texture.

Assessment

To achieve successful skin and wound healing, the clinician must meticulously follow every step of skin and wound management, including assessment, planning, implementation, evaluation, and documentation. Clinicians are responsible for assessing the patient's skin, wounds, and management modality (dressing, drug, or device); implementing wound care orders; selecting and changing the management modality; and preventing infection during procedures. Identifying and addressing systemic factors in wound healing also are important for successful outcomes.

Performing a comprehensive patient assessment is the essential first step toward healing the chronic skin condition or wound. Once the clinician has assessed the patient, identified any underlying conditions affecting healing, performed a complete assessment of the patient's nutritional status, performed the proper tests to provide an accurate diagnosis of the underlying problem, assessed the patient's knowledge of the disease, and documented all factors that affect the learning needs of the patient, a complete skin and wound assessment can be completed.

The assessment is set in motion with a one-on-one discussion between the patient or caregiver and clinicians who have cared for the patient's skin and wound. Understanding the patient's past and current family, social, and medical history may provide important insight into why the wound isn't healing.

Clinical interventions will vary according to the assessment.

Obtaining a history

A thorough review of the patient's medical history, laboratory tests, medications, and diet can help the clinician determine the cause of the skin condition or wound. Chronic wounds, for example, can be caused by a multitude of different diseases. Primary causes include pressure, chronic venous insufficiency, lower-extremity arterial disease, and diabetic neuropathy. To obtain a patient's history, follow these steps:

- Review the patient's medical history, which details allergies, laboratory studies, radiologic studies, vascular studies, medications, past illnesses, surgical procedures, and other pertinent facts related to the patient's illnesses and problems. Ask about allergies to foods or medications, including topical skin and wound care products. Also, ask the patient if his skin's appearance changes with the seasons.
- Review the patient's family history, paying particular attention to the history of parents, siblings, grandparents, and natural children, and detailing the age and general health information of living relatives, the death and cause of death of all deceased family members, and any chronic diseases that occur in the immediate family. This information will alert you to the presence of inherited or congenital conditions or diseases.
- Review the patient's social history, including age-appropriate information regarding past and current activities, such as marital status, living arrangements, current employment and occupational history, sexual history, level of education, and use of drugs, alcohol, or tobacco. Ask about other social factors that may influence the patient's activities of daily living.
- Ask about the patient's bathing routines and about the different soaps, shampoos, conditioners, lotions, oils, and other topical products he uses routinely. Any such products may lead to changes in skin, appearing as xerosis, pruritus, wounds, rashes, or a change in skin color.
- Obtain a list of past and current medications and dressings, including all medications and dressings that have been used, have been effective, or have failed.
- Review previous treatments, dressings, drugs, adjunctive modalities (such as physical therapy, skin replacements, and growth factors) and determine their effectiveness.
- Review all laboratory, radiology, and vascular studies that have been performed.
- Review the patient's nutritional status and supportive therapies.
For the patient who has a wound, obtain the following information:
- Review all clinician consultations related to specialty management programs for skin and wound care.
- Review (if indicated) all support surfaces and positioning devices used to manage the patient's tissue load.
- Review (if indicated) any use of devices, such as compression stockings, custom shoes or braces, and assistive devices.

- Assess the patient's knowledge of the disease, and document all factors that affect learning needs.

This comprehensive patient assessment will provide the clinician with the four W's she needs to know for skin and wound caring:

1. When did the skin condition or wound occur?
2. Who has taken care of the skin condition or wound?
3. What strategies have been used to facilitate healing of the skin condition or wound?
4. What documented findings (for example, written information, laboratory text results, and vascular or radiology test results) can be reviewed to support the care of the skin condition or wound?

Answers to these questions will provide the clinician with a strong foundation upon which to manage the patient's skin and wound. An incomplete assessment may delay the skin- or wound-healing process.

PERFORMING A PHYSICAL ASSESSMENT

Differential assessment of the skin condition or wound is essential to understanding its cause and development. First, assess the patient's skin temperature, dryness, itching, bruising, and changes in texture of skin and nail composition. Also, assess the skin for color and uniform appearance, thickness, symmetry, and primary or secondary lesions. (See *Identifying primary and secondary lesions,* page 24.)

Examine the patient's nails for changes in thickness, splitting, discoloration, breaking, and separation from the nail bed. Question the patient about changes in his nails, which may be a sign of a systemic condition.

Document all the findings of the skin assessment. Note, too, any presence of a skin condition: erythema, itching, scratching, skin weeping, skin blistering, bruising, primary lesions, secondary lesions, and open wounds.

Wound assessment

After completing the patient assessment and physical assessment, a comprehensive wound assessment is the next important step. The wound assessment helps define the status of the wound and helps identify impediments to the healing process. A clear understanding of the anatomy of the skin is essential for assessing and classifying the wound and defining the level of tissue destruction. (See chapter 1, Skin care and wound prevention strategies.) A detailed assessment of the patient's wound status includes, but isn't limited to, the following parameters:

- *Location.* Anatomic location describes the lesion and the nearest bony prominence or another anatomic landmark. Detailing each wound's location is imperative for accurate documentation and consistent care by each provider working with the patient.
- *Size (length, width, depth, undermining).* Accurate wound measurements can assist the clinician in designing an appropriate care plan. Size is determined by length, width, and depth. Consistent vocabulary and units

Identifying primary and secondary lesions

These guidelines will help you differentiate between primary and secondary lesions.

Primary lesions
Primary lesions are those present at the initial onset of the disease.

■ *Bulla*—a vesicle greater than 5 mm in diameter

■ *Cyst*—an elevated, circumscribed area of the skin filled with liquid or semisolid fluid

■ *Macule*—a flat, circumscribed area; brown, red, white or tan in color

■ *Nodule*—an elevated, firm, circumscribed, and palpable area; can involve all layers of the skin; greater than 5 mm in diameter

■ *Papule*—an elevated, palpable, firm, circumscribed lesion; generally less than 5 mm in diameter

■ *Plaque*—an elevated, flat-topped, firm, rough, superficial papule; greater than 2 cm in diameter (papules can coalesce to form plaques)

■ *Pustule*—an elevated, superficial area that's similar to a vesicle but filled with pus

■ *Vesicle*—an elevated, circumscribed, superficial, fluid-filled blister; less than 5 mm in diameter

■ *Wheal*—an elevated, irregularly shaped area of cutaneous edema; solid, transient, and changing, with a variable diameter; red, pale pink, or white in color

Secondary lesions
Secondary lesions are the result of changes over time caused by disease progression, manipulation (scratching, rubbing, picking), or treatments.

■ *Crust*—slightly elevated; variable size; consists of dried serum, blood, or purulent exudate

■ *Excoriation*—linear scratches on the skin, which may or may not be denuded

■ *Lichenification*—rough, thickened epidermis; accentuated skin markings caused by rubbing or scratching (for example, chronic eczema, lichen simplex)

■ *Scale*—heaped-up keratinized cells; flaky exfoliation; irregular; thick or thin; dry or oily; variable size; silver, white or tan in color

of measure are essential when documenting or describing the wound (See *Measuring wound depth.*)

■ *Color and type of wound tissue.* Wound bed description and wound color provide a consistent approach in defining the tissue in the base of the wound. Descriptors such as granulation tissue, slough, and eschar are generally used to define tissue type. Color of the tissue also has been used to distinguish viable tissue from nonviable tissue and is another descriptor that assists in the management process.

Measuring wound depth

To properly evaluate healing, the health care professional must measure the wound initially and regularly during treatment. One method is to use a sterile, flexible applicator and follow the procedure below.

■ Put on gloves. Gently insert the applicator into the deepest portion of the wound that you can see.

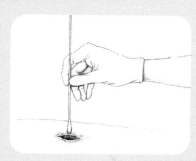

■ Grasp the applicator with the thumb and forefinger at the point corresponding to the wound's margin.

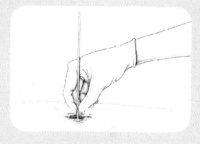

■ Carefully withdraw the applicator while maintaining the position of the thumb and forefinger. Measure from the tip of the applicator to that position.
■ According to your facility's policy, record the depth (in centimeters) on a tracing of the wound, showing the actual position of the deepest parts of the wound.

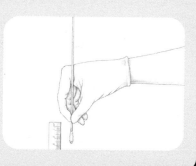

- *Exudate or drainage amount and type.* The amount of wound exudate or drainage is assessed and described with each dressing change. The number of dressing changes needed per week can help with estimating the amount of exudate present. Large amounts of exudate may indicate an infection and a barrier to healing.
- *Odor.* Odor helps define the presence and type of bacteria in the wound and is assessed only after the clinician has cleaned the wound.
- *Periwound skin condition.* Periwound skin is assessed for color and temperature. Inflammation or erythema may indicate wound infection or dermatitis. Assessing the periwound skin for maceration or denuded tissue is also important. Macerated periwound skin should prompt the clinician to assess the topical wound dressing for its ability to manage exudate. Macerated or denuded periwound skin is also a concern when the clinician needs to anchor a dressing.
- *Wound margins.* The condition of the wound margins can provide the clinician with information about the wound's chronicity or healing ability. Newly formed epithelium along the wound edge, commonly flat and pale pink to lavender in color (termed the *edge effect*), indicates stimulated healing.
- *Pain.* The presence, absence, or type of pain may indicate infection, underlying tissue destruction, neuropathy, or vascular insufficiency.
- *Adjunctive therapies.* Adjunctive therapies and support—such as negative-pressure wound therapy, support surfaces for bed and chair, and rehabilitation services—play a vital role. The patient's wound should define the level of therapy needed.
- *Patient knowledge of the disease and wound management.* The educational needs of the patient must be evaluated on an individual basis, beginning with the nonjudgmental assessment of the patient's knowledge relevant to the care plan. An experienced clinician should direct the educational activities.
- *Dressing management.* A moist wound-healing environment requires a proper dressing. Considerations for choosing proper primary and secondary dressings are based on wound characteristics, including size, undermining or tunneling, and amount of exudate. (See *Measuring wound tunneling.*)

    A thorough wound assessment includes:
- condition of the skin around the wound
- status of the wound (whether acute or chronic)
- amount of wound exudate, if any
- presence or absence of necrosis
- appearance of the wound, such as whether the wound is red, yellow, or black
- evidence of possible infection or lack thereof
- degree of cleaning and packing required
- nature of the dressings needed
- management of the drainage.

Measuring wound tunneling

The health care professional should document both the direction and depth of tunneling, as outlined below.

Direction of tunneling

To determine the direction of tunneling, perform the following steps:

■ Put on gloves and gently insert the applicator into the sites where tunneling occurs.

■ View the direction of the applicator as if it were a hand of a clock (12 o'clock points in the direction of the patient's head).

■ Progressing in a clockwise direction, document the deepest sites where the wound tunnels (for example, 3 o'clock).

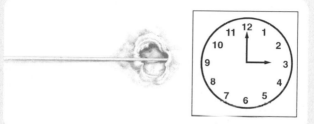

Depth of tunneling

To measure the depth of tunneling, perform the following steps:

■ Insert the applicator into the tunneling areas.

■ Grasp the applicator where it meets the wound's edge.

■ Pull the applicator out, place it next to a measuring guide, and document the measurement (in centimeters).

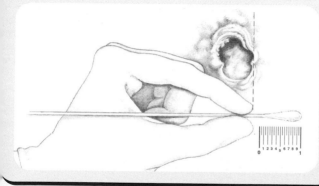

Additional qualifying factors for wound management

Body measurements

To ensure accuracy, patient stature (height and weight) must be measured by the clinician rather than reported by the patient.

If standing height can't be measured, knee height calipers may be used. These calipers measure the length of the lower leg from the bottom of the foot to the top of the patella, and a mathematical formula is then used to determine the patient's height.

Other body measurements—such as triceps skin-fold measurement, mid-arm circumference, and mid-arm muscle circumference—have limited usefulness in most wound care settings.

Any changes in the patient's weight, as well as a history of the weight change, need further evaluation to provide information about the patient's normal weight. Interview family members if the patient is unable to provide a history because of illness or mental deficiency.

LABORATORY TESTS

Laboratory tests help evaluate the patient's nutrition and hydration status. A complete nutritional assessment includes an evaluation of both a standard multiple analysis and a complete blood count as well as protein stores, electrolyte and fluid balance, renal function, liver function, glucose levels, anemias, and immune status. It may also include other specific nutritional laboratory values, such as prealbumin, folic acid, vitamin B_{12}, ferritin, and transferrin levels, and lymphocyte count. The accompanying table indicates the levels of mild, moderate, and severe depletion for common protein status laboratory values. (See *Markers of malnutrition;* see also chapter 4, Laboratory values in chronic wound management.) Many laboratory assays, such as albumin, are affected by hydration status. It's important to repeat laboratory tests after a patient has been rehydrated.

NUTRITIONAL ASSESSMENT

Performing a complete assessment of the patient's nutritional status is critical to making sure that his diet is optimal for the healing process.

Such an assessment includes body measurements, evaluation of laboratory test results, physical examination, and a dietary interview. Based on the information collected in these four areas, the clinician can then determine a patient's nutrient needs, evaluate the adequacy and appropriateness of his diet, and recommend changes.

Physical examination for nutritional status

The physical examination provides evidence of nutritional deficiencies and signs of malnutrition. It also provides insight into the patient's functional status, including the ability to self-feed. This physical examination includes:

■ hair—dry, sparse, brittle, or easily plucked

Markers of malnutrition

Marker	Normal value	Mild depletion	Moderate depletion	Severe depletion
Percent of usual body weight	100%	85 to 95	75 to 84	<75
Albumin, g/dl	≥3.5	2.8 to 3.4	2.1 to 2.7	<2.1
Prealbumin, mg/dl	16 to 30	10 to 15	5 to 9	<5
Transferrin, mg/dl	>200	150 to 200	100 to 149	<100
Total lymphocyte count, mm^3	2500	<1500	<1200	<800

From *Understanding Normal and Clinical Nutrition*, 5th edition, by Whitney/Cataldo/Rolfes. 1998. Reprinted with permission of Brooks/Cole, a division of Thomson Learning: www.thomsonrights.com. Fax (800) 730-2215.

- skin—turgor, bruises, tears, pressure ulcers, xerosis, or other skin integrity problems
- lips—cheilosis or angular fissures
- gums—swelling or bleeding
- teeth—condition of natural teeth or denture fit and acceptance
- tongue—glossitis, pallor, atrophy, or sores
- nails—brittle or spoon nails
- mucous membranes—dry
- hands—arthritis and inability to open food containers
- vision—inability to see food on the plate
- mental status—inability to communicate food preferences and understand diet instruction
- height and weight—visual confirmation of anthropometric data obtained
- motor skills—extent of hand-to-mouth coordination and any inability to hold utensils and self-feed.

Dietary interview

A thorough dietary history can provide important details with regard to writing the care plan. The extent of this history depends on the clinical setting.

A basic history may include a food frequency list or a 3-day diet recall. Understanding the patient's usual eating pattern and the typical food consumed on a daily basis is important. Ask the patient about food preferences, cultural favorites, food allergies, and lactose intolerance. Inquire about digestive problems, such as nausea, constipation, diarrhea, vomiting, chewing problems, swallowing trouble, and any flavor or taste changes.

In outpatient and clinical settings, obtain additional details about grocery shopping and food preparation. Isolation and lack of socialization commonly result in poor intake and nutritional deficiencies.

After collecting the data, evaluate the patient's nutritional status and needs. The four components of the nutrition assessment (body measurements, laboratory test results, physical examination, and dietary interview) provide sufficient information on which to base clinical judgments.

Nutrient needs

Understanding the patient's nutrient needs for calories, protein, and fluids helps determine whether daily intake is meeting those needs. Dietitians calculate caloric needs using the Harris-Benedict equation to predict basal energy expenditure (BEE):

Females: 655 + 9.56 W + 1.85 H - 4.68 A

Males: 66.5 + 13.75 W + 5.0 H - 6.78 A

(W = weight in kilograms; H = height in centimeters; A = age in years)

After calculating the patient's BEE, dietitians modify it for level of activity and extent of illness and injury. Activity factors add 20% to 30% to the BEE for most patients. Injury factors can add an additional 50% or more. Clinical judgment must be used to best estimate the patient's daily total energy expenditure (TEE); many different systems exist for arriving at this estimate. For example, a 75-year-old woman weighing 108 lb and standing 5' tall has a BEE of 1,055 calories per day (655 + 469 + 282 − 351). If she's confined to bed, an activity factor of 1.2 is added. If she has a stage 3 wound, an additional injury factor of 1.3 is added. The resulting TEE is 1,055 × 1.2 × 1.3 = 1,646 calories per day. If this patient has a history of losing weight or shows signs of malnutrition, an additional injury factor is added. Some clinicians simply add 250 calories per day to the TEE for weight gain of about ½ lb per week.

An alternate system to the Harris-Benedict formula is calculating needs based on calories per kilogram of body weight. The accompanying table outlines guidelines for calculating calories, protein, and fluid needs based on this system. (See *Nutrient needs based on body weight.*)

After collecting and evaluating the data, the clinician can begin to formulate the treatment plan, starting with the least invasive and least costly interventions and progressing to more invasive and higher-cost interventions as needed. The accompanying treatment algorithm demonstrates how interventions should advance in a logical fashion. (See *Nutrition screening and assessment,* page 32.)

Nutrient needs based on body weight

Nutrient	Requirement
Calories	
Normal	25 to 30 kcal/kg/day
Protein-calorie malnutrition (PCM)*	30 to 35 kcal/kg/day
Critically ill or injured*	35 to 40 kcal/kg/day
Protein	
Recommended daily allowance	0.8 g/kg/day
PCM	1.5 g/kg/day
Critically ill or injured*	1.5 to 2 g/kg/day
Fat	<30% kcal
Water	30 cc/kg body weight or 1 L/1,000 kcal

*Nutrient supplementation required.

Documentation

Developing documentation guidelines, whether for pen-and-paper or computerized records, is a prerequisite to evaluating the clinical efficiency and cost-effectiveness of your facility. Proper documentation provides guidance for appropriate treatment decisions, evaluation of the healing process, support for reimbursement claims, and a defense for litigation. Once established, the documentation system should become the framework of clinical practice for all members of the wound care team.

DOCUMENTATION CHECKLIST

Skin and wound care documentation combines various information-gathering tools that reflect the wound's status. When assessing the patient with a skin condition or wound as it heals, documentation should include:

- chief complaint
- history of present illness
- medical, family, and social history
- review of systems
- physical assessment
- risk assessment
- manual assessment
- skin and wound assessment

Nutrition screening and assessment

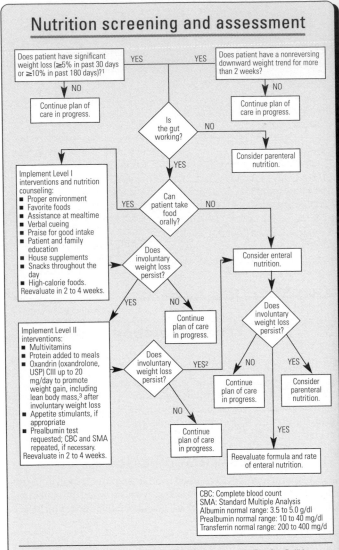

Does patient have significant weight loss (≥5% in past 30 days or ≥10% in past 180 days)?[1]

— YES — YES → Does patient have a nonreversing downward weight trend for more than 2 weeks?

NO ↓

Continue plan of care in progress.

NO ↓

Continue plan of care in progress.

Is the gut working? — NO → Consider parenteral nutrition.

YES ↓

Implement Level I interventions and nutrition counseling:
- Proper environment
- Favorite foods
- Assistance at mealtime
- Verbal cueing
- Praise for good intake
- Patient and family education
- House supplements
- Snacks throughout the day
- High-calorie foods.

Reevaluate in 2 to 4 weeks.

Can patient take food orally? — YES — NO → Consider enteral nutrition.

Does involuntary weight loss persist?

YES ↓   NO → Continue plan of care in progress.

Does involuntary weight loss persist? — YES → Consider enteral nutrition.

NO → Continue plan of care in progress.

YES → Consider parenteral nutrition.

Implement Level II interventions:
- Multivitamins
- Protein added to meals
- Oxandrin (oxandrolone, USP) CIII up to 20 mg/day to promote weight gain, including lean body mass,[3] after involuntary weight loss
- Appetite stimulants, if appropriate
- Prealbumin test requested; CBC and SMA repeated, if necessary.

Reevaluate in 2 to 4 weeks.

Does involuntary weight loss persist? — YES[2] →

NO ↓

Continue plan of care in progress.

YES → Reevaluate formula and rate of enteral nutrition.

CBC: Complete blood count
SMA: Standard Multiple Analysis
Albumin normal range: 3.5 to 5.0 g/dl
Prealbumin normal range: 10 to 40 mg/dl
Transferrin normal range: 200 to 400 mg/d

1. American Health Care Association, Resident Assessment Instrument for Long Term Care Facilities. Version 2.0.
2. Strawford, A, et al. "Resistance exercise and supraphysiologic androgen therapy in eugonadal men with HIV-related weight loss: A randomized controlled trial." JAMA, 281:1282–90, 1999.
3. If, at any time, patient can't receive adequate nutrient intake, reevaluate gut function and consider nutritional support.

Adapted with permission from BTG Pharmaceuticals, Iselin, N.J. (2001).

- procedures performed
- supplies and tests ordered
- patient education provided
- care plan
- discharge plan.

Chief complaint

The chief complaint—the specific reason the patient has sought care, record-ed in his own words—links the reason for the patient's visit to the detailed history and physical assessment obtained by the clinician.

History of present illness

The clinician reviews the history of present illness information in con-junction with reviewing symptoms, physical examination, risk assessments and screening tools, and skin and wound assessments. The history of pre-sent illness should include a complete chronological account of the chief complaint to date. Most of this information is subjective because it's based on the patient interview. If multiple chronic conditions are discussed—for example, lower leg pain and headaches—make sure to document this in the history of present illness to justify orders for tests or medications or treatments prescribed. Symptoms, such as pain, and current care of the pre-senting wound or skin care problem should be documented here.

Medical, family, and social history

Many elements affect wound healing, such as chronic illnesses or diseases, medications, allergies, diet, and activities of daily living. Review the pa-tient's medical history, family, and social activities with particular atten-tion to:

- autoimmune diseases, blood disorders, bowel disorders, cancer, car-diovascular disease, cerebral vascular disease, diabetes, heart disease, hy-pertension, kidney disease, liver disorders, malignancies and associated treatments, musculoskeletal disorders, neurologic infections, peripher-al vascular disease, prior hospitalizations, renal failure, venous insuffi-ciency; ostomy surgeries, revisions, or diversions; and chronic illnesses, including accidents or injuries that lead to chronic insufficiencies
- medications used, such as chemotherapeutic agents, steroids, or corti-costeroids
- allergies, such as to dressings and securement products, medications, or the environment
- vascular tests, such as palpation of pulses, ankle-brachial index (ABI), and transcutaneous oxygen tension
- radiologic tests, such as X-rays, bone scan, magnetic resonance imaging, and angiography
- dressing history, including products used effectively and ineffectively, and ostomy history, if any
- modality history, including products used effectively in the past and products that inhibited healing rate; laboratory values; nutritional val-

ues (such as albumin, prealbumin, and transferrin levels, and total lymphocyte count), chemistry values (blood urea nitrogen, creatinine, and liver enzyme levels; hepatitis panel; hemoglobin A_{1C} level; and lipid panel), hematologic values (complete blood count, sedimentation rate, C-reactive protein, protein S, and protein C), immunologic values (rheumatoid factor and immune complexes), and microbiology values (biopsy and quantitative cultures)

- activities of daily living, such as alcohol use, recreational drug use, modality use, smoking, and eating patterns.

Thorough documentation provides the information the clinician needs to accurately and effectively assess and treat the patient with a chronic wound.

Review of systems

A review of systems is generally a question-and-answer session intended to provide the clinician with a full description of the patient's complaints. The systems addressed during the review include:

- constitutional signs and symptoms, such as fatigue, fever, weakness, or weight loss
- eye problems, such as double vision, pain, eye strain, or impaired vision
- ears, nose, mouth, or throat signs and symptoms, including ear pain, sinus drainage, pain when swallowing, impaired hearing, and mouth pain or sores
- cardiovascular signs and symptoms, including chest pain, claudication, edema, heart or circulatory problems, hypertension, or pain while resting
- respiratory signs and symptoms, such as shortness of breath or wheezing
- GI signs and symptoms, such as appetite changes, bloating, fecal incontinence, or stomach pain; question the patient about his bowel habits
- genitourinary signs and symptoms, such as burning upon urination, discharge, hematuria, or incontinence
- musculoskeletal signs and symptoms, such as muscle or joint pain, stiffness, swelling, or edema
- integumentary (skin) signs and symptoms, such as previous wound sites, previous ostomy sites, pigmentation changes, pruritus, lumps, or rashes
- neurologic signs and symptoms, including loss of sensation, headaches, tremors, seizures, numbness, or paralysis
- psychologic signs and symptoms, such as change in sleeping patterns, ability to comply with treatment plan, and attitudes toward health
- endocrine signs and symptoms, such as excessive thirst or hunger, excessive sweating, and disorders such as diabetes or thyroid conditions
- hematologic and lymphatic signs and symptoms, such as bleeding, bruising, or anemia; inquire about past transfusions
- allergic and immunologic signs and symptoms, such as allergies, reactions, immune symptoms or problems, and autoimmune disorders.

Physical assessment

A thorough physical examination includes the following:

- determination of constitutional signs and symptoms: temperature, pulse, blood pressure, height, and weight
- examination of the eyes for such signs and symptoms as dry, pale, discolored conjunctiva and edema of eyelids
- evaluation of the ears, nose, mouth, throat, and neck for signs and symptoms such as impaired hearing, dry mouth, dry throat, loss of teeth, inflammation of the tongue, and so forth
- cardiovascular assessment of pulses, temperature gradient, color changes, skin turgor, and lower-extremity circulation changes, edema, or venous filling
- respiratory evaluation for such signs and symptoms as shortness of breath and wheezing
- GI evaluation for the appearance of stoma, wounds, or skin conditions
- genitourinary evaluation, including assessment of the appearance of stoma, wounds, or the presence of skin conditions
- musculoskeletal evaluation, including the appearance of digits and nail beds, presence of limited joint mobility, muscular appearance and strength, orthopedic deformities, gait evaluation, and plantar pressure assessment
- integumentary (skin and/or breast) evaluation, including temperature changes that may indicate a "hot spot" or decrease in circulation, and skin appearance, the presence of calluses or fissures, and the absence or presence of hair
- neurologic assessment, including results of Semmes-Weinstein test, deep tendon reflex testing, Babinski test, and vibration perception threshold assessment
- psychologic evaluation, including body image and orientation to person, place, present surroundings, and time
- endocrine findings
- lymphatic assessment, including groin, lymph nodes, axillae, and neck
- allergy and immunology evaluation, including assessment of the patient's skin for skin dryness, macules, papules, or rashes.

Risk assessment tools

Risk assessment tools are used to predict of a patient's level of risk and prevent various disease states. Some risk assessment tools are specific to particular areas of risk, such as pressure ulcers or diabetic foot ulcers. Nutritional risk assessment tools enable the clinician to calculate the patient's risk for nutritional deficits. Other factors—such as laboratory values, radiologic studies, and vascular studies—should also be considered when evaluating a patient's level of risk.

Examples of risk assessment tools and the parameters evaluated include:

- Braden scale for pressure ulcers evaluates sensory perception, moisture, activity, mobility, nutrition, and friction and shear (see Appendix C, *Braden scale*, pages 572 to 573.)

Norton scale

Assess the following five conditions and assign appropriate scores. A total score of 14 or less indicates risk of pressure ulcer. A score below 12 indicates high risk.

Name _____ Date _____

PHYSICAL CONDITION		MENTAL CONDITION		ACTIVITY		MOBILITY		CONTINENCE	
Good	4	Alert	4	Walks	4	Full	4	Good	4
Fair	3	Apathetic	3	Walks		Slightly		Occasional	
Poor	2	Confused	2	with help	3	limited	3	incontinence	3
Very poor	1	Stuporous	1	Sits in		Very		Frequent	
				chair	2	limited	2	incontinence	2
				Remains in bed	1	Immobile	1	Urine and	
								fecal	
								incontinence	1
TOTAL		**TOTAL**		**TOTAL**		**TOTAL**		**TOTAL**	

TOTAL SCORE _____

- Norton scale for pressure ulcers evaluates physical condition, mental status, activity, mobility, and incontinence (see *Norton scale*)
- International Working Group of the Diabetic Foot risk categorization system evaluates risk for development of diabetic foot ulcers.

Nutritional status plays a significant role in establishing a patient's level of risk; nutritional assessment is a comprehensive process that includes:

- body measurements, including height, weight, body mass index, and degree of variation from usual body weight
- evaluation of laboratory test results to assess the patient's nutritional and hydration status, including complete blood count, protein stores, electrolyte and fluid balance, renal function, glucose levels, anemias, and immune status
- physical examination of hair, skin, lips, gums, teeth, tongue, nails, mucous membranes, hands, vision, mental status, and motor skills
- dietary interview, including food frequency and preferences; a 3-day diet recall; and digestive process concerns, such as nausea, constipation or diarrhea, chewing problems, swallowing trouble, or flavor or taste changes.

The information collected from the dietary interview will enable the clinician to determine the patient's nutrient needs and recommend any dietary changes.

Manual assessment

Manual screening tools, used to assist the clinician in making an accurate diagnosis, include the following:

- ABI is used to screen and help assess arterial vascular disease. It is calculated by a ratio of pressure at the ankle to pressure in the arm. The reference range for ABI is 0.9 to 1.1.
- Cultures identify whether infection is present. A wound infection is caused by colonization of viable wound tissue by microorganisms whose presence causes local tissue damage. Identifying the microorganisms that are inhibiting wound healing enables the clinician to develop a care plan. Culture types include swab, tissue biopsy, punch biopsy, and needle aspiration.
- Lower-leg and foot assessments evaluate vascular and neuropathic risk factors. Lower-leg pulses usually include palpation and auscultation of right and left femoral, right and left popliteal, right and left posterior tibial, and right and left dorsalis pedis. Foot pulses usually include right and left posterior tibial and right and left dorsalis pedis. Other parameters evaluated include skin temperature changes, color and circumference of the lower leg, sensory level of the feet, capillary refill time, and toe pressures.
- Palpation of pulses and Doppler readings assist the clinician in determining the degree of blood flow. Doppler ultrasound is a noninvasive screening tool used to determine the patient's vascular status.
- Segmental blood pressures assist in locating possible obstructions. These readings are taken at the ankle, below the knee, above the knee, and high up on the thigh, using a Doppler probe and blood pressure cuff. Segmental blood pressures shouldn't vary more than 20 to 30 mm Hg between segments.
- The Semmes-Weinstein monofilament test helps to quantify the degree of neuropathy in patients with diabetes. This test is performed using a standard monofilament. A foot that is insensate to the monofilament, typically a 5.07 monofilament (10 g), is considered at risk for skin ulcerations (part of the neurologic examination).
- Vibration perception threshold assessment (part of the neurologic examination) is useful when evaluating a patient with diabetes who is at risk for skin ulceration.
- Transcutaneous oxygen tension ($TcPO_2$) provides a measurement of oxygenation at skin level. The reference value for $TcPO_2$ is 55 mg or greater.

Skin and wound assessment

Wound care documentation includes a variety of information that reflects the skin and wound status across the healing continuum. Providing an accurate description of the skin and wound characteristics is critical during each patient visit. These findings assist the clinician in mapping the care during the wound management process. Wound classification establishes a common language for wound assessment and wound healing. It helps to foster sound clinical judgments, provides a universal scheme for documentation, and allows better evaluation of treatments.

Accurate measurements of wound length, width, depth, and tunneling complement and complete the classification of a wound (see page 41). Other essential documentation elements include a description of the skin around the wound, the wound's surface (intact, exuberant granulation tissue, or necrotic tissue), and the drainage or exudate found in the wound.

Three main types of classification systems are used; two are based on the degree of tissue layer destruction, and the other is based on the color of the wound bed. The values obtained include cause, qualitative information, and quantitative information.

Cause
Establishing the cause of the wound or skin condition will help identify the correct classification and management process. Underlying medical conditions—such as poor nutrition, diabetes, or neuropathy—may explain why the wound may be healing slowly. These underlying conditions need to be treated concurrently. Finally, treatment history is significant because the clinician may learn which management modalities have been tried and either succeeded or failed.

The anatomic location of existing skin breakdown (for example, left hip, right lateral malleolus, or right ischial tuberosity) should be documented consistently. A documentation form with diagrams of different anatomic sites is a helpful tool. (See *Wound and skin assessment tool*, pages 118 and 119.) One way to use this form is to circle the areas involved and assign a different letter for each location to ensure consistency of documentation.

Qualitative information
Qualitative information includes the following:
- Anatomic location describes the extremity and nearest bony prominence or anatomic landmark.
- Classification describes the degree of tissue layer destruction. Wound classification establishes a common language for wound assessment and wound healing, helps foster sound clinical judgments, provides a universal scheme for documentation, and allows better evaluation of treatments. Staging systems identify certain types of wounds by stage. Wounds also may be classified by thickness or color. (See *Other criteria for classifying wounds*.)
- Edema, or swelling, of tissues may indicate vascular compromise.
- Document exudate describing the amount, color, and consistency. Amount is documented as light, moderate, or heavy or as scant, moderate, large, or copious. Drainage color and consistency can be described as serous (clear, watery plasma), sanguineous (bloody [fresh bleeding]), serosanguineous (plasma and red blood cells), or purulent (thick drainage, white blood cells and living or dead organisms, possibly with a yellow, green, or brown color that suggests the type of infecting organism).
- Odor defines the presence or absence of high bacteria counts in the wound and should be assessed only after the clinician has cleaned the

Other criteria for classifying wounds

Wounds can also be classified by thickness and color, as described here.

Thickness

Partial thickness and *full thickness* are terms commonly used to classify wounds whose primary cause is something other than pressure. Partial-thickness wounds extend through the first layer of skin (the epidermis) and into, but not through, the second layer of skin (the dermis). Partial-thickness wounds heal by reepithelialization. Full-thickness wounds extend through both the epidermis and the dermis and may involve subcutaneous tissue, muscle and, possibly, bone. Full-thickness wounds primarily heal by granulation, contraction, and reepithelialization. Examples of wounds that may be partial- or full-thickness wounds include skin tears, lacerations, surgical wounds, and vascular (venous and arterial) ulcers.

Describing a wound as partial thickness or full thickness identifies the depth of the wound. However, it doesn't identify the condition of intact skin, the identifiable layers of tissue exposed (for example, bone), or the color of the exposed wound bed.

Color

A three-color concept of wound classification was adapted by Marion Laboratories for use with traumatic, surgical, and other wounds that heal by secondary intention (open wound bed). The system can be used as a component of wound assessment and as a tool to help direct treatment. The three-color concept classifies wounds as red, yellow, or black.

- Red may indicate clean, healthy granulation tissue. When a wound begins to heal, a layer of pale pink granulation tissue covers the wound bed, which later becomes beefy red.
- Yellow may indicate the presence of exudate or slough and the need for wound cleaning. Exudate can be whitish yellow, creamy yellow, yellowish green, or beige.
- Black may indicate the presence of eschar (necrotic tissue), which slows healing and provides a site for microorganisms to proliferate.

If a wound displays two or even all three colors at once, intervention strategy is based on the least desirable color present. For example, if a wound is both yellow and black, intervention strategy is the type used for a black wound. Some facilities classify mixed wound colors by percentages, for example, 75% black and 25% yellow.

wound. A pungent, strong, foul, fecal, or musty odor suggests critical colonization or infection.

- Periwound skin is assessed for color and temperature. When checking for potential skin breakdown or assessing the skin around an existing pressure ulcer or other wound, begin with temperature. Warmth may indicate pressure ulcer formation, if the skin is intact, or the presence of an underlying infection.

- Type of tissue exposed, including wound bed description and wound color, provides a consistent definition of the tissue in the base of the wound. Descriptors—such as granulation tissue, slough, or eschar—are generally used to define the tissue types. Color of the tissues also has been used to distinguish viable tissue from nonviable tissue and is another descriptor that aids the management process.

A description of the wound margin condition may provide the clinician with information related to the wound's chronicity or wound-healing ability. Pain, if present, may indicate infection, swelling, or edema; underlying tissue destruction that isn't visible; or vascular insufficiency. Document the presence of severe pain or tenderness within or around the wound, and report it to the primary care clinician. Document the absence of pain, which may indicate nerve destruction or neuropathy. Work with the patient who can't communicate verbally but can understand commands to locate the site of any pain. If the patient is unable to respond verbally or with simple hand gestures, watch for signs of pain, such as facial grimaces, retraction of a body part, or tenseness during the procedure. Document the patient's nonverbal as well as verbal responses because both are important descriptors. Specific information related to pain, tolerance of the dressing change procedure, the patient's ability to provide self-care, and response to adjunctive therapies and treatments (such as rehabilitation) assist in developing a proactive care plan.

The Joint Commission has developed evidenced-based pain management standards that have been incorporated into the requirements for Joint Commission accreditation. To comply with these standards, facilities must implement policies and procedures to inform patients of their right to pain relief and demonstrate that pain is being routinely addressed, reassessed, treated, and managed effectively. Assessment data collected to determine the patient's pain level include:

- Pain intensity: Use a pain-intensity rating scale appropriate for the patient population. Document pain intensity at present, worst, and least levels. If possible, use the same pain rating scale consistently in the organization and among disciplines.
- Location: Ask the patient to mark the site on a diagram or to point to the site of pain.
- Quality, patterns of radiation, and character: Elicit and record the patient's own words whenever possible.
- Onset, duration, variations, and patterns
- Alleviating and aggravating factors
- Present pain management regimen and effectiveness
- Pain management history: Include a medication history, presence of common barriers to reporting pain and using analgesics, past interventions and response, and patient's manner of expressing pain.
- Effects of pain: Ask about pain's impact on everyday issues, such as work, sleep, appetite, relationships with others, emotions, and concentration.
- Patient's pain goal: Include goals for managing pain intensity and goals related to function, activities, and quality of life.

■ Physical examination and observation of the pain site.

Quantitative information

Quantitative assessment elements are objective rather than subjective and include precise measurements.

Ankle and calf circumference

Ankle and calf circumference (for vascular parameters) provides the measurement around the extremity. Ulcerations, particularly on the lower legs or feet, commonly occur from arterial insufficiency, venous hypertension, neuropathy, or a combination of these conditions. A common cause is a decrease in blood supply to the area. Predisposing factors, such as the anatomic location of the ulcer and distinctive wound characteristics, help to distinguish among ulcers of the lower extremities. (See *Differentiating arterial, diabetic, and venous ulcers,* pages 98 and 99.)

Photograph

Wound documentation is usually supplemented with a photograph of the wound when needed for legal or clinical purposes. Photographic documentation helps the clinician assess the wound and measure changes over time. Typically, the wound is photographed in color on initial assessment and then at select intervals according to facility policy.

Surface area of wound

Surface area includes wound depth and undermining. Depth describes the distance from the visible surface to the deepest point in the wound base. Undermining, or tunneling, describes the tissue destruction underlying intact skin.

Wound measurements

Accurate wound measurements assist the wound care team in designing an appropriate care plan. Size of the wound is determined by measuring length, width, and depth, usually in centimeters, or by measuring volume. Several methods exist for measuring wounds, including linear measurement, wound tracings, and wound molds. The direction and depth of any tunneling also should be described. Use consistent vocabulary and consistent units of measure when documenting and describing wound measurements.

The length and width of any wound are measured as linear distances from wound edge to wound edge. To ensure accurate and consistent measurements, establish landmarks for wound measurements. For example, look at the wound as if it were a clock face. The top of the wound— 12 o-clock—is toward the patient's head. Conversely, the bottom of the wound—6 o'clock—is in the direction of the patient's feet. Therefore, length can be measured from 12 to 6 o'clock, using the patient's head and feet as guides. Width can be measured from side-to-side or hip-to-hip or from 3 to 9 o'clock.

Length and width can also be documented by making a tracing of the wound on transparent paper with a permanent marker. The tracing should be placed in a plastic bag (for infection control) and may be kept in the patient's chart for reference throughout treatment. If the wound is healing normally, subsequent tracings will show a progressive decrease in size.

The depth of a wound can be described as the distance from the visible surface to the deepest point in the wound base. If the depth varies, measure different areas of the wound bed to confirm the deepest site. Document your findings according to your facility's policy. (See *Measuring wound depth*, page 25.)

When assessing a pressure ulcer, also document the depth of tissue loss by staging it on a scale of 1 to 4. Stages 3 and 4 are the most serious, sometimes requiring surgical closure or grafting.

An alternative method for measuring a wound cavity is to determine wound volume. This can be done by filling the wound cavity with an amorphous material (such as dental alginate paste), allowing the material to solidify, removing the resulting mold of the wound, and submerging the mold in a calibrated container that contains a set amount of water. The amount of water displaced is the wound volume. This technique is used mainly in research and laboratory studies, rather than daily clinical practice.

Tunneling, also referred to as rimming or undermining, is tissue destruction underlying intact skin. Both the direction and the depth of tunneling should be documented. (See *Measuring wound tunneling*, page 27.)

When documenting partial- and full-thickness wounds, include length, width, and depth, as well as tunneling (if present) in full-thickness wounds. All partial-thickness wounds have depth because the wound has penetrated through the epidermis. Because measuring superficial wounds is difficult, some clinicians choose to document the depth as less than 0.1 cm. Any depth equal to or greater than 0.1 cm can be measured with a measuring device. Other parameters to use when describing partial- and full-thickness wounds are the color of the wound bed, appearance of the skin around the wound (periwound skin), and the presence of tunneling, drainage, and odor.

Wound classifications
Information on pressure ulcers is documented using the four-part classification system. (See *Staging pressure ulcers*, pages 52 and 53). For diabetic foot ulcers, the University of Texas classification system can be used. (See *University of Texas diabetic foot classification system*.)

Procedures
Components of the procedure performed include, but aren't limited to:
- consent for the procedure
- physical examination completed and updated in the last 7 days
- name of the physician or clinician performing the procedure
- preoperative diagnosis
- procedure description
- anesthesia
- complications

University of Texas diabetic foot classification system

Stage	Grade 0	Grade I	Grade II	Grade III
A	Prelesion or postlesion completely epithelialized	Superficial wound, not involving tendon, capsule, or bone	Wound penetrating to tendon or capsule	Wound penetrating to bone or joint
B	Infected	Infected	Infected	Infected
C	Ischemic	Ischemic	Ischemic	Ischemic
D	Infected and ischemic	Infected and ischemic	Infected and ischemic	Infected and ischemic

Reprinted with permission from Inlow, S, et al: "Best Practices for the Prevention, Diagnosis, and Treatment of Diabetic Foot Ulcers," *Ostomy/Wound Management* 46(11):55-68, November 2000.

- postoperative diagnosis
- procedure performed (for example, techniques used and tissues removed).

The body of documentation should detail every aspect of the procedure performed. Procedures include debridement, application of a biologic skin substitute, or application of a multilayer sustained graduated compression system.

Ordering of supplies and tests
The clinician must supply an order for all the care the patient receives related to the treatment. Product supplies, tests, and modalities to be documented may include:

- wound care supplies such as alginates, collagens, composites, contact layers, foams, hydrocolloids, hydrogels, specialty absorptive dressings, surgical supplies (miscellaneous), transparent films, and wound fillers
- drugs such as topical steroids, debriding agents, and growth factors
- modalities such as lower-limb immobilizers, total contact cast, foot casts or boots, removable walking braces with rocker-bottom soles, crutches, walkers, or canes
- adjunctive therapies and support, such as negative pressure wound therapy pumps or support surfaces for bed and chair
- noninvasive tests, such as segmental blood pressures, Doppler waveform analysis, toe pressures, and transcutaneous oxygen tension
- vascular tests

- laboratory tests, such as fasting or random blood glucose level, glyco-hemoglobin (hemoglobin A_{1C}) level, complete blood count with or without differential, erythrocyte sedimentation rate, wound cultures, blood cultures, urinalysis, prealbumin and transferrin levels, and blood chemistries
- support surfaces, such as mattress overlays, mattress replacements, total bed replacements, and chair cushions
- referrals, such as rehabilitation management, wellness programs, and diabetes education.
   When documenting an order for dressings, remember to include:
- cleanser
- anatomic location
- primary dressing
- secondary dressing, if applicable
- securement device, if applicable
- duration of need
- frequency of change.
   When documenting an order for prescription drugs, remember to include:
- name of drug and unit of measure
- route
- frequency
- duration of use
- prescriber's name and signature
- number of refills.
   When ordering radiology, vascular, and laboratory tests, remember to:
- order the exact name of the test performed in your facility
- select the ICD-9 code that supports the medical necessity of the test.
   When ordering a support surface, remember to speak with your support surface representative to clearly understand the guidelines set forth for your care setting.

   When ordering a referral for your patient, remember to ask the referring department if any specific information is required so that the patient's appointment can be scheduled without delay.

Patient education

Patient education and compliance are the cornerstones of successful wound and skin care. The educational needs of the patient should be evaluated to determine his current knowledge base relevant to the care plan determined. A clinician familiar with the care plan should direct the educational activities. Principles of adult learning should be used to develop, implement, and evaluate the effectiveness of the educational activity. Measuring the patient's retention of the material also is important for a successful plan.

   The Joint Commission and the Panel for the Prediction and Prevention of Pressure Ulcer in Adults have identified patient education as a critical element of care delivery.

   Effective patient education includes:

- identifying the barriers to learning, including cultural, physical (pain), learning style, and environmental barriers
- performing a needs assessment of the patient and his caregiver to determine their knowledge levels, beliefs, and compliance practices as well as perceived educational needs
- assessing the patient's and caregiver's readiness to learn
- identifying patient and caregiver learning styles, including an assessment of the patient's reading and comprehension abilities
- identifying the patient's and caregiver's overall learning goals
- identifying and managing physical stressors that affect learning, such as pain
- documenting and reevaluating the patient's skin and wound care skills at each visit.

Care plan

The Joint Commission defines a *care plan* as:

a plan, based on data gathered during patient assessment, that identifies the patient's care needs, lists the strategy for providing services to meet those needs, documents treatment goals and objectives, outlines the criteria for terminating specified interventions, and documents the individual's progress in meeting specified goals and objectives. The format of the 'plan' in some organizations may be guided by patient-specific polices and procedures, protocols, practice guidelines, clinical paths, care maps, or a combination of these. The care plan may include care, treatment, habilitation, and rehabilitation.

The care plan answers the following questions:

- Have all of the ICD-9 codes been chosen to support the clinical documentation?
- Have the short-term goals accurately reflected the patient's condition?
- Have the long-term goals accurately reflected the patient's status?

Discharge plan

The discharge summary provides a synopsis of all patient events during the course of care. All the events, assessments, and diagnoses found in the discharge summary should be easily found in the previous documented visits.

Documenting care takes time and coordination of efforts from all team members for a complete and accurate portrayal of the care performed. Given the fast pace of our society as well as the clinical and regulatory constraints to date, it's prudent for clinicians to record assessment, documentation, clinical, and financial outcome data in an electronic database. The data collected can then be used to advance critical pathways, improve product formularies, validate contract fees with payers, and improve patient and physician satisfaction, which in turn increases business opportunities. (See *Top 20 strategies for effective skin and wound documentation,* page 112.)

TYPES OF CHRONIC WOUNDS

Venous, arterial, and diabetic ulcers (often referred to as *lower-extremity ulcers*), as well as pressure ulcers, are commonly encountered. Managing these frequently problematic wounds can be difficult, exacting a costly toll on the patient's well-being. In addition, health care expenditures in the United States related to the evaluation and management of vascular wounds are estimated to run into the billions of dollars.

Management of vascular, diabetic, and pressure ulcers has improved over the past decade as clinicians have realized the importance of proactive measures and a multidisciplinary team approach. The introduction of newer treatment modalities, such as growth factors and biologic skin replacements, holds the promise of treating difficult wounds, accelerating the wound-healing process, and preventing new wound formation to a degree not previously thought possible.

Pressure ulcers

A pressure ulcer is a localized site of cell death that occurs most commonly in areas of compromised circulation secondary to pressure. These ulcers may be superficial, caused by local skin irritation with subsequent surface maceration, or deep, originating in underlying tissue. Deep ulcers may go undetected until they penetrate the skin.

Pressure ulcers are most likely to develop in patients who experience sustained pressure over bony prominences. Patients who spend most or all of their time in a bed or alternative seating device such as a wheelchair without shifting their body weight properly are at great risk. Risks increase with various cofactors, such as partial or total paralysis and malnutrition. (See *Patients at risk for pressure ulcers.*)

PATHOGENESIS

Most pressure ulcers develop when soft tissue is compressed between a bony prominence (such as the sacrum) and an external surface (such as a mattress or the seat of a chair) for a prolonged period. (See *Common pressure ulcer sites*, pages 48 and 49.) Pressure—applied with great force for a

Patients at risk for pressure ulcers

At greatest risk for pressure ulcers are patients compromised by the following conditions:
- chronic illness that requires bed rest
- dehydration
- diabetes mellitus
- diminished pain awareness
- fractures
- history of corticosteroid therapy
- immunosuppression
- incontinence
- malnutrition
- mental impairment, possibly related to coma, altered level of consciousness, sedation, or confusion
- multisystem trauma
- paralysis
- poor circulation
- previous pressure ulcers
- significant obesity or thinness.

short period or with less force over a longer period—disrupts blood supply to the capillaries, impedes blood flow to the surrounding tissues and deprives tissues of oxygen and nutrients. This leads to local ischemia, hypoxia, edema, inflammation and, ultimately, cell death. The result is a pressure ulcer, also called a *bed sore, decubitus ulcer,* or *pressure sore.*

Shear, which separates the skin from underlying tissues, and friction, which abrades the top layer of skin, also contribute to pressure ulcer development. Contributing systemic factors include infection, malnutrition, edema, obesity, emaciation, multisystem trauma, and certain circulatory and endocrine disorders.

ASSESSMENT

Blanching erythema, which is verified by finger compression, is an early sign that an ulcer may be forming over a bony prominence. The condition may resolve without tissue loss if pressure is reduced or eliminated. Nonblanchable erythema, a more serious sign, suggests that tissue destruction is imminent or has occurred. The skin may appear bright red to dark red or purple. If deep tissue damage is also present, the area may be indurated or boggy when palpated. Wound management effectiveness and duration depend on wound severity.

Several classification systems identify pressure ulcers by stages, identifying wounds by the tissue layers involved. These systems don't describe a

(Text continues on page 50.)

Common pressure ulcer sites

These figures show the anatomic locations that are susceptible to pressure ulcer formation.

Lateral position

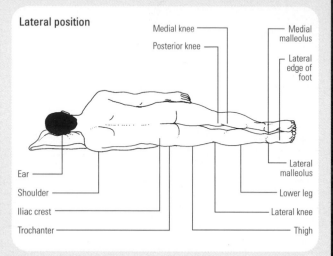

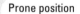

Prone position

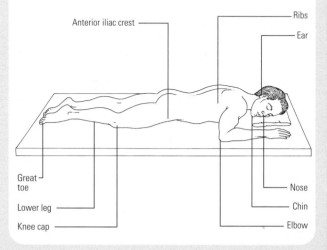

Common pressure ulcer sites *(continued)*

Posterior position

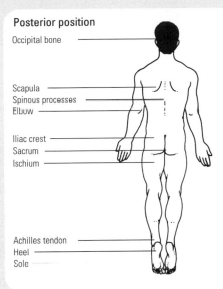

Occipital bone

Scapula
Spinous processes
Elbow

Iliac crest
Sacrum
Ischium

Achilles tendon
Heel
Sole

Sitting position

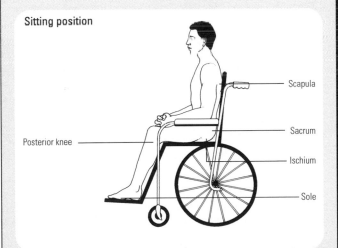

Scapula

Sacrum

Ischium

Posterior knee

Sole

wound completely; rather, they provide an anatomic description of the wound's depth. The National Pressure Ulcer Advisory Panel (NPUAP) system for describing pressure ulcers is a combination of the most commonly used staging systems and is also used to classify other wound types. (See *Staging pressure ulcers,* pages 52 and 53.)

When documenting the stages of pressure ulcers, the health care professional should be familiar with the vocabulary necessary for accurate description and measurement.

Research indicates that there are several stages to the severity and condition of pressure ulcers. Treatment of these ulcers must acknowledge these differing stages. The following stages are adapted from the Agency for Health Care Policy and Research (1994) (AHCPR, now known as Agency for Healthcare Research and Quality [AHRQ]) guidelines:

- *Stage 1:* Nonblanchable erythema of intact skin, the heralding lesion of skin ulceration. In individuals with darker skin, discoloration of skin, warmth, edema, induration, or hardness may also be indicators. The definition according to the National Pressure Ulcer Advisory Panel (NPUAP) states "Intact skin with nonblanchable redness of a localized area usually over a bony prominence. Darkly pigmented skin may not have visible blanching; its color may differ from the surrounding area."
  - Stage 1 pressure ulcer staging is difficult in patients with dark skin. In lighter-skinned people, a stage 1 pressure ulcer may change skin color to a dark purple or red area that doesn't become pale under fingertip pressure. In dark-skinned people, this area may become darker than normal. The affected area may feel warmer than surrounding tissue. When eschar is present, accurate staging is impossible.
  - Document and describe only the length and the width. No measurable depth exists because the epidermis is intact, although underlying tissue may be damaged.
  - Keep in mind that assessment of stage 1 pressure ulcers may be difficult in patients with darker skin.
- *Stage 2:* Partial-thickness skin loss involving epidermis, dermis or both (such as abrasion, blister, or shallow crater).
  - Document and describe length, width, and depth. All stage 2 pressure ulcers have depth because the wound has penetrated the epidermis.
  - For superficial pressure ulcers, remember that the depth may be documented as less than 0.1 cm. Any depth equal to or greater than 0.1 cm can be accurately measured with a measuring device.
- *Stage 3:* Full-thickness skin loss involving damage to or necrosis of subcutaneous tissue that may extend down to, but not through, underlying fascia (deep crater with or without undermining). The ulcer presents clinically as a deep crater with or without undermining adjacent tissue.
  - Document and describe length, width, depth, and tunneling, if present.
  - Be aware that when necrotic tissue is present, accurate staging of the pressure ulcer isn't possible until the slough or eschar has been debrided and the wound base is visible.

- *Stage 4:* Full-thickness skin loss with extensive destruction, tissue necrosis, or damage to muscle, bone, or supporting structures (such as tendon or joint capsule).
  - Document and describe length, width, depth, tunneling (if present), and underlying support structures (fascia, muscle, and bone).
  - Be aware that when necrotic tissue is present, accurate staging of the pressure ulcer isn't possible until the slough or eschar has been debrided and the wound base is visible.
- *Unstageable:* The definition according to the NPUAP is "Full thickness tissue loss in which the base of the ulcer is covered by slough (yellow, tan, gray, green, or brown) and/or eschar (tan, brown, or black) in the wound bed. Until enough slough and/or eschar is removed to expose the base of the wound, the true depth, and therefore stage, cannot be determined. Stable, dry adherent, intact (without erythema or fluctuance) eschar on the heels serves as the body's natural (biological) cover and should not be removed."

Deep tissue injury

Health care practitioners have been classifying pressure ulcers using the existing four-part staging system. A pressure ulcer, as redefined by the National Pressure Ulcer Advisory Panel (NPUAP), is "localized injury to the skin and/or underlying tissue, usually over a bony prominence, as a result of pressure or pressure in combination with shear and/or friction."

The purpose of the staging system is to provide clinical documentation of a pressure ulcer using anatomical depth as the determining factor. But at times, the clinician is confronted with wounds that don't fit in the existing staging system. Purple wounds or bruised areas over bony prominences are just a couple of examples. So, what recourse does the health care professional have in this situation? It would probably be safe to say that most health care professionals document these purple wound types as stage 1 or stage 2 pressure ulcers in an effort to best describe and complete their documentation in the medical record. This begs the question: Is that the best thing to do? If you stop to reflect on the given definitions of these stages, you will see that a definition doesn't exist for all of the anomalies found on the skin nor may it fit the wound description.

In 2007, the NPUAP added a definition for suspected deep tissue injury to assist the health care practitioner in the pressure ulcer assessment process: Deep tissue injuries have been documented as intact skin on the first assessment but rapidly deteriorate to a full-thickness wound shortly thereafter. It has also been documented that the location of deep tissue injuries are in the muscle or subcutaneous fat.

The health care practitioner must carefully assess the patient and document the true appearance of the skin condition or wound in the medical record. Reassessment of the skin condition or wound is paramount to further defining changes to the patient's skin.

Staging pressure ulcers

The following staging system is consistent with the recommendations of the National Pressure Ulcer Advisory Panel (Consensus Conference, 1991) updated 2007.

Stage 1
Intact skin with nonblanchable redness of a localized area, usually over a bony prominence, characterizes stage 1 of a pressure ulcer. Darkly pigmented skin may not have visible blanching, but its color may differ from that of the surrounding area.

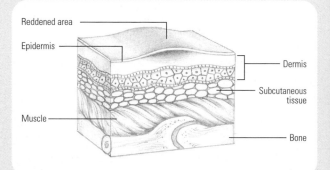

Stage 2
Stage 2 is defined as a partial-thickness loss of dermis appearing as a shallow open ulcer with a red-pink wound bed, without slough. This stage of pressure ulcer may also appear as an intact or open, ruptured serum-filled blister.

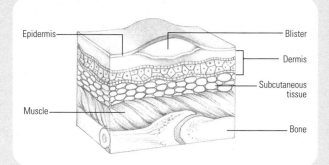

Staging pressure ulcers *(continued)*

Stage 3

In stage 3 pressure ulcers, there's full-thickness tissue loss. Subcutaneous fat may be visible, but bone, tendon, or muscle isn't exposed. Slough may be present but doesn't obscure the depth of tissue loss. Undermining and tunneling may occur.

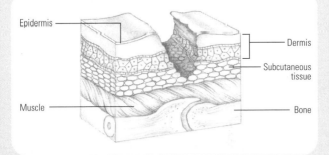

Stage 4

Stage 4 pressure ulcers feature full-thickness tissue loss with exposed bone, tendon, or muscle. Slough or eschar may be present on some parts of the wound bed. Undermining and tunneling are common.

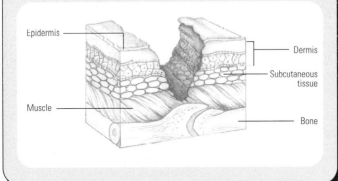

Reverse staging

Staging is intended to describe the amount of tissue destroyed rather than the amount of tissue healed. Reverse staging rests on the misconception that a *stage 4* ulcer becomes a *stage 3* ulcer and proceeds upward through the staging system as it heals. However, original tissue that was destroyed by the wound (such as subcutaneous tissue, muscle, and bone) is instead replaced with granulation tissue and new epithelium. Review the NPUAP position statements about reverse staging by visiting www.npuap.org.

Because tools to measure pressure ulcer healing didn't exist until after 1900—and because it's essentially required for reimbursement (in areas such as in the long-term, home health and outpatient care settings)—some clinicians continue to use reverse staging. More efficient methods to describe wound healing include tools such as the Pressure Sore Status Tool, the Pressure Ulcer Scale for Healing, the Sessing scale, and the Sussman tool. Alternatively, the clinician may simply document:

- dimensions of size (length and width)
- dimensions of depth
- dimensions of tunneling or undermining
- tissue amount and type (eschar, slough, or granulation)
- amount and qualitative description (color, thickness, and odor) of exudate.

Regular comparisons between the current depth of the wound at its worst point and the depth at the same point as documented on admission allow an accurate evaluation of wound healing. Health care professionals should develop specific wound care policies and procedures based on standard guidelines, such as those of the Agency for Health Care Research and Quality; the Wound, Ostomy and Continence Nurses Society; or the NPUAP.

MANAGEMENT

As an aid to risk assessment and management, the Agency for Health Care Research and Quality (formerly the Agency for Health Care Policy and Research), a branch of the U.S. Department of Health and Human Services, published two booklets for health care professionals: *Pressure Ulcers in Adults: Prediction and Prevention,* and *Treatment of Pressure Ulcers.* The agency also published a handbook for patients, available in English and Spanish, titled *Preventing Pressure Ulcers: A Patient's Guide to Treating Pressure Sores.* Although these resources were published respectively in 1992 and 1994, they continue to provide the basic guidelines needed to develop a sound program. Additionally, the Wound, Ostomy, and Continence Nurses Society published guidelines for pressure ulcer care, titled *Prevention and Management of Pressure Ulcers.*

All stages of pressure ulcers require topical wound care, and surgical intervention may be required for stages 3 and 4. Topical wound care varies with the management modalities used and the ulcer's stage. (See *Topical management algorithm for wound care,* pages 56 and 57.) Interventions to reduce pressure over bony prominences, such as the use of support surfaces, are vital to the success of the care plan.

If infection develops or the patient is immunocompromised, immediate surgical debridement may be necessary. In stage 3 pressure ulcers, spontaneous closure may take months and may cause scar tissue that can predispose the patient to recurrent pressure ulcers. For these reasons, surgical excision and closure may be used to manage these ulcers. Stage 4 ulcers are handled similarly, but debridement may be more radical when a bony prominence is involved.

Tissue flaps are commonly used for surgical management of pressure ulcers. They involve the transfer of skin and underlying structures to fill a defect. Tissue flaps are classified according to the tissue layers included and the surgical methods used to transfer the tissue. All flaps require partial detachment of the tissue from its original site (with the base remaining attached).

An accurate assessment of the skin and wound type will assist the clinician in designing and implementing an effective care plan.

Mobility

For most patients, maintaining current activity level, mobility, and range of motion is sufficient to prevent pressure ulcers or for their early treatment. If a patient has a mobility or activity deficit, implement the interventions listed below to help protect him from the adverse effects of pressure, friction, and shear. (See "Tissue load management modalities," page 121.)

Venous ulcers

Venous ulcers are believed to account for 70% to 90% of chronic leg ulcers. These ulcers can be difficult to heal. The incidence of venous ulceration increases with age, with women being three times more likely than men to develop venous leg ulcers. In some studies, 50% of patients had venous ulcers that persisted for more than 9 months, and 20% had ulcers that didn't heal for more than 2 years. After healing, more than 60% of patients experienced a recurrence of venous ulcers.

PATHOGENESIS

The proper diagnosis and management of venous ulcers begins with a basic understanding of the venous system of the lower extremities. The venous circulation consists of the superficial veins (greater and lesser saphenous) and their branches, the deep veins (popliteal and femoral), and the perforating veins (which connect the superficial and deep veins). During calf muscle contraction, such as that which occurs with normal ambulation, the veins empty from the superficial veins, to the perforating veins, to the deep veins, and back to the heart. Retrograde blood flow is prevented by venous valves, which exist in all three venous components mentioned above. In the presence of healthy veins and calf muscles, standing deep vein pressure is about 80 to 90 mm Hg. With ambulation, the calf squeezes the blood toward the heart and the venous pressure drops to 30 to 40 mm Hg.

Chronic venous insufficiency is the result of deep vein obstruction, incompetent venous valves, and inadequate calf muscle function. Partial or complete deep vein obstruction may occur from thrombosis, scar tissue,

(Text continues on page 58.)

Topical management algorithm for wound care

Use this chart to help you effectively assess, plan, intervene, and evaluate wounds. You'll need to exclude patients with diabetic or neurotrophic ulcers and those with stages 3 and 4 osteomyelitis, systemic infection, or venous stasis ulcers.

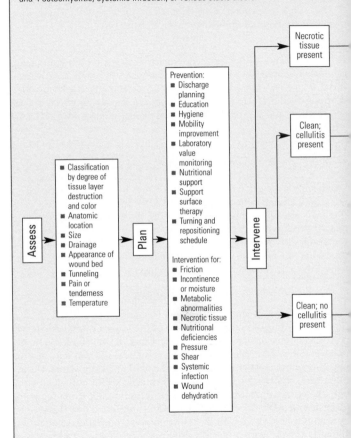

Assess
- Classification by degree of tissue layer destruction and color
- Anatomic location
- Size
- Drainage
- Appearance of wound bed
- Tunneling
- Pain or tenderness
- Temperature

Plan

Prevention:
- Discharge planning
- Education
- Hygiene
- Mobility improvement
- Laboratory value monitoring
- Nutritional support
- Support surface therapy
- Turning and repositioning schedule

Intervention for:
- Friction
- Incontinence or moisture
- Metabolic abnormalities
- Necrotic tissue
- Nutritional deficiencies
- Pressure
- Shear
- Systemic infection
- Wound dehydration

Intervene
- Necrotic tissue present
- Clean; cellulitis present
- Clean; no cellulitis present

*Debridement performed according to practitioner's state practice, professional regulation standards, and competency validation

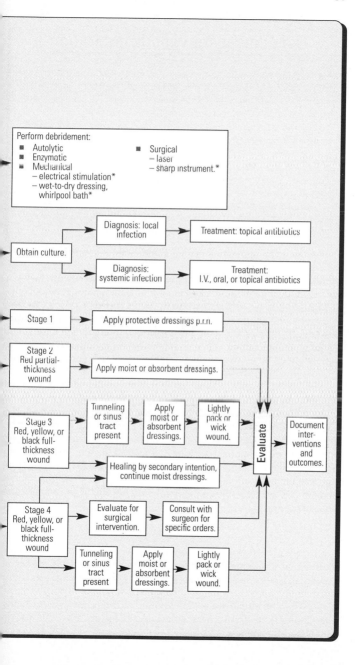

Perform debridement:
- Autolytic
- Enzymatic
- Mechanical
  – electrical stimulation*
  – wet-to-dry dressing, whirlpool bath*
- Surgical
  – laser
  – sharp instrument.*

Obtain culture. → Diagnosis: local infection → Treatment: topical antibiotics

Obtain culture. → Diagnosis: systemic infection → Treatment: I.V., oral, or topical antibiotics

Stage 1 → Apply protective dressings p.r.n.

Stage 2 Red partial-thickness wound → Apply moist or absorbent dressings.

Stage 3 Red, yellow, or black full-thickness wound → Tunneling or sinus tract present → Apply moist or absorbent dressings. → Lightly pack or wick wound.

→ Healing by secondary intention, continue moist dressings.

Stage 4 Red, yellow, or black full-thickness wound → Evaluate for surgical intervention. → Consult with surgeon for specific orders.

→ Tunneling or sinus tract present → Apply moist or absorbent dressings. → Lightly pack or wick wound.

Evaluate → Document interventions and outcomes.

Hypotheses for venous ulceration

Fibrin cuff hypothesis: High venous pressures lead to distention of the capillary bed and leakage of macromolecules, such as fibrinogen, into the tissue. The fibrinogen polymerizes to fibrin, which then forms a barrier around the capillaries, preventing oxygen and nutrients from reaching the tissue. This leads to ulceration.

White blood cell hypothesis: Flow through the capillary is decreased due to high venous pressures. White blood cells, quite large when compared to red blood cells, plug the capillary, leading to local ischemia. The trapped cells release proteolytic enzymes and oxygen metabolites that damage the endothelium, making it more permeable to leakage of macromolecules into the tissue. These activated white cells also cause a local inflammatory reaction.

Trap hypothesis: Macromolecules, such as fibrin, trap growth factors and other important proteins making them unavailable for tissue repair and maintenance of tissue integrity.

obesity, pregnancy, or malignancy. Valves may be incompetent due to lower-leg trauma, deep vein thrombosis, or congenital anomalies. Poor calf muscle function may be secondary to paralysis, decreased ankle joint mobility (as seen with fractures or arthritis), decreased activity, or muscle atrophy. Abnormalities in the veins, valves, and calf muscle result in impaired venous return and abnormally high venous pressure, both at rest and with ambulation. In other words, the venous pressure doesn't drop with ambulation as seen in normal venous and calf function; it remains high at 80 to 90 mm Hg. This leads to edema and altered microcirculation in the skin, which results in impaired healing.

Venous ulcers are commonly precipitated by trauma. The patient may have experienced the trauma weeks to months before, and the wound never healed. The patient may also report that he had a pruritic rash (stasis dermatitis), and the ulcer started after he scratched the skin. Finally, a spontaneous blister may form in the presence of severe edema and, after rupture, result in a chronic wound. Once the wound occurs, the high venous pressure and resulting edema interferes with healing. (See *Hypotheses for venous ulceration.*)

ASSESSMENT

A thorough history and physical examination is essential for the diagnosis of venous ulceration. In obtaining the history, the clinician should focus on risk factors, such as a history of deep vein thrombosis, leg trauma (crush injury, fracture, or surgery), congenital venous abnormality, limited mobility with impaired calf muscle pump (arthritis, paralysis, or a muscular disorder), pregnancy, heart failure, family history of venous disease, obesity, gender, and advanced age.

Clinical findings associated with venous leg ulcers

Assessment parameter	Assessment finding
Wound location	30% to 40% of wounds occur superior to the medial malleolus (near the saphenous vein); the remainder occur primarily in the lower one-third of the calf.
Appearance of wound bed	Wound bed appears "ruddy" or "beefy" red and granular.
Wound shape and margins	Wound has flat, irregular margins without undermining.
Drainage or exudate	Drainage or exudate may be moderate to heavy, depending on the amount of edema.
Surrounding skin	Surrounding skin will exhibit venous dilation, including submalleolar venous flare (typical of venous insufficiency), telangiectasias, reticular veins, varicose veins, edema (typical of more advanced venous disease), atrophie blanche, maceration, hyperpigmentation (from hemosiderin staining), dermatitis, and lipodermatosclerosis; scarring from prior healed ulcers is also possible.
Pain	Presence of pain with venous leg ulcers is controversial. Many believe that pain usually isn't present; however, several studies have reported severe pain occurring in as many as 76% of patients with venous ulcers. Deep ulcers, particularly around the malleoli, or small venous ulcers surrounded by atrophie blanche are the most painful. Generally, patients report that pain occurs with leg dependence (for example, sitting or standing) and diminishes with leg elevation.

Characteristic clinical findings include the presence of varicosities, hyperpigmentation, lipodermatosclerosis, and dermatitis. The shape of the leg may also provide a clue—for example, the "inverted bottle shape" is a sign of lipodermatosclerosis. Venous ulcers tend to have flat wound edges, without undermining. (See *Clinical findings associated with venous leg ulcers*.)

CEAP classification of venous disease

The American Venous Forum's CEAP system is used to categorize venous disease according to **c**linical signs, **e**tiology, **a**natomic distribution, and **p**athologic condition.

- Class 0: No visible or palpable signs of venous disease
- Class 1: Telangiectasias, reticular veins, malleolar flare *(noted below the malleolus)*
- Class 2: Varicose veins
- Class 3: Edema without skin changes
- Class 4: Skin changes ascribed to venous disease (pigmentation, eczema, lipodermatosclerosis)
- Class 5: Skin changes as defined above, with healed ulceration
- Class 6: Skin changes as defined above, with active ulceration

Reprinted with permission from Porter, J.M., and Moneta, G.L. "An International Consensus Committee on Chronic Venous Disease," *Journal of Vascular Surgery* 21(4):635-45, April 1995.

The American Venous Forum has developed a system, known by the acronym CEAP, for classifying venous disease based on:

- Clinical signs
- Etiology of venous disease (congenital or primarily or secondarily acquired)
- Anatomic distribution (superficial, perforating, and deep veins)
- Pathologic condition (obstruction or reflux). (See *CEAP classification of venous disease.*)

The use of non-invasive vascular testing facilitates identification of the anatomic and pathologic aspects of this system. Use of the CEAP classification system improves documentation, assists in planning treatment strategies, and facilitates insurance approval of various treatment and surgical intervention.

When assessing the patient with venous disease, it's crucial to rule out coexisting peripheral arterial disease (PAD). If normal pulses can't be felt due to edema, a Doppler examination will reveal biphasic or triphasic sounds, in the absence of PAD. If the pulses are abnormal, an ankle-brachial index (ABI) must be performed to quantify arterial flow at the ankle. The ABI is a reimbursable procedure that can be easily done at the bedside. If the ABI indicates decreased arterial flow, further noninvasive vascular testing should be done before treatment.

Although most leg ulcers are venous ulcers, the clinician should suspect other causes when the wound looks atypical (presence of necrotic tissue, exposed tendon, livedo reticularis on surrounding skin, or a deep, "punched out" ulcer), has been present for longer than 6 months, or hasn't responded to good care. Don't hesitate to take a biopsy when in doubt. (See *Differential diagnosis of lower-extremity ulcers.*)

Differential diagnosis of lower-extremity ulcers*

- Inflammatory disorders
  - Granuloma annulare
  - Necrobiosis lipoidica
  - Pyoderma gangrenosum
  - Sweet's
- Malignancy
  - Malignant transformation of long-standing ulcer (Marjolin's)
  - Metastatic malignancies
  - Primary skin malignancies
  - Ulcers associated with hematologic or internal malignancies
- Pressure ulcers
- Infectious disorders
  - Bacterial (*Pseudomonas,* staphyloccocal scalded skin syndrome, streptococcal necrotizing fasciitis)
  - Fungal (blastomycosis, chromomycosis, Madura foot)
  - Mycobacterial (*M. leprae, M. tuberculosis, M. ulcerans*)
  - Parasitic (Chagas disease, leishmaniasis)
  - Viral (herpes simplex, herpes zoster)
- Trauma (burns, postsurgical trauma)
- Factitial ulcers
- Bites (dog, snake, spider)
- Medication-related ulcers
  - Drug reactions leading to blisters and large-scale wounds (erythema multiforme, Stevens-Johnson syndrome, toxic epidermal necrolysis)
  - Ulcer-causing medications used to treat malignancies (doxorubicin, hydroxyurea, radiation)
- Autoimmune disorders
  - Blistering (epidermolysis bullosa, pemphigoid, pemphigus)
  - Nonblistering (dermatomyositis, lupus, rheumatoid arthritis, scleroderma)

- Atherosclerotic arterial ischemic ulcers
- Nonatherosclerotic ischemic ulcers
  - Hypertensive ulcers (Martorel's)
  - Sickle cell disease
  - Thromboangiitis obliterans
  - Vasculitis
    • Churg-Strauss syndrome
    • Henoch-Schönlein purpura
    • Leukocytoclastic vasculitis
    • Microscopic polyangiitis
    • Polyarteritis nodosa
    • Urticarial vasculitis
    • Wegener's granulomatosis
  - Vasculopathy
    • Cryoagglutination (cryoglobulins, cryfibrinogens)
    • Embolic (cholesterol emboli, hyperoxaluria)
    • Thrombotic
      - Antiphospholipid antibody syndrome, Sneddon's
      - Coumadin necrosis
      - Dego's disease
      - Disseminated intravascular coagulation, purpura fulminans
      - Factor 5 Leiden deficiency
      - Heparin necrosis
      - Homocysteinuria
      - Livedoid vasculitis
      - Polycythemia vera
      - Protein C/S deficiency
      - Thrombotic thrombocytopenic purpura
  - Vasospastic/Raynaud's disease
  - Venous ulcers
- Neuropathic disorders
  • Diabetes
  • Leprosy

*See Appendix I, *Laboratory tests to rule out atypical causes of leg ulcers,* page 579, for screening laboratory tests for these diagnoses.

Complications associated with venous ulceration include the development of dermatitis, wound infection (bacterial and fungal), osteomyelitis, squamous cell carcinoma, and basal cell carcinoma. Venous ulceration can be further complicated by the presence of acute or chronic lipodermatosclerosis, or arterial insufficiency.

DIAGNOSTIC TESTING

Performing the appropriate diagnostic tests is paramount when evaluating the patient with a suspected venous ulcer. The results of the tests will provide the basis for proper interventions and patient management. Recommended tests include:

- *ABI* is a simple, noninvasive test that determines the difference in blood pressure between the upper and lower extremities. ABI is important when checking for arterial insufficiency, which is present in about 25% of patients with venous disease. An ABI less than 0.9 contraindicates the use of compression therapy until further evaluation for the presence of arterial disease is performed. (See Appendix J, *Ankle-brachial index use in patients with diabetes,* pages 580 and 581.)
- *Contrast venogram* is a radiographic picture of the venous system obtained using radiopaque dye injected into a dorsal pedal vein. This test is less desirable than ABI because it's invasive. In addition, the test places the patient at risk for inducing local thrombophlebitis and deep vein thrombosis. Nonionic dye should be used in patients with renal insufficiency.
- *Doppler ultrasonography* is a qualitative, noninvasive test to establish the absence or presence of venous reflux. Excellent sensitivity and specificity is obtained when the test is done at the saphenofemoral or saphenopopliteal junctions; other sites may not accurately reflect venous status.
- *Air plethysmography* provides a quantitative assessment of calf venous reflux and calf muscle pump function. It measures venous filling index, which is the best determinant of the clinical severity of venous disease. It also assists in identifying patients who are suited for venous reconstruction. However, this test doesn't provide information about the venous status above the knee.
- *Photoplethysmography* is a quick, easy test that uses a photoelectrode to measure blood flow and blood volume changes in the skin at rest and after calf muscle exercise to determine venous refill time, a determinant of severity of venous reflux.

MANAGEMENT

The key to treating any chronic wound is to address the underlying problem. Because elevated venous pressure and resulting edema is the problem with venous ulcers, compression therapy to control this is crucial to successful management. Leg elevation, dressings, and debridement all play important roles in managing venous ulcers.

New technologies—such as skin substitutes and biologics, growth factors, and gene therapy—provide greater choices for the treatment of chronic venous ulcers.

Compression therapy

The mainstay of treatment of venous ulcers, compression therapy has been shown to improve the rate of ulcer healing, reduce the incidence of recurrence, and prolong the interval to a first recurrence. Between 50% and 60% of patients heal with compression therapy alone within 6 months. Some of the physiologic changes that have been reported to occur using compression therapy include improvement of lymphatic drainage, reduction of superficial venous pressure, improvement of blood flow velocity through unoccluded deep and superficial veins, and reduction of reflux in the deep veins. Studies have shown that venous ulcers that demonstrate healing after 4 weeks of compression therapy are likely to be completely healed by 24 weeks. In contrast, venous ulcers that don't show healing after 4 weeks of compression therapy tend to remain problematic. Compression products are described in Part 3 of this book.

Compression can be safely applied to patients with an ABI less than 0.9. Cautious use is necessary for patients with an ABI between 0.7 and 0.9. Compression is contraindicated if the ABI is at or below 0.7. A low ABI warrants referral to a vascular surgeon for further testing and evaluation. Uncompensated heart failure may also be a contraindication for compression therapy.

Consider the patient's desires regarding the type of device used for compression therapy. It doesn't matter if a particular device is best for a patient if he won't wear it. Available products can be categorized into two main types: rigid compression or elastic compression.

Using compression therapy

Paste bandages or multilayer wraps are typically used for ulcer treatment. Once these devices are applied, the patient should be seen again in 3 to 4 days to assess the wound and the patient's ability to tolerate compression therapy. If he has significant edema and exudate, twice-weekly changes may be necessary until the edema and exudate decrease. In addition, if the patient is having pain related to edema, the initial wraps should be applied with less compression to decrease pain and help him become accustomed to the therapy. Sufficient analgesia should be provided so that the compression therapy can be used comfortably.

Once the edema is reduced, the pain and exudate typically decrease. The wrap should then be applied with the recommended stretch and changed weekly. Once the wound is healed, the patient will be anxious to be out of the device; however, it's prudent to maintain the compression (with weekly changes) for an additional 2 to 4 weeks after healing to allow the scar to mature and strengthen. Many ulcers have rapidly recurred from a simple friction injury secondary to stocking application and removal over weak scar tissue. Once the ulcer has healed, stockings, wraps, or leggings are used for long-term compression. For patients with mild venous disease, a stock-

ing with 20 to 30 mm Hg compression can be used; for patients with severe disease, a stocking with 30 to 40 mm Hg compression may be necessary. Also, it must be consistently reinforced to the patient that the key to
preventing ulcers from recurring is lifelong compression therapy. The patient must regularly replace his device. A typical Ace wrap, for example,
may need to be replaced after 1 month; a pair of quality stockings will
maintain compression for 4 to 6 months.

Rigid compression

Rigid, or inelastic, compression is effective at reducing edema in the ambulatory patient. It provides low resting pressure and high ambulatory pressure. This type of wrap or legging doesn't stretch, so when the calf muscles
contract during ambulation, they press against this rigid "container" and
are forced to contract inward, massaging the veins and pumping blood toward the heart. Because a competent calf muscle pump is essential for the
efficacy of rigid compression, this modality is less effective with patients
who are nonambulatory, have limited ankle joint mobility, or have a muscular disorder.

Examples of rigid compression devices include paste bandages, Circ-Aid
leggings, and low-stretch bandages. Paste bandages, traditionally called
Unna's boot, are composed of gauze bandages impregnated with a gelatinous substance and zinc oxide paste. They provide a moist wound-healing environment, and many will hydrate dry skin. A disadvantage of the
paste bandage is its inability to conform to the changing volume of the leg
as edema decreases; when used alone, the paste bandage will maintain
compression only for about 48 hours. Typically, an elastic wrap is applied
over the paste bandage component to maintain compression for longer
periods. Dressings can be used over the wound or gauze, and can be added
between the paste bandage layer and the elastic wrap for exudate absorption. Caution should be used with patients with a history of contact sensitivity because they may react to the ingredients in the paste bandage.

Elastic compression

Elastic compression provides high resting pressure and moderately high
ambulatory pressure (lower than rigid compression during walking). Because of sustained pressure at rest, it is ideal for nonambulatory patients
or patients who don't have a competent calf muscle pump. However, its
sustained high pressure at rest can lead to pain and pressure areas, especially in a patient with mild arterial disease (those with an ABI of 0.7 to
0.9).

Compression stockings, elastic wraps, and multilayer wraps are examples of elastic compression devices that aid venous return when used in
conjunction with leg elevation. Compression stockings are available with
different grades of pressure, and they can be applied often, even though
they may be difficult to apply. Patients who desire daily showers may ap-
preciate use of a stocking for ulcer treatment.

Elastic wraps are inexpensive products that maintain pressure at about
20 to 30 mm Hg, depending on how they are applied, their thickness, and

their age. They also allow the patient to shower. After being washed, however, these wraps lose some of their compression capability. Newer elastic wraps with printed rectangles that stretch to squares when applied correctly are available. These wraps will maintain compression through 20 washings.

Multilayer wraps, consisting of three to four dry layers, are high-stretch bandages that stay in place for up to 1 week at a time. This compression system, made up of several different components, has been clinically proven to achieve pressures of 30 to 40 mm Hg at the ankle, graduating to 12 to 17 mm Hg below the knee. Padding is applied as the initial layer to assist in redistributing the pressure around bony prominences and absorbing wound exudate. The remaining layers are elastic, cohesive bandages that achieve sustained graduated compression. The multilayer system is appropriate for both ambulatory and nonambulatory patients. It's flexible and comfortable and can control heavy drainage. These bandages may slip down the leg and wrinkle more often than paste bandages, but they have the advantage of not causing sensitivity reactions.

Compression pumps facilitate venous return, decrease edema, and enhance fibrolytic activity. They function by inflation and deflation of select chambers on a given cycle, providing the "pumping" action needed to assist in resolving venous hypertension. Although this process may prove to be effective for some patients, it may be too time-consuming for some patients and caregivers. In addition, it may lead to lymphatic congestion in the upper thigh and pelvic region, further worsening lymphatic return.

Dressings

Topical wound management varies according to the wound's characteristics, including amount of exudate, size of the wound, presence or absence of infection, and the characteristics of the surrounding skin. Moisture-retentive dressings, such as hydrocolloids and certain foams, should be selected for wounds with light to moderate drainage. Absorbent dressings—such as foams, alginates, and specialty absorptive dressings—should be selected for wounds with moderate to heavy exudate. Some dense foam dressings will also provide local compression under wraps, especially important if the ulcer is located in a concave area, such as inferior or posterior to the malleolus. (See Part 2 of this book.)

Debridement

Wound debridement classically has been considered the first step in treating venous ulcers. Debridement can be accomplished using autolytic, chemical, mechanical, or biological methods; however, evidence supporting the efficacy of many of these methods is sparse.

■ Autolytic debridement is accomplished by using occlusive dressings. These dressings help maintain a moist wound environment, thereby promoting reepithelialization. They have also been shown to reduce pain, enhance autolytic debridement, and provide a barrier to infection. There are five basic types of occlusive dressings: hydrogels, alginates, hydrocolloids, foams, and films. Because venous ulcers tend to have moderate to high exudate, the use of film or hydrogel dressings isn't a common choice.

- Chemical debridement involves the use of enzyme debriding agents, including fibrinolysin, deoxyribonuclease, papain, collagenase, and trypsin. Compelling clinical evidence for the use of these agents for venous ulcers is limited. Because some patients with venous insufficiency have contact sensitivities to products, use these agents with caution.

- Mechanical debridement can be accomplished by several methods, including application of wet-to-dry dressings, hydrotherapy, and irrigation. The major disadvantage of mechanical debridement is that it's nonselective, frequently removing viable tissue with necrotic tissue.

- Sharp debridement involves the use of instruments to remove necrotic tissue or debris. Venous ulcers may benefit from curettage to remove fibrin and senescent cells. This is especially important when preparing the wound for the application of bioengineered skin.

Arterial ulcers

Arterial ulcers fail to heal due to impaired blood flow to the wound, possibly as a result of disruption in microvascular blood flow, such as in vasculitis, microthrombosis, Raynaud's phenomenon, and sickle cell anemia. More commonly, macrovascular flow is disrupted due to atherosclerosis. Atherosclerosis, caused by deposits of cholesterol, lipids, and calcium in the lumen of vessels, may affect any artery in the body and lead to impaired arterial flow. Peripheral arterial disease (PAD) is atherosclerosis of the large and medium-sized vessels of the lower extremities.

The incidence of atherosclerosis increases in the elderly. Patients with arterial ulcers are typically older than age 50. The reported incidence of PAD ranges from 2.2% in patients ages 50 to 59 to 7.7% in patients ages 70 to 74. The patient with PAD may present with a history of coronary artery disease, cerebrovascular disease, hyperlipidemia, diabetes, hypertension, and cigarette smoking. He may have undergone prior revascularization procedures and amputation.

PATHOGENESIS

Arterial insufficiency is the impairment of arterial blood flow leading to tissue ischemia and, potentially, necrosis. Such impairment can occur acutely (trauma or thrombosis) or chronically (atherosclerosis). Both acute and chronic arterial insufficiency can lead to the formation of lower-extremity ulcers. Arterial insufficiency can occur at any level, from large arteries, to arterioles and capillaries. Tissue ischemia that leads to leg ulcers tends to occur more in large vessel or mixed disease.

Obstruction of arterial flow can be classified as anatomic or functional. Anatomic causes of obstruction include thrombosis, emboli, atherosclerosis, and vasculitis. Functional impairment occurs with conditions such as Raynaud's phenomenon, in which abnormal vasomotor function leads to reversible obstruction. Reversible ischemia tends to cause pain and, infrequently, results in ulceration. Other potential causes of impaired arterial flow include disruption (trauma), fistulas, and aneurysms. Nonatherosclerotic or vasculitic causes should be considered in the patient with signs of tissue ischemia but normal pulses.

The most common cause of arterial ulcers is atherosclerosis. Risk factors for the development of atherosclerosis include age, smoking, diabetes mellitus, hypertension, dyslipidemia, family history, obesity, and sedentary lifestyle. It's estimated that 5% to 20% of leg ulcers are caused by ischemia due to PAD. These ulcers typically result from trauma—for example, the patient may have developed a blister from a shoe. Regardless, in the presence of severe PAD, if blood flow is insufficient to meet the metabolic demands of tissue repair, a chronic wound results.

Arterial insufficiency may also act with other pathologic mechanisms, leading to tissue necrosis and ulceration. Diabetic foot ulcers, for example, may result from the combination of neuropathy, trauma, and arterial insufficiency.

ASSESSMENT

The initial assessment of any ulcer begins with a thorough history and physical examination. Although most leg ulcers are caused by venous insufficiency, one must carefully assess the patient for the presence of arterial insufficiency as well because concomitant arterial disease can delay or prevent healing. In addition, compression therapy—the cornerstone of treatment for venous insufficiency—can cause tissue necrosis and ulceration in patients with underlying arterial disease.

The history should include screening for risk factors for atherosclerosis—especially smoking, diabetes, hyperlipidemia, and hypertension. A medical history of coronary artery disease (angina pectoris or myocardial infarction) and carotid disease (transient ischemic attacks or ischemic stroke) increases the likelihood of PAD. Claudication, a burning sensation of the calf muscles exacerbated by ambulation and relieved by rest, is the physical manifestation of arterial insufficiency of the large arteries of the legs.

Arterial ulcers tend to have a "punched-out" appearance, being small and round, with smooth, well-demarcated borders. The wound base is typically pale and lacks granulation tissue. Wet or dry necrotic tissue may be present. Arterial ulcers tend to occur over the distal part of the leg, especially the lateral malleoli, the dorsum of the feet, and the toes. They can be shallow or deep and are frequently painful. Typically, the patient complains of pain when the feet are elevated, especially at night, and states that the pain is reduced with leg dependence. In addition to these common features, the physical examination may reveal a decrease in peripheral pulses, lack of hair over the distal leg, and cyanosis, pallor, and atrophy of the surrounding skin. Lifting the leg greater than 60 degrees can induce pallor in the ischemic limb. When dropped to a dependent position, the limb may become very red.

Vasculitic ulcers have some characteristics similar to arterial ulcers, including their location, size, and shallow depth. There are several typical differences, however; for example, many vasculitic ulcers have irregular shapes and borders. In addition, the base of the wound tends to be necrotic with significant vascularity. The surrounding skin is usually hyperemic rather than pale. Vasculitis may also feature other cutaneous manifestations, including palpable purpura, petechiae, and persistent urticaria.

DIAGNOSTIC TESTING

Testing should be done to obtain anatomic and physiologic data. Noninvasive testing is crucial to determine arterial functioning. Angiography is performed to plan the revascularization procedure after noninvasive testing has indicated a functional problem. It makes no difference whether an angiogram demonstrates a severe stenosis if the noninvasive testing indicates adequate functional flow. Tests that can be performed to assess the patient with a suspected arterial ulcer include the following:

- *ABI* is a simple calculation that can be performed in the clinic to assess the patient for arterial insufficiency. Blood pressures are measured over the brachial artery and the posterior tibial artery. The ankle pressure, measured using a handheld Doppler device, should be the same as or slightly higher than the brachial pressure. Arterial insufficiency is likely to present if the ABI (the ankle pressure divided by the brachial pressure) is 0.9 or less. Claudication typically occurs when the ABI is less than 0.8. An ABI of 0.5 to 0.75 represents severe arterial disease, whereas an ABI less than 0.5 is limb threatening. The ABI has the advantages of being inexpensive, noninvasive, and a reported high sensitivity and specificity. (See Appendix J, *Ankle-brachial index use in patients with diabetes,* pages 580 and 581.)
- *Segmental pressures,* obtained in a noninvasive test, can be used to confirm arterial insufficiency. Supine systolic pressures are recorded at the high thigh, low thigh, below the knee, and above the ankle. These segmental pressures should be about the same, and similar or slightly higher than the brachial systolic pressure. A drop in the segmental pressure of more than 20 to 30 mm Hg indicates arterial occlusion. Abnormally high pressures, especially in the presence of dampened waveforms, indicate medial calcification of the arteries, which leads to noncompressibility. When this is present, segmental pressures can't be used to assess arterial disease.
- *Toe pressures* are measured by a small pneumatic cuff placed around the toe; this cuff monitors blood flow using a photoelectrode. As the cuff is inflated, the photoelectrode records absence of flow; as the cuff is deflated, it records the pressure when flow returns. The reference value for a toe-brachial index is greater than 0.8. A toe pressure of less than 30

mm Hg indicates poor healing potential. This measurement is rarely affected by medial calcification.

■ *Arterial waveforms* can be obtained using pulse volume recording or Doppler waveform analysis. The normal arterial waveform is triphasic. A monophasic waveform is indicative of moderate arterial occlusive disease, whereas severe disease is indicated by a severely blunted waveform.

■ In *color duplex scanning*, ultrasound provides anatomic and physiologic data about arterial flow. This test determines extent of arterial disease.

■ *Transcutaneous oxygen measurements (TcPO$_2$)* can be used to assess the patient for microvascular insufficiency. A measurement greater than 30 mm Hg indicates adequate perfusion, whereas a value less than 20 mm Hg indicates disease. If the tissue surrounding an ulcer has a TcPO$_2$ less than 20 mm Hg, the wound typically won't heal.

■ *Skin perfusion pressure (SPP)* is measured by a pneumatic cuff with a laser Doppler flow sensor. The cuff is placed around the toe, foot, ankle, calf, or thigh and attached to a monitor that records capillary blood flow. As the cuff is inflated, pressure is exerted on the skin, which causes capillary flow to cease. As the cuff is deflated, the sensor notes the point at which flow returns; this is the skin perfusion pressure. The reference value for SPP is 80% of brachial systolic pressure. SPP above 30 mm Hg indicates good potential for healing; SPP below 20 mm Hg, poor potential for healing.

■ *Lower extremity angiography* is the gold standard for diagnosing arterial vascular disease. This procedure is indicated for patients who are candidates for revascularization procedures. The test has associated risks, including cholesterol plaque embolization, acute vascular occlusion, arterial damage, and contrast-induced nephropathy.

■ *Magnetic resonance angiography (MRA)* is a noninvasive means of determining the presence and severity of arterial obstruction. It has become an increasingly important tool in the diagnosis of PAD, and may ultimately supplant lower extremity arteriography as the gold standard. Because of the strong magnetic field, patients whose bodies contain metallic objects, such as a cardiac pacemaker or a vascular clip, can't undergo magnetic resonance angiography. In addition, many patients who suffer from severe claustrophobia are unable to tolerate the small confines of the magnetic resonance imaging machine, which is used to perform the test.

MANAGEMENT

Revascularization is the key to treating arterial ulcers secondary to PAD. Other measures include topical therapy, conservative debridement, and pain control. Treatment is also directed at the pathogenic causes of arterial disease. For example, the management of atherosclerosis includes exercise therapy, reduction of cholesterol levels, smoking cessation, and control of blood pressure and blood glucose levels. Antiplatelet agents (aspirin, ticlopidine, and clopidogrel) and xanthine derivatives (such as pentoxifylline) are commonly used to treat the symptoms associated with PAD. However, medical treatment alone has been of limited efficacy in treating arterial ulcers. Newer modalities, including human growth factors and bioengineered skin substitutes, hold significant promise in treating these commonly difficult-to-heal wounds.

Management of vasculitic ulcers and other conditions that cause arterial insufficiency is typically directed at correcting the underlying condition; however, these conditions won't be discussed here.

Diabetic ulcers

About 16 million people in the United States have diabetes, with 798,000 new cases reported annually. Of those with diagnosed and as-yet-undiagnosed diabetes, 15% will develop at least one foot ulcer during the chronic state of the disease. The leading risk factor for ulceration is previous ulceration. Diabetes is responsible for 56% to 83% of the estimated 125,000 lower-extremity amputations performed annually.

The financial and emotional costs and the potential complications associated with the effects of diabetic foot ulcers are overwhelming. Preventing the loss of limb and function is the goal of the multidisciplinary team caring for the patient with a diabetic foot ulcer. To achieve this end, clinicians must understand the scope and severity of diabetes and its physiologic results.

As diabetes progresses, underlying clinical conditions—such as neuropathy, vascular disease, foot deformity, and infection—become more prevalent. These conditions may occur alone or with other factors. An estimated 60% to 70% of patients with diabetes have peripheral neuropathy, 15% to 20% have peripheral vascular disease, and 15% to 20% have both.

PATHOGENESIS

The pathogenesis of diabetic ulcers varies according to their etiology. A diabetic ulcer may arise due to diabetic neuropathy, peripheral arterial disease, or diabetic foot structure.

Diabetic neuropathy

Diabetic neuropathy, which commonly accompanies long-term diabetes, is commonly overlooked and undiagnosed until an ulcer or pain in the extremity develops. However, early diagnosis and an aggressive ulcer prevention plan can be very successful. Both are imperative to decreasing the number of amputations in this population.

Diabetic neuropathy involves components of the sensory, motor, and autonomic nervous systems. Sensory damage causes the patient to lose the sensation of pain; he may, in fact, lose all sensation, which results in partial or total numbness of the foot. Because of this loss of sensation, also known as a loss of protective sensation, the patient may be unaware of trauma or a damaging process in the foot region. The patient can discover blisters, wounds, or infections only by doing a visual foot check or experiencing systemic signs of infection.

Motor neuropathy, another facet of diabetic neuropathy, can cause changes in the biomechanics of the weight-bearing foot. Imbalances of the foot occur when some muscles atrophy and opposing muscles are unchecked in their action. This can lead to changes in which particular surfaces bear weight in phases of the gait cycle. Deformities such as claw toes, which aren't accommodated in normal shoes, can result and may produce areas of pressure or friction.

Diabetic neuropathy may also affect the autonomic nervous system, which controls the functions of smooth muscle, glands, and visceral organs. Possible effects include changes in the vascular tone, which result in abnormal blood flow, and anhidrosis, which leads to fragile, dry skin that's easily damaged and difficult to heal. Autonomic neuropathy also leads to a decreased flame reaction, in which vasodilation in response to injury or infection is impaired.

Damage associated with diabetic neuropathy is irreversible; however, controlling blood glucose levels can prevent or delay further damage. Pain that may accompany diabetic neuropathy can be treated in various ways. Some risk factors for developing diabetic neuropathy are modifiable, such as hyperglycemia, hypertension, smoking, cholesterol levels, and heavy alcohol use. Patient education about these risk factors and the benefits of controlling these areas is imperative.

Peripheral arterial disease

Peripheral arterial disease is a serious medical problem for patients with and without diabetes. In those with diabetes mellitus, the process of atherosclerosis is accelerated and involves vessels of the entire body. Treatment for narrowing of the arteries and thrombosis includes antiplatelet therapy, surgery for the damaged and blocked vessels, and noninvasive techniques for better evaluation of the vascular status.

Diabetic foot structure

When the physiologic processes of diabetic neuropathy occur in the lower extremity, structural and functional changes in the foot result. Most diabetic foot ulcers result from mechanical forces that exceed what the tissue is able to bear and repair. Because diabetic neuropathy causes loss of protective sensation, the patient can't feel the overloaded tissue. Diminished blood flow and the skin's weakened state mean that the tissue may have difficulty bearing normal stress, much less increased stress to particular areas due to muscle imbalance, poor footwear, and gait changes.

Several structural changes can occur in the diabetic foot. The most severe cases are seen in those who develop Charcot foot (neuroarthropathy). Charcot foot usually first presents with erythema, increased local skin temperature, swelling, bounding pulses and, sometimes, moderate pain. Distinguishing Charcot foot from cellulitis can be difficult. However, the patient with Charcot foot doesn't have a fever or an elevated white blood cell count, which would be present with infection.

In patients with long-term Charcot foot, actual osseous destruction can be viewed on X-rays. This bony destruction occurs at the distal ends of the metatarsals and the ankle bones. Because the patient usually has neuropathy and decreased sensation, chronic cases generate little pain. Continued ambulation results in further bony destruction and stress fractures. Resulting bony fracture changes cause the arch structure to collapse. The foot then takes on a new weight-bearing rocker-bottom shape. The major pressure area of the gait cycle now becomes the arch, an area of ulceration for many patients with Charcot foot.

Ulcerations are common in patients with diabetes, even without Charcot factors. The heads of the metatarsals are major areas of ulceration. Although pressure is known to increase on the tissue in the area of eventual ulceration, the cause of this increased pressure is under investigation. One theory holds that weakness of the intrinsic muscles results in the claw toe deformity and the displacement of the fatty pads that normally cushion the metatarsal heads. This loss of cushioning results in easier ulceration. However, some studies have examined the integrity of the plantar fascia as the source of the claw toe deformities.

Weakness of the musculature responsible for dorsiflexion and plantarflexion of the foot and ankle complex is another effect of long-term diabetes and may play a role in load patterns on the plantar surface. Changes also occur in the joint mobility of foot structures. The first ray (the first metatarsal and phalange) may lose mobility, thus increasing pressure on the first metatarsal head. Other areas of limited joint mobility are associated with increased ulcerations. These include the subtalar joint with increased plantar pressure and the fourth and fifth metatarsals and phalanges.

Plantar callus formation in diabetic feet is commonly the focus of treatment. Callus formations occur in weight-bearing and non–weight-bearing areas of the diabetic foot. Although some clinicians believe that the callus is a response to increased pressure on the specific point, it may also stem from the autonomic effects of neuropathy and the resulting skin changes. Once present, the callus causes increased pressure and can lead to an underlying blister or hematoma. It should be trimmed off regularly to avoid ulceration. In addition, shoe gear should be adjusted to offload weight from the area of increased pressure.

ASSESSMENT

Wound care team members should be proactive when assessing and managing a patient with a diabetic foot structure. For clinical management to be effective, the team must have a keen understanding of the disease state and the patient's current overall health, not just the status of the foot as well as an awareness of his actual and potential risk factors.

Assessment questions

- When was the patient diagnosed with diabetes?
- What is the medication regimen for this patient?
- Does the patient have a clear understanding of the disease process and potential complications?
- How often does the patient self-monitor his blood glucose level?
- Has the patient had a blood test to check the glycosylated hemoglobin levels (a measure of glycemic control) in the past 3 months?
- Has a licensed professional, that is a certified diabetic educator, dietitian, counseled the patient?
- Does the patient complain of lower limb or foot pain (indicative of claudication)?
- Has the patient ever experienced foot ulcers?
- Has the patient suffered any known heart disease?

Hess, C.T. *Clinical Wound Manager Manual Series for the Wound Care Department.* © Wound Care Strategies, Inc., 2001.

Patient history

Clinical team members must ask specific questions with regard to patient history to determine the status of the patient's diabetes. (See *Assessment questions.*)

The clinician can't take for granted the patient's ability to care for himself. Rather, the patient should be asked to provide both verbal descriptions of self-care techniques (including foot care, foot checks, and insulin administration) and physical demonstrations of self-care (for example, the ability to assess the feet and between the toes). The clinician's responsibility is to accurately document the goals that the patient achieves.

PHYSICAL EXAMINATION

Obtaining a verbal patient history provides the clinician with only half of the clinical picture—a thorough evaluation of the patient's lower legs, feet, and toes for muscular tone, skin and tissue integrity, and vascular status is also essential. (See *Physical assessment checklist,* page 74.)

Assessment to evaluate the diabetic foot should include the following:
- Perform the Semmes-Weinstein test.
- Obtain the patient's ABI to assess blood flow, or refer the patient for more advanced arterial vascular studies. ABI should be interpreted with caution in patients with diabetes secondary to a high degree of calcified or stenotic vessels, which give falsely elevated values.
- Examine the patient's feet for ulcers, especially the plantar aspect of the toes, laterally to the foot, between the toes, and the tips of the toes.
- Evaluate the patient's footwear. Does it protect the feet, or does it promote rubbing?

Physical assessment checklist

- Has the team member performed a general physical examination that assesses the patient for signs of neuropathy and muscle wasting?
- Has the team member evaluated the patient's popliteal and pedal pulses?
- Has the team member described the condition of the patient's foot or feet? Is there evidence of Charcot foot, healed or existing areas of breakdown, or poor nail condition?
- Has the team member noted the overall status of the skin and presence of any scars from previous ulcers or surgery?
- Has the team member noted any other lower-extremity conditions such as venous insufficiency, which may complicate treatment?

Hess, C.T. *Clinical Wound Manager Manual Series for the Wound Care Department.* © Wound Care Strategies, Inc., 2001.

Semmes-Weinstein test

The most widely used test for identifying loss of protective sensation in a diabetic foot is the Semmes-Weinstein test. Annual screening with this test is recommended for all patients with diabetes. (See *Monofilament test to assess protective sensation.*)

After completing a thorough patient history and physical assessment, the clinician should document the findings in detail. The next step is to educate the patient about the disease process and the importance of his role in the care plan. This also involves assessing the patient's preferred learning style and accommodating that style in the teaching plan. Providing the patient with the proper skills and products needed to prevent foot ulceration is a team approach.

Risk factor evaluation

Evaluating the patient's foot ulcer risk is part of assessment. Risk factors for patients with diabetes include:

- absent protective sensation
- autonomic neuropathy causing fissure and integument and osseous hyperemia
- foot deformity causing high-pressure focal points
- history of foot ulceration
- history of lower-extremity amputation
- impaired vision
- limited joint mobility
- obesity
- poor control of blood glucose levels, resulting in advanced glycosylation and impaired wound healing

Monofilament test to assess protective sensation

A Semmes-Weinstein monofilament is commonly used to assess protective sensation in the feet of patients with diabetes. A 10-g (5.07 log) monofilament wire is applied to each foot at 10 sites — the plantar aspect of the first, third, and fifth digits; the plantar aspect of the first, third, and fifth metatarsal heads; the planter midfoot medially and laterally; the plantar heel; and the dorsal aspect of the midfoot.

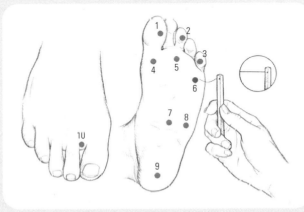

Loss of protective sensation is indicated when a patient can't feel the monofilament at 4 or more sites. These pointers ensure that the procedure is done correctly:

■ Place the patient in a supine or sitting position with legs supported and shoes and socks removed. Touch the Semmes-Weinstein monofilament to the patient's arm or hand to demonstrate what it feels like. During the test, the patient should respond "yes" each time he feels the pressure of the monofilament on his foot.

■ Make sure the patient's feet are in a neutral position, with toes pointing straight up. Have the patient close his eyes. Hold the Semmes-Weinstein monofilament perpendicular to the patient's foot, then press it against the first site, increasing the pressure until the monofilament wire bends into a C shape. Make sure it does not slide over the skin. The device should be held in place for about 1 second. After the patient responds, record the response on a foot screening form. Use a "+" for a positive response and a "−" for a negative response. Then move to the next site.

■ Test sites in random order and vary the time between applications so that the patient can't guess the correct response. If the patient has an ulcer, scar, callus, or necrotic tissue at the test site, apply the monofilament along the perimeter of the abnormality, not directly on it.

(continued)

> ## Monofilament test to assess
> ## protective sensation *(continued)*
>
> ■ If results show a loss of protective sensation, the patient should be taught self-assessment with the Semmes-Weinstein monofilament, although this doesn't replace a professional evaluation.
>
> Adapted with permission from Sloan, H.L., and Abel, R.J. "Getting in touch with impaired foot sensitivity," *Nursing98* 28(11):50-51, November 1998.

- poorly designed or poorly fitting footwear, causing or inadequately protecting the foot from tissue breakdown
- vascular insufficiency.

DIABETIC FOOT ULCER CLASSIFICATION

Diabetic ulcers are described according to their depth and are classified using a grading system. The most commonly used system is the Wagner Ulcer Grade Classification, developed by Wagner and Meggitt. (See Appendix B, *Wagner ulcer grade classification*, page 571.) According to this scale, the lower-grade ulcer is less complex and may respond to medical intervention. Higher grades may need surgery or amputation.

Some difficulties in using the Wagner scale have led to the development of several other assessment scales. One example is the Brodsky scale, which combines depth and ischemia. The University of Texas diabetic foot classification system is also used to classify diabetic foot ulcers. (See *University of Texas diabetic foot classification system*, page 43.)

Infection in the diabetic foot

Diabetic foot infections are always serious and should be considered limb threatening. A patient with diabetes may be unaware of the presence of an infection, resulting in delayed diagnosis and management. Diabetes itself, diabetic neuropathy, vasculopathy, and lack of proper wound healing mechanisms all contribute to the problem of infection in patients with diabetes. The disease compromises the immune system, which results in decreased function of defense mechanisms. Patients with diabetes also have increased problems with nail fungi and skin infections, which can damage the skin and allow access for bacteria.

Infection spreads easily in the foot because of its compartmentalized structure. Edema associated with infections can cause elevated compartmental pressures, leading to ischemia and further foot damage. This problem of compartmental spread is commonly seen in ulcerative infections that move rapidly through the plantar fascial plane and compartment.

A diagnosis of infection requires the presence of two or more signs of infection, including purulent drainage, crepitus, fluctuance, loss of glycemic control, and systemic signs. Because the diabetic patient's response to infection may be impaired, white blood cell count and erythrocyte sedimentation rate may not be elevated, further complicating diagnosis.

Bone infection results in destructive bone changes that may mimic those of neuropathy or Charcot disease. Bone infections are difficult to diagnose with X-rays, bone scans, or other procedures; destructive changes may not be visible on an X-ray, for example, for 3 to 4 weeks. Hence, the clinician should always suspect the presence of osteomyelitis when bone can be palpated through a chronic open wound. Correlation with localized wound status, drainage, systemic signs, and location supports a diagnosis of bone infection. Identifying the organism that has invaded the bone requires a bone culture because it may not be the same organism that appears on the swab cultured from the surrounding wound.

Treatment of the ulcer infection centers on debridement of the necrotic wound tissue, glycemic control, administration of systemic antibiotics, and good local wound care. If the patient has peripheral vascular disease, achieving adequate antibiotic levels in the area of tissue damage may be difficult because of poor tissue perfusion. If the patient has osteomyelitis, the treatment is usually prolonged 6 weeks or more to allow for the poor penetration of antibiotic into the bone. In some cases, the only way to eliminate the infection is to remove the bone.

MANAGEMENT

Key elements of the management regimen developed by the wound care team, which should always include the patient and his family, include preventing future damage, minimizing current damage, and ensuring maximum function and quality of life. This means preventing amputation and loss of life associated with the diabetic foot.

Interventions to achieve these goals include both nonsurgical and surgical options. Patient education, prevention, and management programs are also essential in managing diabetic foot ulcers.

Nonsurgical options

Nonsurgical management of the diabetic foot includes maximizing wound care by maintaining an appropriate wound environment, debriding necrotic tissue, eliminating pressure areas on the foot, and improving the muscular strength and length of the lower extremity.

Relieving pressure areas on the foot, or offloading, sounds easier than it is. It relies on patient compliance, clinician understanding of biomechanics, and availability of the appropriate products or materials.

Total contact casting is widely considered the best way to offload diabetic foot wounds. The pressure is redistributed across the rest of the plantar surface and away from the wound through careful cast application. Casting materials are available in most clinics, and patient compliance is relatively high because the cast is applied and removed by the clinical team.

Other methods of offloading include custom-molded ankle-foot orthoses, posterior splints, orthotic dynamic splints (which are bivalved and similar to a total contact cast), and custom-molded healing sandals. Prefabricated products, such as cast walkers, are also available. These walkers may be more appropriate for patients with vascular compromise or wounds that require frequent care. Other options include customizable postoperative shoes and shoe materials provided through trained professionals.

Whatever the options for offloading available in a facility, they all require a complete education plan for the patient, a level of commitment on the patient's part—compliance is key to successful wound healing—and close monitoring, with any necessary modifications made promptly.

Physical therapy can also assist in diabetic wound healing with programs that address muscular imbalances in the lower extremity and foot, gait changes, offloading, and exercise programs to assist in glycemic control. Electric stimulation, another modality widely available through physical therapy, is highly effective in assisting the wound-healing process. In addition, physical therapists in many states are able to perform sharp debridement and are active members of the wound care team in both inpatient and outpatient settings.

Surgical options

Many patients need surgery to aid in healing the diabetic foot ulcer. Such intervention may involve addressing nail issues, debridement to remove necrotic tissue, or changing the wound from a chronic, nonhealing state to an active, inflammatory (acute) state to jump-start the healing process. When osteomyelitis is present, the infected section of the bone must usually be removed to allow the ulcer to heal. Osteotomy—partial bone removal—may be necessary if the bone is a source of pressure during weight bearing. Osteotomies and tendon releases to address structural changes are occasionally performed as preventive measures in foot areas that are highly prone to breakdown. However, these approaches are controversial.

Vascular issues in the diabetic foot should be assessed for possible surgical intervention. If the foot doesn't have adequate blood supply, healing won't occur despite the wound care team's best efforts. Vascular assessment and frequent reassessment are imperative throughout the patient's care. The incorporation of risk assessment tools can complement this reassessment process (see "Risk assessment tools," in chapter 2, page 35).

Identifying and treating wound infections

After assessing the patient and the wound, the clinician can develop a care plan that focuses on preparing the wound bed for healing. The goals of wound bed preparation include removing necrotic or fibrinous tissue, reducing the total number of senescent or abnormal cells, decreasing exudate and bacterial load, and increasing granulation tissue. These goals are achieved through a multistep process, using strategies designed to improve wound status. (See *Managing bacterial bioburden,* pages 80 to 85.)

BACTERIAL BALANCE

Most wounds contain various organisms. The notion of bacterial balance stresses the clinician's need to recognize when the bacterial load has increased via a change in granulation tissue appearance and exudate amount.

Contamination or colonization

In a chronic wound that's healing, the level of the bacterial load present is called contamination or colonization. This is a steady state of replicating organisms in the wound that don't cause injury or delay wound healing.

For a patient with contamination or colonization, the clinician should select topical therapies that can create and maintain a moist wound environment. Adjunctive therapies, in combination with absorbent topical management products, may assist wound healing. For example, compression therapy may be combined with a moist wound dressing in a patient with a venous ulcer. Patient education for the care of the chronic wound is paramount to achieving and maintaining a healed wound.

Critical colonization

The next level of bacterial load is critical colonization. This level is characterized as replicating (infectious) organisms that cause a change in the wound's status. The clinician may observe understated clinical features in the wound's appearance, including:
- absent or abnormal granulation tissue
- change in color of the wound bed from previous evaluations
- delayed healing
- excessive or increased serous exudate
- foul or excessive odor
- friable granulation tissue
- serous exudate with concurrent redness of periwound edges
- severe or increased pain at the wound site
- tunneling or pocketing of the wound.

The clinician should select topical therapies that will reduce the bacterial load, manage exudate, and improve the qualities of the wound's granulation tissue. The patient may benefit from adjunctive therapies, such as compression therapy in combination with absorbent topical management products. Teach the patient to help achieve and maintain a healed wound.

Infection

A wound infection can be characterized as an invasion of organisms into the wound and surrounding soft tissue that results in a host response and leads to nonhealing or worsening of the wound. Classic signs and symptoms include:
- raised white blood cell count with increased newly developed cells (bands)
- excessive or purulent drainage

(Text continues on page 86.)

Managing bacterial bioburden

Use this algorithm and the explanation of its 10 steps (pages 88 to 91) to guide you through the wound management process.

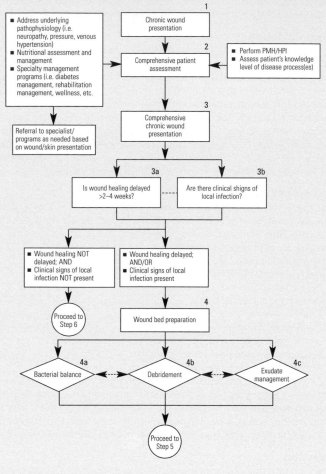

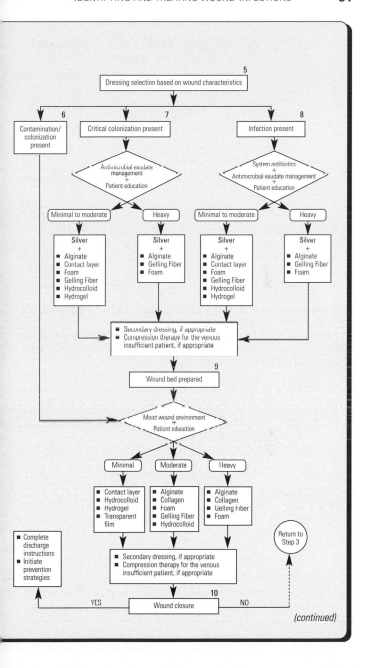

(continued)

Managing bacterial bioburden *(continued)*

1   Chronic wound

An insult or injury that has "failed to proceed through an orderly and timely process to produce anatomic and functional integrity, or proceeded through the repair process without establishing a sustained anatomic and functional result" as described by Lazarus, et al.

2   Comprehensive patient assessment

- Obtain a detailed assessment of the patient's past and current family, social, and medical.
- Obtain a medication list of current and past medications and dressings that have failed.
- Review all laboratory, radiology, vascular studies that have been obtained.
- Review the patient's nutritional status and supportive therapies.
- Review all support surfaces and positioning devices used to manage the patient's tissue load.
- Address all underlying pathologies compromising the wound healing process (neuropathic, pressure, vascular, venous hypertension).
- Review all physician and non-physician consults related to specialty management programs for skin and wound care.
- Correct all underlying pathologies compromising the wound healing process. Assess the patient's knowledge level relative to the disease process and document any and all factors that affect learning needs.

3   Comprehensive wound assessment

- A detailed assessment of the patient's wound status should include but isn't limited to:
  - location
  - size (length, width, depth, undermining)
  - color and type of wound tissue
  - exudate/drainage amount or type
  - odor
  - periwound skin condition
  - wound margins
  - pain
  - dressing management
  - adjunctive therapies
  - patient knowledge level of disease process and wound management.

3a   Is wound healing delayed > 2 to 4 weeks?

- One assessment parameter predictive of delayed wound healing is the lack of wound closure or decrease in wound size. Validated research suggests the level of bacteria could be a causative factor for delay or impairment of wound healing.

3b Are there clinical signs of local wound infection?

The clinical signs and symptoms of local wound infection include:

- abnormal odor
- absent or abnormal granulation tissue
- change in color of the wound bed
- delayed healing
- friable granulation tissue
- increased pain at the wound site
- increased serous exudate
- serous exudate with concurrent inflammation
- tunneling or pocketing of the wound.

4, 4a, 4b, 4c Wound bed preparation

- Multi-step processes/strategies employed to improve the wound status through:
  - Bacterial balance:
    - Understanding that all wounds are contaminated with a variety of organisms, bacterial balance stresses the need for the clinician to recognizing an increase bacterial load through a change in granulation tissue appearance and exudate amount.
  - Debridement
    - Senescent and non-migratory cells in the wound may be removed during the removal of devitalized tissue and foreign matter from a wound.
    - Techniques: autolytic, biosurgical, enzymatic, and mechanical.
  - Exudate management

    Controlling the amount of exudate has been shown to improve healing through improving migration of key cells (such as keratinocytes, fibroblasts and endothelial cells) as well as matrix metalloproteinases (MMPs) and proteases.
    - Uses of exudate management devices employed are dependent on the etiology of the wound occurrence and may include compression therapy, absorptive dressing management, and/or mechanical devices/products.

5 Dressing selection based on wound characteristics

- More than 2,000 wound products are available to assist the clinician in achieving successful wound healing. Clinician's should choose a dressing based on the following:

(continued)

Managing bacterial bioburden *(continued)*

5　Dressing selection based on wound characteristics *(continued)*

- Wound and skin-related factors, such as etiology, classification, anatomical location, wound size and depth, presence of undermining or tunneling, type of tissue present (i.e., granulation, slough, eschar), appearing of wound edges, condition of periwound skin, volume of exudate, presence of odor. Other considerations include:
    - patient-related factors, such as odor control requirements, comfort and preferences; and cost benefit ratio
    - dressing related factors, such as availability, durability, adaptability, and uses.

6　Contamination or colonization

- Most chronic wounds that heal have bacteria present. This level of bacteria is called contamination/colonization and can be characterized as steady state of replicating organisms that maintain a presence in the wound but do not cause injury or delay the wound healing process.
- At this juncture, select topical therapies can be employed to create and maintain a moist wound environment.
- Adjunctive therapies, in combination with absorbent topical management products, may assist the patient in achieving wound healing. These therapies may include compression therapy.
- Patient education for the care of the chronic wound is paramount to achieving and maintaining a healed wound.

7　Critical colonization

- Critical colonization can be characterized as replicating (infectious) organisms present in the wound that begin to cause a change in the wound's status. At this time, the clinician may see understated clinical features in the wound's appearance which include:
    - foul or excessive odor
    - absent or abnormal granulation tissue
    - change in color of the wound bed from successive evaluations
    - delayed healing
    - friable granulation tissue
    - severe or increased pain at the wound site
    - excessive of increased serous exudate
    - serous exudate with concurrent redness of surrounding periwound wound edges
    - tunneling or pocketing of the wound.
- At this juncture, select topical therapies can be employed to decrease the bacterial load, contain exudate, and improve the qualities of the wound's granulation tissue.

- Adjunctive therapies, in combination with absorbent topical management products, may assist the patient in achieving wound healing. These therapies may include compression therapy.
- Patient education for the care of the wound is paramount to achieving and maintaining a healed wound.

8   Infection

- Infection can be characterized as organisms present in the wound and surrounding soft tissue that result in a host response, and lead to non-healing or decline of the wound (increase in size, pain). Classic clinical signs and symptoms include:
  - periwound and soft tissue edema (swelling)
  - periwound and soft tissue erythema
  - fever
  - foul odor
  - severe or increasing pain at the wound's site
  - tenderness at the wound, periwound site, and surrounding soft tissue
  - excessive and/or purulent drainage
  - warmth of the surrounding soft tissue and periwound skin.
- At this juncture, appropriate systemic antibiotics in conjunction with select topical therapies can be employed to treat the bacterial infection, contain exudate, and improve the qualities of the wound's granulation tissue.
- Adjunctive therapies, in combination with absorbent topical management products, may assist the patient in achieving wound healing. These therapies may include compression therapy.
- Patient education for the care of the wound is paramount to achieving and maintaining a healed wound.

9   Wound bed prepared

- Organized and holistic approaches/processes employed to optimize wound healing. Goals to maintain bacterial balance, remove necrotic debris and excessive exudates have been met.

10   Wound closure

- The final phase of wound healing. Wound healing is defined as a restored epithelial covering but maturation of the epithelium may take weeks to occur. In tandem, wound remodeling (collagen and other matrix materials) occurs over a period of many months, and the healed wound is never as strong as the previously unwounded skin. Prevention of wound recurrence through patient education of risk factors and behavior modification are critical.

- fever
- foul odor
- periwound and soft tissue edema and erythema
- severe or increasing pain at the wound site
- tenderness at wound and periwound site and surrounding soft tissue
- warmth of the surrounding soft tissue and periwound skin.

Systemic antibiotics can be used with topical therapies to treat the bacterial infection, contain exudate, and improve the quality of the wound's granulation tissue.

DEBRIDEMENT

Through the process of removing devitalized tissue and foreign material from a wound, the clinician may also remove senescent and nonmigratory cells in and around the wound. Removing these materials may contribute to the release of available growth factors in the wound. (See chapter 5, Developing a skin and wound care formulary.)

Debridement techniques include autolytic, biosurgical, enzymatic, mechanical, and surgical. The type of debridement and the frequency with which it's used depend on the patient's condition and care plan.

EXUDATE MANAGEMENT

Chronic wound fluid inhibits cell growth in culture and is interconnected with barriers to healing, including necrotic tissue and bacterial imbalance. Controlling the amount of exudate may improve healing by improving migration of key cells, such as keratinocytes, fibroblasts, and endothelial cells.

The type of exudate management device used depends on the cause of the wound and may include compression therapy, mechanical devices or products, or absorptive dressing management.

LABORATORY VALUES IN CHRONIC WOUND MANAGEMENT

Wound healing is a complex process that uses specific cellular and biochemical actions to achieve wound closure. These processes—homeostasis, inflammation, proliferation, and maturation—occur over defined periods of time. They are often taken for granted as the wound innately granulates, contracts, and epithelializes under optimal conditions.

A wound begs the clinician's attention when the healing processes stall and the wound doesn't progress to closure. This type of wound is deemed chronic; it's defined as an insult or injury that has failed to proceed through an orderly and timely process to produce anatomic and functional integrity, or that has proceeded through the repair process without establishing a sustained anatomic and functional result.

Despite advances in wound care over the last few decades, many chronic wounds continue to be affected by local and systemic factors that impair the healing process. Local factors include bacterial load and infection, trauma, edema, pressure, and moisture. Systemic factors include age; chronic medical conditions, such as anemia, diabetes mellitus, and renal or hepatic dysfunction; stress; medications; tissue oxygenation; and nutritional status, such as vitamin, protein, or fluid deficiencies.

Clinicians commonly evaluate and manage the typical chronic wounds, such as pressure ulcers, vascular ulcers, and diabetic ulcers. However, many unusual wounds mimic these common chronic wounds. Because these *unusual wounds* are often incorrectly assessed, they're also misdiagnosed. Examples of conditions featuring unusual wounds include pyoderma gangrenosum, calciphylaxis, toxic epidermal necrolysis, epidermolysis bullosa, polyarteritis nodosa, antiphospholipid antibody syndrome, cryoglobulinemia, cholesterol emboli, disseminated intravascular coagulation/ purpura fulminans, bullous pemphigoid, and necrotizing fasciitis.

Misdiagnosis

Misdiagnosis of a wound prolongs the patient's suffering by delaying healing; increasing the emotional and financial toll on the patient, caregiver, and facility; and increasing medical liability. It also leads to improper medication delivery and improper topical treatments, which further exacerbates the patient's condition, covers up symptoms, prolongs the wrong diagnosis, and increases the patient's morbidity or mortality.

This point is well illustrated in an article by Weening and associates on skin ulcers misdiagnosed as pyoderma gangrenosum. The authors reviewed 8 years' worth of charts (240 from their facility and 157 from another one) in which wounds were diagnosed as pyoderma gangrenosum, but 10% of these were found to be misdiagnosed for a median of 10 months. The authors concluded that misdiagnosis exposes patients to substantial risks associated with the wound's treatment, and a thorough workup is needed to rule out diagnoses that mimic pyoderma gangrenosum.

TOOLS TO AVOID MISDIAGNOSIS

Clinicians can reduce the chance of misdiagnosing a wound by using the following tools:

- the medical record, to accurately describe the wound's characteristics at each patient visit
- risk assessment tools, which ensure systematic evaluation of individual risk factors
- nutritional risk assessment tools
- manual screening tools, including the ankle-brachial index, lower leg and foot assessments, palpation of pulses and Doppler ultrasound, segmental blood pressures, Semmes-Weinstein monofilament testing, transcutaneous oxygen pressure ($TcPO_2$), and vibration perception threshold assessment
- other diagnostic tests, such as laboratory values, bacterial swab cultures, tissue cultures, skin biopsies, and radiologic and vascular studies.

Tracking laboratory values

Laboratory values can be used to evaluate and monitor chronic underlying medical conditions and to determine the patient's nutritional status. These values should be assessed on the first patient visit to establish a baseline for care. In addition, if healing hasn't occurred as expected, certain laboratory values can be monitored to ensure that local and systemic factors aren't contributing to poor healing. Important parameters to evaluate include protein levels, complete blood count, erythrocyte sedimentation rate, liver function tests, glucose and iron levels, total lymphocyte count, blood urea nitrogen and creatinine levels, lipoprotein levels, vitamin and mineral levels, and urinalysis. (See *Monitoring selected laboratory values*.) Even if only one deterrent is present, healing can't occur.

IN PRESSURE ULCERS

Careful interpretation of a number of laboratory values can help the clinician accurately manage a patient with a pressure ulcer. Because the results

Monitoring selected laboratory values

Listed below are laboratory tests that can help assess the patient's condition during wound and skin therapy. Levels should be monitored, as appropriate, based on the care plan related to the clinical presentation for the patient and the wound.

Laboratory test	Normal range*
Alanine aminotransferase	10 to 40 U/L
Albumin	3.5 to 5.5 g/dl
Alkaline phosphatase	90 to 130 U/L
Aspartate aminotransferase	10 to 40 U/L
Blood urea nitrogen	8 to 25 mg/dl
Calcium	9 to 11 mg/dl
Cholesterol	100 to 200 mg/dl
Copper	70 to 140 µg/dl
C-reactive protein	2.6 to 7.6 µg/dl
Creatinine	0.6 to 1.4 mg/dl
Erythrocyte sedimentation rate	<10 mm/hr
Folate	3 to 16 ng/ml
Glucose	70 to 120 mg/dl
Hematocrit	42% to 52% men; 37% to 48% women
Hemoglobin	13 to 18 g/dl men; 12 to 16 g/dl women
Hemoglobin A1C	<6%
Iron	50 to 150 µg/dl
Magnesium	1.5 to 2.5 mEq/l
Prealbumin	16 to 40 mg/dl
Total protein	5 to 9 g/dl
Total lymphocyte count	2,000 cells/mm^3
Transferrin	200 to 400 mg/dl
Triglycerides	100 to 200 mg/dl
Vitamin A	30 to 95 µg/dl
Vitamin B$_1$	10 to 60 ng/ml
Vitamin B$_6$	5 to 30 ng/ml
Vitamin B$_{12}$	200 to 900 pg/ml
Vitamin C	>2 mg/dl
Vitamin E	5 to 20 µg/ml
Zinc	60 to 150 µg/dl

*Values vary among laboratories.

of many laboratory assays, such as albumin, are affected by hydration status, tests should be repeated after a patient has been rehydrated. Current laboratory test data must be used to provide the most accurate information on the patient's condition.

Common laboratory tests to consider in patients diagnosed with pressure ulcers include albumin, prealbumin, hemoglobin A1C, glucose, and complete blood count. Additional tests may be performed based on the patient's overall condition.

Albumin

Albumin is a protein that acts as a building block for cells and tissues. It's produced by the liver and, therefore, may be reduced in patients with liver disease. The albumin level is also diminished in patients with renal disease, malnutrition, severe burn wounds, and malabsorption syndromes. Adequate intake of protein and essential nutrients is necessary to ensure adequate production of albumin.

The albumin test is the basic screening tool for protein status and a gross indicator of nutritional status and fluid balance. Albumin has a half-life of 18 to 20 days, making it sensitive to long-term protein deficiencies. The lower the albumin level, the greater the risk of edema, because albumin accounts for a large portion of the oncotic pressure of blood plasma.

The albumin value is directly related to the severity of the protein deficiency. The extent to which albumin is decreased can help predict the risk of pressure ulcer formation. Albumin levels less than 3.2 g/dl have been shown to correlate with increased morbidity and mortality in patients admitted to the critical care unit. Elevated levels can be found in patients with dehydration, vomiting, diarrhea, and multiple myeloma.

Prealbumin

Prealbumin, or transthyretin, is another type of protein produced by the liver. It has a half-life of 2 to 3 days, making it a better indicator of acute nutritional status changes than albumin. The level can be diminished in patients with liver disease, widespread tissue damage, malnutrition, protein wasting, or inflammation, as well as in patients taking estrogen or a hormonal contraceptive.

The lower the prealbumin level, the greater the risk of mortality. Prealbumin carries thyroxine and vitamin A throughout the body; thus, lower prealbumin levels decrease transport of these substances. Elevated prealbumin levels have been found in patients with Hodgkin disease and in those taking a steroid and a nonsteroidal anti-inflammatory drug.

Hemoglobin A_{1C}

Hemoglobin A_{1C} (A_{1C}) is composed of hemoglobin A with a glucose molecule, which is attached through a process called glycosylation. It's an indicator of long-term glucose control, and its value depends on the amount of serum glucose available. A_{1C} is mainly used as a measure of the efficacy of diabetic therapy. An elevated A_{1C} level carries the same implications as an elevated serum glucose level, including impaired wound healing and decreased ability to fight infection. A level above 8% increases the risk of long-term complications.

Glucose

Glucose is formed from dietary carbohydrates and is stored in the liver and muscles as glycogen. A fasting blood glucose level gives the best indication of overall glucose homeostasis. Insulin allows transport of glucose into the cells for storage as glycogen. Glucagon stimulates conversion of glycogen to glucose for use by the cells as energy. Hypoglycemia results from malnutrition, cirrhosis, alcoholism, and excess insulin. The serum glucose level is elevated in patients with diabetes mellitus, burns, crush injuries, or renal failure and in those using a steroid. A chronically elevated glucose level causes microvascular damage, which inhibits oxygen and nutrient perfusion and hampers wound healing. An elevated glucose level also affects polymorphonuclear lymphocytes, causing decreased chemotaxis, diapedesis, and phagocytosis, which in turn leads to a diminished ability to fight infection. Finally, an elevated glucose level is a risk factor for the development of arterial and neuropathic ulcers in patients with diabetes mellitus.

Complete blood count

A complete blood count (CBC) measures the number of red blood cells (RBCs), white blood cells (WBCs), total amount of hemoglobin in the blood, the fraction of the blood composed of RBCs (hematocrit), and the mean corpuscular volume (MCV). It also provides information about the mean corpuscular hemoglobin (MHC) and mean corpuscular hemoglobin concentration (MCHC), which are calculated from other measurements in the CBC. The platelet count is usually included in the CBC.

It's important to review these blood components because they map directly to the wound-healing process. For example, hemostasis occurs immediately after initial injury. The primary cell responsible for this function is the platelet, which causes the body to form a clot to prevent further bleeding. Platelets also release key cytokines, such as platelet-derived growth factor, that call in cells to participate in later phases of healing. Without the proper platelet count, wound healing is delayed.

These and other tests, such as renal and liver function tests and electrolyte levels, should be monitored based on the care plan related to the clinical presentation of the patient and the wound.

IN VENOUS ULCERS

To accurately evaluate and manage a patient with a venous ulcer, the clinician should obtain a CBC plus laboratory values for various nutritional elements. Other tests to consider when evaluating a patient with venous insufficiency are venography, Doppler ultrasound, ankle-brachial index, plethysmography, and tissue biopsy.

Protein

Protein is responsible for the growth and maintenance of tissue, fluid balance, and antibody and T-cell formation, as well as for hormone and enzyme production. It can be influenced by various factors, such as diminished dietary intake; decreased protein production; increased metabolic rate; or excessive loss through the skin, kidney, or GI tract. The protein level also can be affected by stress, hormones, infection, and organ dysfunction, however, so it isn't a specific indicator of nutritional status. Total protein is primarily composed of albumin and globulin.

The presence of a wound and the body's attempt to heal it may increase the patient's baseline metabolic rate. The liver catabolizes protein to support the wound's increased demands on the body. If the patient doesn't consume enough protein to compensate for the increased catabolism, protein deficiency results.

Protein deficiency impedes wound healing for various reasons, including a reduced ability to repair the wound and to fight infection. Reduced wound repair capability is caused by decreased DNA production, neovascularization, fibroblast proliferation, collagen synthesis, and wound remodeling that result from protein deficiency. Weakened resistance to infection is caused by decreased antibody and complement production, leukocyte phagocytosis and intracellular killing, and macrophage phagocytosis.

Protein deficiency also causes edema, which decreases oxygen and nutrient transport to the wound. In addition, decreased thymic hormone secretion causes thymic atrophy, which leads to decreased T-lymphocyte production.

Total lymphocyte count

Lymphocytes are part of the immune system. T-lymphocytes, which develop in the thymus, are involved in cell-mediated immunity, such as bacterial death and tumor immunity. B-lymphocytes develop in the bone marrow and are responsible for humoral immunity. They synthesize immunoglobulins, which react to specific antigens.

Measurement of lymphocytes aids in the diagnosis of immunosuppression and autoimmunity. A decrease in the total lymphocyte count (indicating impaired immunity) can result from decreased protein intake. The lower the count, the higher the risk of morbidity and mortality. A decreased total lymphocyte count has also been associated with surgery, lupus erythematosus, lymphoma, malnutrition, immunodeficiency, and the use of immunosuppressants. An increased total lymphocyte count has been associated with alcohol use, smoking, and autoimmune disorders.

Blood urea nitrogen

Urea, a byproduct of protein metabolism, is excreted by the kidneys. Blood urea nitrogen (BUN) is an indicator of renal function and fluid status. Men usually have a slightly higher BUN level than women.

Elevated urea levels (uremia) have been associated with delayed wound healing. Causes of uremia include GI bleeding; prerenal failure due to reduced blood flow to the kidneys or crush injuries; intrinsic renal failure due to glomerulonephritis or nephrotic syndrome; postrenal failure due to obstruction of the ureter or urethra by stones or tumor; and use of nephrotoxic drugs (such as cyclosporin), diuretics, certain antibiotics, or salicylates.

Concurrently elevated levels of BUN and creatinine suggest kidney disease, whereas an elevated BUN level alone may indicate dehydration or a breakdown of blood products in the GI tract, which may occur with intestinal bleeding. With declining renal function, doses of certain medications and antibiotics should be decreased to avoid toxic buildup. Electrolyte abnormalities can occur with worsening renal function. Decreased urea levels result from overhydration, liver damage, malnutrition, and phenothiazine use. Patients should ingest 30 to 35 ml/kg of fluids, preferably water, daily.

Liver function tests

Liver function tests measure the enzymes alanine aminotransferase (ALT), aspartate aminotransferase (AST), and alkaline phosphatase. These enzymes are produced by liver cells and are effective for diagnosing liver dysfunction. The transaminases, AST and ALT, catalyze the transfer of an amino group between an amino acid and an alpha-keto acid, which aids in the production of amino acids for protein synthesis in the liver. ALT is found almost exclusively in the liver, whereas AST can also be found in skeletal muscle, the kidneys, and the brain. Alkaline phosphatase is an enzyme produced in the liver and bones.

Extreme elevations in ALT and AST levels are characteristic of acute hepatitis; mild elevations are indicative of chronic liver disease, commonly caused by medications or chronic hepatitis. The longer the duration of liver disease, the more likely that liver failure or cirrhosis is imminent. If the ALT level is more elevated than the AST level, acute hepatitis or liver necrosis is likely. However, an AST level greater than the ALT level suggests chronic hepatitis, cirrhosis, or myocardial necrosis.

The alkaline phosphatase level is significantly elevated in acute hepatitis, with slightly elevated levels characterizing chronic hepatitis. Paget disease, fractures, rheumatoid arthritis, and bone malignancy also lead to elevated levels. Malnutrition, hypothyroidism, and vitamin C deficiency can decrease the alkaline phosphatase level. The more severe and the longer the insult to the liver, the greater the decrease in alkaline phosphatase production. This liver dysfunction can also lead to toxic levels of certain antibiotics, which are metabolized through the liver.

Hemoglobin

Hemoglobin, a protein, gives blood its red color. It's composed of a protein globin envelope and heme, which uses iron to bind and transport oxygen. Any deficiency of vitamins, minerals, or amino acids can decrease hemoglobin production.

The lower the hemoglobin level, the less oxygen is carried to tissues and the less capacity wounds have to heal properly. Oxygen plays a role in enzymatic and cellular metabolic reactions needed for cell growth and proliferation. A low hemoglobin level can result from anemia, cirrhosis, hemorrhage, renal disease, volume overload, or use of medications such as penicillin, tetracycline, aspirin, sulfonamides, indomethacin, and vitamin A. An artificially low level of hemoglobin occurs when blood is drawn from the same arm through which intravenous (I.V.) fluids are being given. A truly decreased hemoglobin level is a risk factor for pressure ulcer formation. Hemoglobin level can increase from dehydration, polycythemia, severe burns, high altitudes, and use of gentamicin.

Hematocrit

Hematocrit is the volume of packed RBCs in 100 ml of blood. A low hematocrit has a direct effect on wound healing and is associated with blood loss, anemia, malignancies, protein malnutrition, liver and renal disease, lupus erythematosus, rheumatoid arthritis, and the use of antineoplastics and penicillin. An artificially low hematocrit can occur if blood is drawn from the same arm through which I.V. fluids are given. Hematocrit increases with dehydration, diarrhea, polycythemia, or burns.

IN ARTERIAL ULCERS

To accurately manage the patient with an arterial ulcer, the clinician should obtain laboratory values for glucose, lipoproteins, CBC, cryoglobulins, antiphospholipid antibodies, antinuclear antibodies, and rheumatoid factor. The laboratory tests, in tandem with diagnostic tests, help the clinician make a more accurate and specific arterial diagnosis.

Glucose

A chronically elevated glucose level causes microvascular damage, which inhibits oxygen and nutrient perfusion and hampers wound healing. An elevated glucose level also affects polymorphonuclear lymphocytes, causing decreased chemotaxis, diapedesis, and phagocytosis, which in turn leads to a decreased ability to fight infection. An elevated glucose level is a risk factor for arterial and neuropathic ulcers in patients with diabetes mellitus.

Lipoproteins

Lipoproteins, such as cholesterol and triglycerides, are lipids bound to protein, absorbed in the intestines. Cholesterol is an important component of cell membranes, bile acid, and steroid hormone synthesis. Triglycerides are manufactured by the liver and provide energy to the heart and muscles. They are transported in blood as chylomicrons.

Hyperlipidemia is a risk factor for peripheral arterial disease and subsequent ischemic ulcer formation. Elevated cholesterol levels are associated with diabetes mellitus, hypothyroidism, atherosclerosis, excess dietary intake of cholesterol, renal failure, alcoholism, familial hyperlipidemia, and the use of aspirin, steroids, sulfonamides, vitamins A and D, and hormonal contraceptives). Artificially elevated levels can result from food consumption 12 hours before obtaining the blood specimen. Decreased levels can be found in the presence of malnutrition; infection; hyperthyroidism; malabsorption; anemia; inflammation; and the use of neomycin, hypoglycemics, estrogens, and tetracycline.

Decreased triglyceride levels are found in hyperthyroidism, protein malnutrition, vitamin C excess, and use of metformin. Increased levels occur in hypothyroidism, nephritic syndrome, atherosclerosis, cirrhosis, diabetes, hypertension, excess dietary intake of triglycerides, alcoholism, familial hyperlipidemia, and hormonal contraceptive use. Artificially elevated levels can occur if patients don't fast for 12 hours before having a blood specimen drawn.

Cryoglobulins

Cryoglobulins are abnormal immunoglobulins. At temperatures below normal body temperature (98.6° F [37° C]), cryoglobulins no longer stay suspended in the blood. They precipitate out, forming complexes that can block small blood vessels, especially in the face and hands. Although a positive cryoglobulin test result can confirm the diagnosis of cryoglobulinemia, it may also be caused by arterial disease. If arterial disease is suspected, a further workup may be indicated.

Antiphospholipid antibodies

Antiphospholipid antibody syndrome, or *Hughes-Stovin syndrome*, is characterized by the presence of multiple antibodies (systemic lupus erythematosus [SLE] and anticoagulant and anticardiolipin antibodies) associated with arterial and venous thrombosis (clotting). The two main classifications of the antiphospholipid antibody syndrome are primary (in patients with no underlying autoimmune disorder) and secondary (in those with an underlying autoimmune disorder, such as SLE). Because ulcers in patients with antiphospholipid antibody syndrome can mimic ischemic arterial ulcers, a test for these antibodies should be ordered if this disorder is suspected.

Antinuclear antibody panel

This test looks for the presence of antibodies that target components of a cell nucleus. An antinuclear antibody (ANA) panel may be ordered to aid in the diagnosis of autoimmune conditions, such as SLE and drug-induced lupus, scleroderma, Sjögren's syndrome, Raynaud's disease, juvenile chronic arthritis, rheumatoid arthritis, antiphospholipid antibody syndrome, autoimmune hepatitis, and many other autoimmune and nonautoimmune diseases. ANA testing can help the clinician properly diagnose the patient's autoimmune disease.

Rheumatoid factor (RF)

RF is an antibody that attaches to a substance in the body called immunoglobulin G (IgG), forming a molecule known as an immune complex. This immune complex can activate various inflammatory processes in the body. RF test results can help the clinician determine the presence of an inflammatory process, such as rheumatoid arthritis. A positive result, however, doesn't definitively rule out arterial causes for an ulcer.

Diagnostic tests

In addition to laboratory tests, certain diagnostic tests can be performed to assist in accurately diagnosing the patient's wound.

ANGIOGRAPHY

Angiography is the gold standard for diagnosing arterial vascular disease. This procedure is indicated for patients who are candidates for revascularization. The test's associated risks include cholesterol plaque embolization, acute avascular occlusion, arterial damage, and contrast-induced nephropathy.

MAGNETIC RESONANCE ANGIOGRAPHY

Magnetic resonance angiography is a noninvasive test to determine the presence and severity of arterial obstructions such as peripheral arterial disease.

$TcPO_2$

Transcutaneous oxygen measurement can assess for the presence of microvascular insufficiency. A value greater than 30 mm Hg indicates adequate perfusion. If the tissue surrounding an ulcer has a $TcPO_2$ less than 20 mm Hg, the wound typically won't heal.

5 DEVELOPING A SKIN AND WOUND CARE FORMULARY

Clinical decision making for skin and wound management depends on the types of patients managed in the care settings, the skillsets of the clinicians making the decisions for those patients, and the products available in the facility to improve skin and wound care. Skin and wound care requires a process-driven management approach. A process is defined as "a series of actions, changes, or functions bringing about a result." And each process has a specific goal.

Every action managing skin conditions and wounds must be clearly defined as part of a skin and wound care process. Before beginning any new process, define a team that will design, implement, and oversee the process. In this case, establish a multidisciplinary team to manage the complex skin and wound care patients admitted to the facility. This team should be composed of professionals who manage different parts of the process.

In this chapter, we define seven skin and wound care processes and their targeted goals. The processes are as follows:

. Perform a needs assessment.
. Develop an operational formulary.
. Develop a skin and wound care product formulary.
. Develop documentation pathways.
. Develop educational and competency validation pathways.
. Identify levels of practicing professionals.
. Develop patient educational pathways.

Perform a needs assessment

Goal: To accurately capture the types of skin and wound care needs in your facility

When evaluating your patient population, whether patients of your facility or outpatients, you should define fundamental skin and wound types. For example, do you care for patients with pressure ulcers, diabetic ulcers, surgical wounds, or unusual wounds such as those associated with calciphylaxis or antiphospholipid antibody syndrome?

Each specific wound type needs to have its own defined assessment parameters, pathway, and management plan, and all team members must be clinically competent in these areas.

Differentiating arterial, diabetic, and venous ulcers

Arterial ulcers	Diabetic ulcers	Venous ulcers
PREDISPOSING FACTORS		
■ Peripheral vascular disease (PVD) ■ Diabetes mellitus ■ Advanced age	■ Diabetic patient with peripheral neuropathy ■ Long-term uncontrolled or poorly controlled diabetes	■ Valve incompetence in perforating veins ■ History of deep vein thrombophlebitis and thrombosis ■ Previous history of ulcers ■ Obesity ■ Advanced age
ANATOMIC LOCATION		
■ Between toes or tips of toes ■ Over phalangeal heads ■ Around lateral malleolus ■ At sites subjected to trauma or rubbing of footwear	■ On plantar aspect of foot ■ Over metatarsal heads ■ Under heel	■ On medial lower leg and ankle ■ On malleolar area
PATIENT ASSESSMENT		
■ Thin, shiny, dry skin ■ Hair loss on ankle and foot ■ Thickened toenails ■ Pallor on elevation and dependent rubor ■ Cyanosis ■ Decreased temperature ■ Absent or diminished pulses	■ Diminished or absent sensation in foot ■ Foot deformities ■ Palpable pulses ■ Warm foot ■ Subcutaneous fat atrophy ■ Arterial assessment findings if patient also has PVD	■ Firm edema ■ Dilated superficial veins ■ Dry, thin, scaly skin ■ Evidence of healed ulcers ■ Periwound and leg hyperpigmentation ■ Possible dermatitis

Differentiating arterial, diabetic, and venous ulcers *(continued)*

Arterial ulcers	Diabetic ulcers	Venous ulcers
WOUND CHARACTERISTICS		
• Even wound margins • Gangrene or necrosis • Deep, pale wound bed • Blanched or purpuric periwound tissue • Severe pain • Cellulitis • Minimal exudate	• Even wound margins • Deep wound bed • Cellulitis or underlying osteomyolitis • Granular tissue present unless PVD is present • Low to moderate drainage	• Irregular wound margins • Superficial wound • Ruddy, granular tissue • Usually minimal to moderate pain • Frequently moderate to heavy exudate

Lack of competence could lead to misassessment, which leads to misdiagnosis. This can delay the true diagnosis, worsen the patient's condition and, at times, increase patient morbidity. Misassessment or misdiagnosis also is a legal concern. To combat these problems, the health care professional needs to clearly understand the assessment parameters for the skin and wound types managed in the facility, to have proper documentation to support the assessment and interventions performed, and to be familiar with administration's expectation of the clinician's role.

Appropriately managing the skin or wound care patient is an important step in correcting all underlying pathologies compromising the healing process. This step takes teamwork.

REVIEW

- Review the patient's past and current family, social, and medical history.
- Obtain a medication list of current and past medications and dressings, including all medications and dressings that have failed.
- Review all laboratory, radiology, and vascular studies that have been obtained.
- Review the patient's nutritional status and supportive therapies.
- Review all physician and nonphysician consults related to specialty management programs for skin and wound care.
- Review all support surfaces and positioning devices used to manage the patient's tissue load.
- Address all underlying pathologies compromising the wound healing process (for example, neuropathic, pressure, vascular, and venous hypertension). (See *Differentiating arterial, diabetic, and venous ulcers.*)

Develop an operational formulary

Goal: To provide all tests and services needed for your skin and wound care patients

To move your operational formulary forward, you would need to:
- identify diagnostic tests
- identify surgical procedures
- identify modalities and devices.

Diagnostic tests and laboratory values

Patients with chronic wounds can experience significant medical, social, and economic hardships. These hardships also can affect society in general. The interplay of several different local and systemic factors can affect chronic wounds, making them difficult to heal. Local factors include bacterial load and infection, trauma, pressure, and moisture. Systemic factors include age; chronic medical conditions or comorbidities, such as anemia, diabetes mellitus, and renal or hepatic dysfunction; and nutritional status, such as vitamin, protein, or fluid deficiencies.

Laboratory values help assess and monitor chronic underlying medical conditions as well as the patient's nutritional status. These values should be evaluated when the patient is encountered for the first time. In addition, if healing isn't occurring as expected, these values can be tracked regularly to ensure that local and systemic factors aren't contributing to poor healing. Important parameters to evaluate include protein levels, complete blood count, erythrocyte sedimentation rate, liver function tests, glucose and iron levels, total lymphocyte count, blood urea nitrogen and creatinine levels, lipoprotein levels, vitamin and mineral levels, and urinalysis. Even if only one deterrent is present, healing can't occur. (See chapter 4, Laboratory values in chronic wound management.)

Cultures

All wounds are contaminated with various organisms. Infection—as evidenced by purulent exudate, induration, erythema, edema, fever, or leukocytosis—may delay healing. Culturing the wound allows identification of infecting organisms. Culture methods include surface swab culturing (see *Swab-culturing technique*), fluid culturing (through needle aspiration), curettage of the wound base (after cleaning the surface of the wound), and deep-tissue biopsy. It's important to remember that swab cultures identify contamination only on the surface of the wound. The Centers for Disease Control and Prevention recommend either obtaining fluid from the wound through needle aspiration or obtaining tissue through a wound biopsy.

A wound that contains necrotic tissue or sinus tracts requires both an aerobic and an anaerobic culture. A wound that's open and viable needs only an aerobic culture. Bacteria levels greater than 10^5 or colony-forming units (CFUs) above 100,000 organisms/ml indicate that wound healing

Swab-culturing technique

Collect a wound culture when purulent or suspicious-looking drainage or signs of infection—induration, fever, erythema, or edema—are present. When collecting, don't use purulent matter to culture, and don't swab over hard eschar. Use a sterile calcium alginate or rayon swab, not a cotton-tipped swab. To obtain a wound culture with a swab, follow these steps:

■ Thoroughly rinse the wound with sterile saline solution before culturing.
■ Gently rotate the swab.
■ Swab wound edges using 10-point coverage as shown in the illustration.
■ Place the swab in the culture medium and take it to the laboratory as soon as possible.

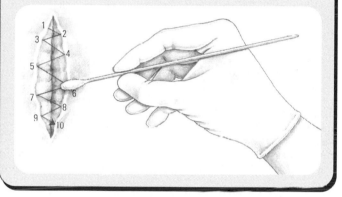

may be delayed. Notify the prescribing health care professional of the culture results so appropriate interventions can be ordered. If the wound doesn't respond to the prescribed antibiotic therapy after 2 to 4 weeks of optimal care, it should be reassessed, generally through tissue biopsy. If the wound is full thickness, evaluate for the presence of osteomyelitis.

SURGICAL PROCEDURES AND DEBRIDEMENT

Through the process of removing devitalized tissue and foreign material from a wound, the clinician may also be removing senescent and nonmigratory cells in and around the wound. Removing these materials may contribute to the release of available growth factors in the wound.

Debridement techniques include autolytic, biosurgery, enzymatic, mechanical, and surgical. The type and frequency of the debridement technique chosen depends on the overall patient condition and treatment plan.

Before performing any type of debridement:

■ Know your professional practice act.
■ Know who can debride in your facility.

- Know your limitations.
- Review policy and procedures for debridement technique with staff.
- Create policy for assessment and implementation of debridement plan of care.

MODALITIES AND DEVICES

All patients in the facility should be screened for the appropriate support surface and off-loading devices (see chapter 6, Tissue load management). According to AHRQ guidelines: "Protect against the adverse effects of external mechanical forces: pressure, friction, and shear." To achieve this goal, the guidelines recommend repositioning the patient, using positioning devices, relieving pressure on the heels, side-lying the patient, using bed positioning, using lifting devices, using pressure-reducing devices for beds, relieving pressure from sitting, using pressure-reducing devices for chairs, and aligning posture. These recommendations are covered in chapter 6.

REVIEW

- Properly identify all lab tests, diagnostic tests, and surgical procedures.
- Provide all modalities and devices needed for your skin and wound care patients.
- Identify all the policies and procedures that support the work performed.
- Create additional policies and procedures to support the facility's work.
- Review all policies and procedures at least annually.

Develop a skin and wound care product formulary

Goal: To provide the proper skin and wound care products to your patients

Once you have performed a needs assessment and developed an operational formulary, you need to build a product formulary so that you can provide the proper skin and wound care products to your patients.

Usually the first step in choosing products is perusing vendor contracts. These contracts house the preferred and non-preferred products provided to the facility. (See *Formulary exceptions*.) When you look at vendor pricing, look beyond the numbers. Ask about other services available to support the product purchased. And remember, the product purchased should be clinically effective, and thus cost-efficient, for the skin condition or wound. In summary, all of the products housed on contract are great, but if the products aren't used appropriately, it's a waste of time and money for the facility and increased wound-healing time for the patient.

Your team should be knowledgeable about the actions, indications, and contraindications of the products provided to the patients. It isn't acceptable to apply the product just because the physician ordered it; you need to understand why the order was written and understand how the product affects the healing process.

Formulary exceptions

Because of the wide variety of wound care supplies, it may be necessary (from time to time) to obtain skin or wound care products not currently on formulary under the skin and wound care program. If a product must be obtained based on the treating physician's orders, the reason for the product needs to be documented in the physician notes, nursing notes, and the care plan. It's the facility's responsibility to obtain the product in a timely fashion.

There are many products on the market from which to choose (see Parts 2 and 3 of this book). Following is an overview of wound dressings and other products by product category. The clinician is responsible for understanding a product's advantages and disadvantages before using it on a patient.

- Alginates—These dry topical wound care products, derived from brown seaweed, can absorb about 20 times their weight. They are composed of soft, nonwoven fibers manufactured in the shape of a pad or rope. When the dressing is placed in the wound, a gel is formed, maintaining a moist environment. When wound drainage has decreased to a minimum level, the alginate is no longer appropriate and may cause the wound bed to dehydrate. Alginate dressings may be used as primary dressings on partial and full-thickness draining wounds, wounds with moderate to heavy exudate, tunneling wounds, and infected and noninfected wounds.
- Antimicrobial dressings are topical wound care products derived from agents such as silver, iodine, and polyhexethylene biguanide. These products combine active ingredients or physical characteristics of a particular active ingredient with a dressing or delivery system in an attempt to deliver an antimicrobial or antibacterial action to the wound. Silver dressings come in various delivery systems as well as shapes and sizes. The silver is activated from the dressing to the wound's surface based on the amount of exudate and bacteria in the wound. Silver dressings are available in foams, hydrocolloids, alginates, barriers layers, and charcoal cloth dressings. Silver dressings may be used with select topical and adjunctive therapies to. among other things. decrease the bacterial load and manage exudate, and as a result optimize the appearance of the wound's granulation tissue.

    Gauze products containing antibacterial properties have been designed to provide a barrier to specific organisms but also inhibit the growth of bacteria within the dressing, thus protecting the wound and potential spread of bacteria from the dressed site.
- Collagens—The most abundant protein in the body, collagen is fibrous and insoluble and is produced by fibroblasts. Its fibers are found in connective tissue, including skin, bone, ligaments, and cartilage. During

wound healing, collagen encourages the deposition and organization of newly formed collagen fibers and granulation tissue in the wound bed. It also stimulates new tissue development and wound debridement, creating an environment conducive to healing. Collagen dressings are manufactured in sheets, pads, particles, and gels. They may be used as primary dressings for partial- and full-thickness wounds, infected and noninfected wounds, tunneling wounds, wounds with minimal to heavy exudate (depending on the form of collagen dressing), skin grafts, donor sites, and red or yellow wounds.

- Composites—Composite dressings combine physically distinct components into a single dressing that provides multiple functions. These functions must include, but aren't limited to, a bacterial barrier; an absorptive layer other than an alginate, foam, hydrocolloid, or hydrogel; and a semiadherent or nonadherent property over the wound site. Composite dressings may be used as primary or secondary dressings for partial- and full-thickness wounds with minimal to heavy exudate, healthy granulation tissue, necrotic tissue (slough or moist eschar), or mixed wounds (granulation and necrotic tissue).

- Contact layers—These dressings provide an interface between the wound and the dressing, which protects the fragile healing tissue. This layer also acts as a liner for deep wounds that need to be packed, allowing for easy removal of the packing material. The nonadherent layer prevents new epithelium from sticking to the dressing and from being inadvertently removed when the dressing is changed. Contact layers also wick exudate or drainage away from the wound. These dressings are generally the first layer of the dressing, which is placed directly over the wound or after the application of a topical medication.

- Foams—Foam dressings are semipermeable and either hydrophilic or hydrophobic with a bacterial barrier. They provide thermal insulation to the wound, create a moist wound-healing environment, are nonadherent, and provide an atraumatic removal. Foams may be used in conjunction with topical antibiotics for infected wounds. Select foam dressings may be manufactured with an adhesive border, which eliminates the need for a securing device. If the foam dressing is to be used as the primary wound contact layer, it's intended to provide absorption and insulation. Foam dressings may also be used as the secondary dressing of choice to absorb moderate to heavy exudate.

- Hydrocolloids—These dressings are occlusive hydroactive wafers, beads, pastes, or granules that promote granulation tissue formation and wound healing within a moist environment. Hydrocolloid dressings protect fragile skin and areas of the body affected by both urinary and fecal incontinence and frictional forces. Most hydrocolloid wafers react with wound exudate to form a gel-like covering to protect the wound and maintain a moist wound-healing environment. Select hydrocolloid wafers facilitate autolytic debridement. Hydrocolloids are contraindicated for use in infected wounds. Secondary dressings aren't needed when hydrocolloid dressings are used as the primary contact layer.

- Hydrogels—Available in three forms—amorphous gels, sheet dressings, and impregnated gauzes—hydrogels are glycerin- and water-based products primarily manufactured for wound hydration. However, because of their high water content, they cannot absorb large amounts of water. They provide a cooling action and may reduce pain. Gel or hydrogel dressings are indicated for infected and noninfected wounds and for minimally draining wounds.

- Specialty absorptives—Specialty absorptives are unitized, multilayered dressings that consist of highly absorptive layers of fibers, such as absorbent cellulose, cotton, or rayon. These dressings, which may or may not have an adhesive border, may be used as primary or secondary dressings to manage moderate to heavy drainage.

- Surgical supplies—When the Statistical Analysis Durable Medical Equipment Regional Carrier and the four Durable Medical Equipment Regional Carriers (DMERCs) perform a Coding Verification Review and fail to reach a consensus coding decision, they sometimes assign the product or procedure to a general category. Therefore, various dissimilar products and procedures are usually assigned to this category. These products in this category don't have a universal definition, use guidelines, or a rate on the DMERC Fee Schedule. Yet, each product listed under this category has an individual action, indication, contraindication, and application and removal process. It remains the clinician's responsibility to understand each product before using it.

- Transparent films—These semipermeable membrane dressings are adhesive and waterproof. They prevent oxygen and water vapor from crossing the barrier while remaining impermeable to bacteria and contaminants. Transparent film dressings maintain a moist environment, promoting granulation tissue formation and autolytic debridement of slough and eschar. They are contraindicated for infected wounds and have little capacity to absorb exudate. Transparent films may be used as a secondary dressing of choice if the wound isn't clinically infected.

- Wound fillers—Also known as *exudate-absorbing products*, wound fillers can be found in a variety of forms—beads, pastes, powders, gels, and pads. These products absorb several times their weight in exudate. Generally, these products are used as primary dressings or wound fillers and must be covered by an appropriate secondary dressing. Used to fill highly exudating, deep wounds and wounds with uneven wound margins, these dressings assist in controlling exudate, cleansing the wound, and reducing odor and bacterial proliferation.

- Therapeutic modalities—These include products such as negative-pressure wound therapy, electrical stimulation, pulsed lavage, ultrasound, and noncontact normothermic therapy.

Skin and wound management order

The prescriber's order for wound and skin management should include:

- specific site
- cleaning solution and method
- primary dressing or drug
- secondary dressing, if applicable
- securement device, if applicable
- frequency of dressing changes
- time frame and clinical parameters for evaluating treatment effectiveness.

These elements must be verified before applying or removing a dressing. For example, a typical wound and skin management order for a wound on the right hip might read as follows: Clean right trochanteric wound with normal saline solution. Loosely pack tunneling areas and base of wound with an alginate rope dressing. Cover with a bordered gauze dressing. Change daily, and reevaluate in 2 days or sooner if the wound declines. Notify the physician for an alternate care plan based on a new assessment if redness, swelling, pain, or increased drainage occurs during the course of care or if the alginate dressing is inappropriate for the amount of exudate in the wound. A change in local or supportive measures is indicated if a wound hasn't decreased in size after 2 to 4 weeks of management. An immediate change in management is indicated if a negative outcome occurs at any time during the course of management.

Managing the wound according to its condition

Once a product or products have been chosen, the health care professional must manage the wound according to its condition. For example, if necrotic tissue is present in the wound, one must evaluate if debridement of the necrotic tissue from the wound is an appropriate next step. For example, you would heed caution to debride arterial wounds and unusual wounds until consulting with the physician for an appropriate plan based on the patient's underlying condition.

Debridement

If debridement is indicated, several options are available.

Debridement techniques include autolytic, biosurgical, enzymatic, mechanical, and surgical. The type of debridement technique chosen and the frequency with which it's used depends on the overall patient condition and care plan.

- Autolytic debridement allows the body to lyse or break down necrotic tissue by using its own enzymes and defense mechanisms. Many dressings are designed to promote autolysis.
- Biosurgical debridement utilizes sterilized bottle fly maggots (*Phaenicia sericata*) to debride wounds. Larval therapy is simple to use and doesn't require extensive medical training. Contraindications to larval therapy

include wounds involving vital organs or exposed blood vessels. The potential for allergic reactions—such as rhinoconjunctivitis, angioedema, and contact dermatitis—exists in susceptible individuals. Aesthetic concerns and wound pain or discomfort are also considerations.

■ Enzymatic debridement harnesses enzymes to break down necrotic tissue without affecting viable tissue. Agents used for enzymatic debridement are available only by prescription and are ordered by the patient's health care provider. The available enzyme preparations differ in efficacy.

■ Mechanical debridement is the use of physical forces to remove necrotic tissue. The three techniques of mechanical debridement include applying a wet-to-dry dressing, using wound irrigation, using a whirlpool bath, and removing the necrotic tissue by a sharp surgical technique. Therapy may range from conservative to aggressive, and depending on the type of injury, debridement techniques may be combined. For example, mechanical methods may be used with enzymatic methods, such as topical agents that absorb exudate and debris.

■ Surgical debridement involves removing dead or devitalized tissue with a sharp instrument or laser, either at the bedside or in the operating room. Surgical excision and skin grafting may be used for certain types of wounds, such as deep burns. Typically, the patient receives a local or general anesthetic. A laser can deliver high energy levels to a small surface area, providing instant hemostasis and sterilization of the wound.

Once the wound is debrided, continue to manage the wound, based on the wound's condition, by assessing the exudate amount, periwound skin condition, and depth of wound, to name a few clinical characteristics.

WHAT IS THE CLINICAL OBJECTIVE FOR THIS WOUND?

The following list describes features of the ideal dressing, drug, or device for the skin and wound care patient:

■ provides an optimal healing environment
■ contours to the wound
■ provides an atraumatic environment upon removal
■ prevents maceration
■ provides nonadherence to the periwound skin
■ debrides autolytically in the presence of necrotic tissue
■ validates your formulary with published evidence.

Each time the health care professional changes the patient's dressing or removes a device, a number of questions should be answered:

■ Is the product providing too little or too much wound hydration?
■ Is the product causing pain and trauma to the wound upon removal of the dressing?
■ Is the product removed easily from the wound bed?

Familiarizing yourself with the major categories of skin and wound care products and their actions, indications, contraindications, advantages, and disadvantages will help you to choose the most appropriate dressing, drug, or device. Also consider the product's availability and its application and removal procedures. In many cases, one product can help you meet more than one therapeutic goal.

REVIEW

- Understand the clinical objectives for each wound care patient.
- Review the patient's history, paying particular attention to the patient's prior medications, dressings, devices, lab results, vascular results, radiology results, etc.
- Address all underlying pathologies compromising wound healing.
- Understand the actions, indications, and contraindications of all the dressings, drugs, and devices ordered for your patient population.

Develop documentation pathways

Goal: To provide an accurate documentation platform to support direct patient care and reimbursement

The focus of documentation has shifted dramatically in the last two decades. Historically, the clinician would document the details of the patient's visit and would file the chart—the physician and his staff were the only people who ever saw the patient's chart.

Now, fast-forward two decades. Documented details that compose a patient's chart aren't used simply to measure clinical outcomes and record your work. That same chart may end up as a piece of evidence in a malpractice claim. It may be used by an insurance company to confirm—or challenge—the level of service for which it's been billed. It may also assure an accreditation body that you have met the standards of care required for employees of your facility. Clinicians have come to understand that today's medical record serves as the instrument for demonstrating their ability to plan, coordinate, and evaluate patient care.

Clinicians someday may view handwritten, pen-and-paper medical records as a distant memory. Today's forms of documentation include telephonic, photographic, and computer-generated information—with the computer taking the lead as the most commonly used medium for maintaining and storing medical records. Computerization has revolutionized the way data are collected, collated, and delivered—at the press of a button.

This electronic medical record (EMR) ties the clinical, functional, and financial information for the patient's visit and is faster proof of the work performed. The EMR tracks the physician's work and his assessment data, as well as the clinician's time and work performed. (See *Computer documentation system*.)

Computer-based documentation systems have emerged to capture the complete medical record for skin and wound care. These systems have the ability to track the clinical activities and outcomes, tie time as a function of the program to determine the cost of care, integrate pathways and al-

Computer documentation system

Shown below is a computerized tool for documenting wound and skin assessment.

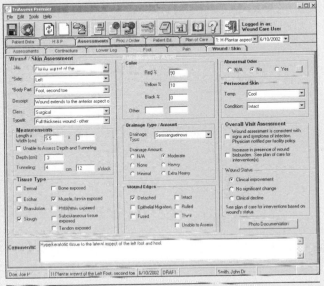

Source: TriAssess Premier Software and the *Clinical Wound Manager Manual Series*, specifically the *Policies and Procedures Manual*. © Wound Care Strategies, Inc., 2003

gorithms to assist in clinical and regulatory compliance, and benchmark the work performed.

Wound care documentation can combine a variety of information that reflects the skin and wound status across the healing continuum. (See *Wound and skin assessment tool,* pages 110 and 111.) Providing an accurate description of the skin and wound characteristics is critical during each patient visit. These findings assist the clinician in mapping the care during the wound management process. Wound classification establishes a common language for wound assessment and wound healing. It helps to foster sound clinical judgments, provides a universal scheme for documentation, and allows better evaluation of treatments. (See *Top 20 strategies for effective skin and wound documentation,* page 112.)

Accurate measurements of wound length, width, depth, and tunneling complement and complete the classification of a wound. Other essential documentation elements include a description of the skin around the

(Text continues on page 112.)

Wound and skin assessment tool

Primary diagnosis _Left CVA_

Secondary diagnosis _Diabetes_

Pertinent medical history _Right-side weakness, depression, IDDM_

WOUND ANATOMICAL LOCATION:

Site _Right heel_   Date of outset _7/18/07_

(circle affected area)

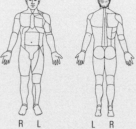
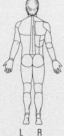

R   L   L   R

L   R —A

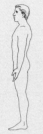
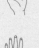
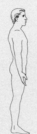

L   R   L   R

DATE (M/D/Y)	TERM	TYPE #	LENGTH, WIDTH (cm)	DEPTH (cm)	TUNNELING (cm, o'clock)	COLOR (R/Y/B/M)	DRAINAGE (amount and type)	ODOR & TYPE (Y/N)	
7/18/07	ST 2	2	4 x 3	< 0.1	Ø	10 serous	Scant,	N	

Patient's Name (Last, Middle, First)	Attending Physician
Brown, Ann	Dr. A. Dennis

Hess, C.T. © Wound Care Strategies, Inc., 2007.

Classification	Terms	Type
Pressure ulcers	**ST1**—nonblanchable redness of intact skin usually over a bony prominence	**1.** Stage 1
	ST2—partial-thickness dermis loss presents as blister or shallow open crater without slough	**2.** Stage 2
	ST3—full-thickness tissue loss that may expose fat but not bone, muscle, or tendon; ulcer presents as a deep crater with slough and possibly undermining and tunneling	**3.** Stage 3
	ST4—full-thickness tissue loss with exposure of muscle, bone, or tendon; slough and eschar posssible, often undermining and tunneling present	**4.** Stage 4
	U—full-thickness tissue loss, wound base covered by slough and/or eschar	**5.** Unstageable
Wound	**PTW** (partial-thickness wound)—loss of epidermis and partial loss of dermis	**6.** Skin tear
	FTW (full-thickness wound)—tissue destruction extending through the dermis and involving the subcutaneous layer; may involve muscle or bone	**7.** Surgical **8.** Vascular ulcer **9.** Other
Color	**R**— clean, healthy, granulating tissue **Y**—presence of slough or fibrinous tissue **B**—presence of eschar **M**—two or more colors present in wound (specify color by letters, such as R/Y)	**10.** Red **11.** Yellow **12.** Black **13.** Mixed
Skin condition	**SC** (skin condition)—an abnormal finding on the surface of the skin	**14.** Rash **15.** Incontinence related **16.** Bruise **17.** Xerosis **18.** Other

PAIN (Y*/N)	PHOTO (Y/N)	ADJUNCTIVE THERAPIES OR PRODUCTS AND ADDITIONAL COMMENTS	SIGNATURE, TITLE
N	Y	☒ Support Surface ☒ Nutritional Intervention ☐ New Orders Obtained T & P 2 hours, heel protectors, heels elevated	B. Carey, RN
		☐ Support Surface ☐ Nutritional Intervention ☐ New Orders Obtained	

Room Number	ID Number
123-2	01726

Top 20 strategies for effective skin and wound documentation

1. Create a comprehensive glossary for your clinical practice setting to ensure accurate documentation.
2. Create clinical pathways and algorithms to ensure consistent care.
3. Declare your clinical strengths and weaknesses. Develop an educational plan to improve your performance.
4. Develop a Quality Improvement plan.
5. Develop policies and procedures for accurate documentation.
6. Discard all "sticky notes" and scrap paper from your department.
7. Document all findings in a consistent place in the medical record.
8. Document concurrently with the patient's visit to accurately record the care provided.
9. Ensure timely and complete documentation. It isn't an option.
10. Establishing complete documentation guidelines can ensure accurate statistical databases, financial planning, clinical staffing, and increased revenues.
11. Investigate your facility's documentation requirements.
12. Organize your thought processes before they're written on paper or in the computer.
13. Perform a documentation audit to ensure accurate documentation.
14. Provide on-going educational seminars to review documentation standards.
15. Review all pertinent local medical review policies.
16. Review all pertinent Medicare coverage decisions.
17. Understand the power of the pen or keystroke.
18. Understand who bears responsibility for clinical documentation in the medical record. Ensure appropriate medical record standards.
19. Validate the competency of each practitioner in the department.
20. Write legibly. If a person can't read the handwriting, it may be interpreted that the service wasn't performed.

Source: TriAssess Premier Software and the *Clinical Wound Manager Manual Series*, specifically the *Policies and Procedures Manual*. © Wound Care Strategies, Inc., 2003.

wound, the wound's surface (intact, exuberant granulation tissue, or necrotic tissue), and the drainage or exudate found in the wound. Three main types of classification systems are used; two are based on the degree of tissue layer destruction, and one is based on the color of the wound bed.

Our technology has come quite far, but our documentation remains the weakest part of the chart for skin and wound care. Whether work is collected on paper or by a computer program, developing a consistent template or database for documentation is necessary to complete this process. Knowledge of the disease process and understanding of what the database means are the equal parts to make a whole medical record and are imperative to using the tools correctly.

Designing a clinical pathway for skin and wound healing begins with a comprehensive patient assessment, which details the patient's medical history inclusive of the wound's status. Appropriate interventions are predicated upon the assessment and documentation outlining the findings. Using a clinical checklist can help to better organize the clinician's time. The clinician's checklist might look as follows:

- The policies and procedures written for skin and wound care should reflect current clinical and operational guidelines approved by the facility. These collective works should be reviewed and updated annually.
- To develop a skin and wound care modality formulary, consider clinically proven efficacy and cost-effectiveness, availability, ease of use, function, and direct cost. Design a supply management system that controls product use, internally or externally, to control costs and waste.
- Technological advancements should be used to reduce the length of stay, the number of dressing changes, the number of professional visits, the time to heal, and the total cost of care.
- Continuing education and validation of staff competency, including physicians, should be performed to ensure their ability to assess, aggressively manage, and appropriately document skin and wound care.
- Customized databases should identify and include all ICD-9-CM, CPT, HCPCS, pass-through and new technology, and local codes representing the diagnosis, evaluation and management service, procedures, and products used by the facility.

Developing documentation guidelines is a critical building block for evaluating the clinical efficiency and cost-effectiveness of the care provided. As discussed, the proper documentation provides guidance for appropriate treatment decisions, evaluation of the healing process, support for reimbursement claims, and a defense for litigation. Once established, the documentation system should become the framework of clinical practice for all wound care team members. The wound care team members should be a part of the quality improvement plan in the facility.

- Develop a Quality Improvement Committee that oversees all skin and wound care policies, procedures, competencies, and educational activities.
- Review all materials and new products for skin and wound care at least annually in a joint meeting through the Quality Improvement Committee.

REVIEW

- Determine if your facility will document on paper or electronically.
- Establish consistent documentation criteria for all team members to use each time they document for a patient with a skin condition or wound.
- Develop policies and procedures to support your facility's documentation practices.
- Review your facility's policies and procedures for skin and wound care documentation at least annually.
- Audit your work. (See chapter 7, Wound care and the regulatory process.)

Develop educational and competency validation pathways

Goal: To support all staff education and competency activities for giving skin and wound care

Competency is the common thread found in the art and science of skin and wound care that directly impacts the overall care of the patient. The Joint Commission defines competency as a determination of an individual's capability to perform per expectations. The Joint Commission further recommends:

- developing a competencies program in your facility
- choosing your annual competencies for validation
- scheduling and assigning annual competencies assessments
- using preceptors and peer review for competency validation
- complying with Joint Commission standards.

Competency affects all health care professionals across the continuum. Providers need to be competent in delivering care, and payers need to be competent in understanding the clinical practices for which they are paying on behalf of the patient. (See *Competency validation form.*)

Skin and wound care competency is mandatory for all professionals delivering care in this disease management approach. These programs need to be monitored, evaluated, and modified as the facility deems appropriate.

One way to improve skin and wound care competency is to structure ongoing education and training that will maintain and improve the clinician's knowledge level. Then, the facility has the responsibility to perform ongoing competency assessment through a defined, continuous process. This ongoing monitoring will identify those professionals who are experts in the art and science of wound care. All facilities benefit greatly from competency testing. It increases patient satisfaction.

The art and science of skin and wound care management directly impacts the patient's clinical and financial outcomes. An outcome is the overall condition of a patient that results from all health care processes performed on or for that patient. It refers not only to the patient's medical condition but also to the resulting quality of life the patient experiences. To achieve the best possible wound care outcomes while controlling costs, a comprehensive wound management system, based on published evidence, validated protocols, and competency programs for staff members should be established.

An effective tool for managing outcomes is the clinical pathway. (See *Venous insufficiency algorithm,* page 116.) Such a pathway can serve as a guideline for the health care team to follow for a specific diagnosis. A wound-healing pathway designed for a specific diagnosis should include accurate assessment, documentation, and intervention processes and the expected outcome.

Competency validation form

COMPETENCY VALIDATION:
Wound Assessment for the Licensed Clinician

Directions:
Assess the clinician's skills for wound assessment. Place a score in the appropriate block not to exceed the point value in the "Points" column. If a low score is achieved, briefly explain why under "COMMENTS." Review this form with the clinician. Upon successfully completing all teaching objectives, both the clinician and the clinical observer must sign this form. A follow-up competency may be administered per facility protocol.

CLINICIAN OBSERVED (please print):

	COMPETENCIES:	MET	NOT MET	COMMENTS
1	Classifies wound types appropriately:			
	• Arterial			
	• Diabetic			
	• Full-thickness wound (FTW)			
	• Partial-thickness wound (PTW)			
	• Pressure			
	• Venous			
2	Classifies pressure ulcers appropriately:			
	• Stage I			
	• Stage II			
	• Stage III			
	• Stage IV			
	• Un-stageable?			
3	Describes and identifies the following terms appropriately:			
	• Epithelialization			
	• Erythema			
	• Eschar			
	• Wound Edges			
	• Granulation Tissue			
	• Non-fused Wound Edges			
	• Peri-wound Skin			
	• Slough			
	• Undermining/Tunneling			
4	Differentiates the following terms appropriately:			
	• Clean Wounds			
	• Contaminated Wounds			
	• Infected Wounds			
5	Explains the goals of wound healing for:			
	• Clean, Granulating Wounds			
	• Necrotic, Infected Wounds			
6	Demonstrates proper technique for:			
	• Cleansing Wounds			
	• Irrigating Wounds			

- Assessment, both initial and ongoing, describes the overall condition of the patient, including wound status.
- Documentation, both written and photographic, lays the foundation for management decisions, evaluation of the wound-healing process, and reimbursement decisions. It also serves as a defense in litigation.
- Interventions, guided by the multidisciplinary wound care team, include topical treatments, use of support surfaces, use of adjunctive therapies and products, and nutritional supplements.
- Expected outcome describes the overall condition of the patient that should result from all the processes performed on or for that patient.

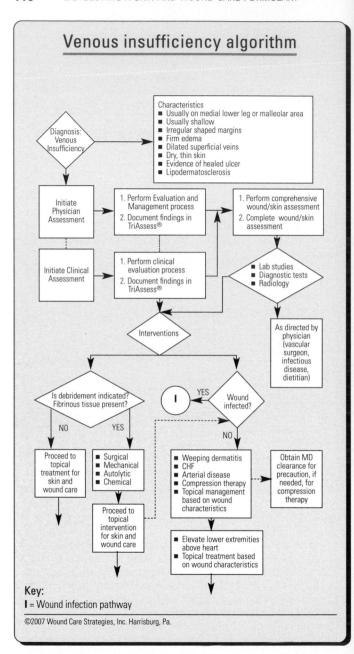

Venous insufficiency algorithm

Diagnosis: Venous Insufficiency

Characteristics
- Usually on medial lower leg or malleolar area
- Usually shallow
- Irregular shaped margins
- Firm edema
- Dilated superficial veins
- Dry, thin skin
- Evidence of healed ulcer
- Lipodermatosclerosis

Initiate Physician Assessment

Initiate Clinical Assessment

1. Perform Evaluation and Management process
2. Document findings in TriAssess®

1. Perform clinical evaluation process
2. Document findings in TriAssess®

1. Perform comprehensive wound/skin assessment
2. Complete wound/skin assessment

- Lab studies
- Diagnostic tests
- Radiology

As directed by physician (vascular surgeon, infectious disease, dietitian)

Interventions

Is debridement indicated? Fibrinous tissue present?

NO — Proceed to topical treatment for skin and wound care

YES
- Surgical
- Mechanical
- Autolytic
- Chemical

Proceed to topical intervention for skin and wound care

Wound infected?

YES → **I**

NO
- Weeping dermatitis
- CHF
- Arterial disease
- Compression therapy
- Topical management based on wound characteristics

Obtain MD clearance for precaution, if needed, for compression therapy

- Elevate lower extremities above heart
- Topical treatment based on wound characteristics

Key:
I = Wound infection pathway

©2007 Wound Care Strategies, Inc. Harrisburg, Pa.

- Monitoring the competency of staff members and patients, evaluating the clinical research for each product used, and assessing outcomes through utilization management tools can help ensure positive outcomes, despite the many variables that can affect wound care outcomes.

Skin and wound care competency is mandatory for all professionals delivering care in your facility. These programs need to be monitored, evaluated, and modified as the facility deems appropriate. Structured ongoing education and training will maintain and improve the clinician's knowledge level, benefiting the clinician, facility, and patient. Some wound competency validation tools that may be appropriate to introduce in your facility are wound assessment and measurement, dressing change, and photographic assessment.

REVIEW

- Incorporate accurate assessment, documentation, and intervention processes based on validated guidelines.
- Review all relevant guidelines at least annually and update your policies, procedures, and facility practices.
- Provide competency validation testing for your staff at least annually to ensure that proper practices support your policies.

Identify levels of practicing professionals

Goal: To establish a multidisciplinary, comprehensive program to manage your complex skin and wound care patient population.

The health care professional's thorough mastery of the assessment and documentation components is imperative. These skills become the link to ensure effective management and healing of wounds. A comprehensive program is linked with a team. The team members may include:

- administrator, head nurse, or designee
- central supply specialist
- board-certified wound, ostomy, and continence nurse or certified wound specialist
- coding specialist
- consulting clinicians
- registered dietitian
- nursing personnel
- occupational therapist
- pharmacist
- physical therapist
- physician
- social worker
- speech therapist.

Each member of the team has defined roles. For example:

- The physician is responsible for the orders that are written to manage the patient. The orders tie directly to the tests and care for the patient. These actions, whether ordering a dressing, drug, device, or test, must tie directly to the plan of care and be realistic and consistent for patients.
- The administrator, head nurse, or designee's role should be clearly defined to oversee the processes put into place and verify that processes are maintained.
- The board-certified wound, ostomy, and continence nurse or certified wound specialist must be able to meet the assessment and documentation needs of your facility and understand the needs of the patient population, to accurately and properly assess, document, refer, and manage the patient within your system.
- The pharmacist makes sure that skin and wound care drugs are dispensed correctly and discontinued when no longer appropriate.
- It's important for the coding and billing specialist to know which products are being purchased and how the products are billed to and paid for by each patient. This step is commonly overlooked until there is a concern or a rejection in the system.
- The central supply specialist maintains the inventory of supplies desired to support the skin and wound care concerns.
- The registered dietitian develops the nutritional instructions for patients and the family or significant others or caregivers. These instructions are necessary for wound healing and the patient's overall well being.
- The social worker's role is integral to evaluate the environmental factors affecting the living conditions of the patient.
- The rehabilitation team—namely, the physical therapist, occupational therapist, and speech therapist—is vital to the care of the wound care patient. The focus of physical therapists and their assistants is to restore and promote the wound patient's optimal strength and physical function. The occupational therapist evaluates the patient for splinting devices to manage contractures and reduce the likelihood of pressure ulcer development, as well as restoring the patient's function. The role of the speech therapist is to evaluate the patient's swallowing ability to maximize the patient's diet.

For the team to operate effectively, it needs to coordinate its activities based on this checklist:

- make skin and wound care rounds
- follow the care of the patient to ensure that all steps of the care plan are appropriate
- oversee policies and procedure to make certain that they reflect the most current clinical and operations guidelines approved by the facility
- annually review and update these policies and procedures
- oversee the design of the formulary management system that controls product utilization to control costs or waste
- evaluate technological advancements presented to the facility in terms of their ability to improve patient outcomes

- provide all team members with ongoing education that improves their ability to prevent wounds and treat existing wounds through better assessment, more aggressive management, and improved documentation.

REVIEW

- Establish a comprehensive team that meets the needs of your skin and wound care patient population.
- Review policies and procedures with team members at least annually.
- Provide competency validation testing for your staff at least annually to ensure proper practices support your policies.

Develop patient educational pathways

Goal: To provide the proper patient-caregiver skin and wound care education across the continuum of care

Patient education and compliance are the cornerstones of successful wound and skin care. The educational needs of the patient should be evaluated on an individual basis beginning with the nonjudgmental assessment of the patient's current knowledge base, relevant to the plan of care determined. An educated clinician should direct the educational activities. Principles of adult learning should be used to develop, implement, and evaluate the effectiveness of the educational activity. Validating the impact of the education by measuring retention of the material is paramount for a successful plan.

While providing patient education, remember:

- Patients have the right to understand their dressing-change order.
- Patients have the right to say no. (Watch for nonverbal cues.)
- Patients have the right to pain assessment and management.

REVIEW

- Principles of adult learning should be used to develop, implement, and evaluate the effectiveness of the educational activity.
- Review all of the policies and procedures with your team members.
- Provide competency validation testing for your staff at least annually to ensure that proper practices support your policies.
- An educated clinician should direct the educational activities.

All of the actions just discussed need to be clearly defined through skin and wound caring processes. Process is defined as a series of actions, changes, or functions that bring about a desired result; and with every process comes defined targeted goals.

Wound care requires a process-driven approach to managing your skin and wound care patients. It's important to define the processes and the goals that you want to achieve.

Incorporate the process steps into your practice

1. Perform a needs assessment to determine the types of skin conditions and wounds admitted to your facility.
2. Develop your operational formulary.
3. Develop your skin and wound care product formulary.
4. Develop your documentation pathways.
5. Develop educational and competency validation pathways.
6. Identify levels of practicing professionals.
7. Develop your patient educational pathways.
   Know the clinical objectives for your skin and wound care patient:
- Provide an optimal healing environment.
- Contour the dressing or drug to the wound.
- Provide an atraumatic environment upon removal of the dressing.
- Prevent maceration to the periwound skin.
- Provide nonadherence to the periwound skin.
- Validate your formulary with published evidence.

To achieve successful skin and wound healing, the practitioner must carefully follow every step in skin and wound management, including critical assessment, planning, implementation, evaluation, and documentation. Practitioners are responsible for assessing the patient's skin, wounds, and dressings; implementing wound care orders; selecting and changing dressings; and preventing infection during procedures. The ultimate objective in clinical practice for skin and wound care is to map the proper product for the skin or wound condition to maximize clinical and patient outcomes.

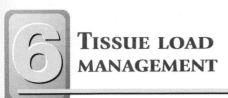

6 TISSUE LOAD MANAGEMENT

Our understanding of how pressure ulcers develop has improved significantly in recent decades. Localized sites of cell death, pressure ulcers occur most commonly in areas where excessive pressure has caused compromised circulation. These ulcers may be superficial, caused by local skin irritation with subsequent surface maceration, or deep, originating in underlying tissue. Deep ulcers may go undetected until they penetrate the skin.

Most pressure ulcers develop when soft tissue is compressed between a bony prominence (such as the sacrum) and an external surface (such as a mattress or the seat of a chair) for a prolonged period. Pressure—applied with great force for a short period or with less force over a longer period—disrupts blood supply to the capillary network, impeding blood flow to the surrounding tissues and depriving tissues of oxygen and nutrients. This leads to local ischemia, hypoxia, edema, inflammation and, ultimately, cell death. The result is a pressure ulcer, also known as a *bedsore, decubitus ulcer, or pressure sore.*

Shear, which separates the skin from underlying tissues, and friction, which abrades the top layer of skin, also contributes to pressure ulcer development. Contributing systemic factors include infection, malnutrition, edema, obesity, emaciation, multisystem trauma, and certain circulatory and endocrine disorders.

The pathophysiology of pressure ulcer development is documented clearly. Successful pressure ulcer management requires a comprehensive approach that includes prevention, relieving pressure, restoring circulation, managing the wound, and minimizing related disorders.

Tissue load management modalities

Support surfaces (or tissue load management surfaces) are a major therapeutic means to managing pressure, friction, and shear on tissues. In addition, many support surfaces control moisture and inhibit bacterial growth. Support surfaces are available in various sizes and shapes for use on beds, chairs, examination tables, and operating-room tables. Used with proper

121

topical skin and wound care, turning, and repositioning, the correct support surface enhances healing of pressure ulcers and helps prevent new ones.

However, the support surface isn't the only intervention that should be employed to prevent pressure ulcers from occurring. As exemplified in the Agency for Health Care Research and Quality (AHRQ, formerly the Agency for Health Care Policy and Research [AHCPR]), effective turning and positioning schedules are the best ways to offset pressure in the immobile patient.

Repositioning
Any individual in bed who is assessed as at risk for developing pressure ulcers should be repositioned at least every 2 hours, if consistent with overall patient goals. A written schedule for systematically turning and repositioning the individual should be used.

Positioning devices
For patients in bed, positioning devices such as pillows or foam wedges should be used to keep bony prominences (for example, knees or ankles) from direct contact with one another, according to a written plan.

Pressure relief for the heels
Patients in bed who are completely immobile should have a care plan that includes the use of devices that totally relieve pressure on the heels, most commonly by raising the heels off the bed. Don't use donut-type devices.

Side-lying positions
When the side-lying position is used in bed, avoid positioning directly on the trochanter.

Bed positioning
Maintain the head of the bed at the lowest degree of elevation, consistent with medical conditions and other restrictions. Limit the amount of time the head of the bed is elevated.

Lifting devices
Use lifting devices such as a trapeze or bed linen to move (rather than drag) patients in bed who can't assist during transfers and position changes.

Pressure-reducing devices for beds
Any individual assessed as at risk for developing pressure ulcers should be placed, when lying in bed, on a pressure-reducing device, such as foam, static air, alternating air, gel, or water mattresses.

Pressure from sitting
Any individual at risk for developing a pressure ulcer should avoid uninterrupted sitting in a chair or wheelchair. The individual should be repositioned, shifting the points under pressure at least every hour, or be put back to bed if consistent with overall patient management goals. Patients who are able should be taught to shift weight every 15 minutes.

Pressure-reducing devices for chairs

For chair-bound patients, the use of a pressure-reducing device such as those made of foam, gel, air, or a combination is indicated. Don't use donut-type devices.

Postural alignment

Positioning of chair-bound patients in chairs or wheelchairs should include consideration of postural alignment, distribution of weight, balance and stability, and pressure relief.

Plans and scheduling

A written plan for the use of positioning devices and schedules may be helpful for chair-bound patients.

Employing these strategies into a comprehensive plan of care addresses the first line of defense for patients at risk for skin breakdown. The Wound, Ostomy, and Continence Nurses Society recently has published additional strategies.

SUPPORT SURFACES

Support surfaces can be divided into two categories: pressure-reducing devices and pressure-relieving devices. A pressure-reducing device for the trochanter or hip lowers pressure below that exerted by a standard hospital mattress or chair surface. A pressure-relieving device relieves pressure at the trochanter or hip below capillary closing pressure (26 to 32 mm Hg). Supportive devices for the heel or special positioning may be needed to eliminate pressure directly on the heel.

Support surfaces can be dynamic, with alternating inflation and deflation, or static, with the pressure load spread over a large area. Static devices maintain constant inflation by use of materials that mold to the body surface, such as foam, gel, and water.

Choose support surfaces carefully, based on the patient's needs. (See *Managing tissue loads,* page 124.) The most common support surfaces are:

- seating devices
- static air-filled overlays
- alternating air-filled mattress overlays
- gel- or water-filled mattress overlays
- replacement mattresses
- low-air-loss replacement mattresses
- low-air-loss specialty beds
- air-fluidized specialty beds. (See *Tissue load management surfaces,* pages 125 to 130.)

Foam mattress overlay or a mattress replacement

Many different types of foam products are available today. These products vary by four parameters: density, thickness or base height, indentation load deflection, and modulus. Density refers to the amount of foam in the product and its ability to support the patient's weight. Thickness or base height

(Text continues on page 130.)

Managing tissue loads

A patient with one or more pressure ulcers may need one of several types of support surfaces and interventions to promote healing. This flowchart shows which ones to choose, based on his condition.

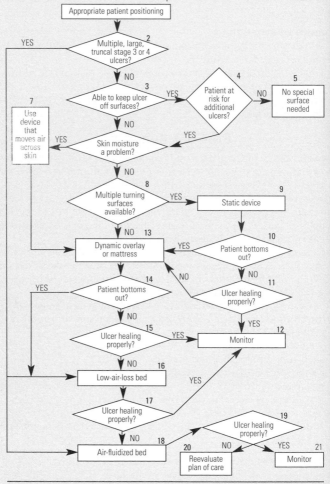

Source: Bergstrom, N., et al. *Pressure Ulcer Treatment*, Clinical Practice Guideline No. 15, AHCPR Publication No. 95-0652. Rockville, MD.: U.S. Department of Health and Human Services, Public Health Service, Agency for Health Care Policy and Research, December 1994.

Tissue load management surfaces

Description	Considerations

BEDS

Air-fluidized bed

- Integrated system of support surface and frame
- Circulates air through silicone-like spheres to create a fluidlike state
- Also known as *bead bed, sand bed,* and *high-air-loss bed*
- Also helps control incontinence and large amounts of wound drainage and body fluids

- Not recommended for mobile patients, patients with pulmonary disease, or patients with unstable spine
- Continuous circulation of warm, dry air may dehydrate patient or desiccate wound bed
- Head of bed cannot be raised
- Weight of product needs to be taken into consideration when placed at a site of service
- Sharp objects may damage product
- Proper inflation necessary for optimal effectiveness

Low-air-loss bed

- Integrated support surface and bed frame
- Distributes the patient's body weight evenly over a sequence of pillows inflated with air by a motor
- Interconnected air cells have a minimum depth of 5″ (12.5 cm)
- Low-air-loss therapy provides a generous amount of dry air flow between the patient and the surface, which controls moisture and heat buildup and prevents maceration and friction
- System has a dedicated power supply unit

- Slippery surface; patient may slide down or out of bed during transfers
- Motor may be noisy
- Sharp objects may damage product
- Proper inflation necessary for optimal effectiveness

Low-air-loss bed with adjuvant features

- Combines other therapies, such as pulsation, percussion, and kinetic therapy, with low-air-loss bed
- Distributes patient's body weight evenly over a sequence of pillows inflated with air by a motor

- Not recommended for patients who have cervical or skeletal traction
- Slippery surface; patient may slide down or out of bed during transfers

(continued)

Tissue load management surfaces *(continued)*

Description	**Considerations**

Low-air-loss bed with adjuvant features (continued)

- Integrated support surface and bed frame
- Interconnected air cells have a minimum depth of 5"
- Low-air-loss therapy provides a generous amount of dry air flow between the patient and the surface, which controls moisture and heat buildup and prevents maceration and friction
- System has a dedicated power supply unit

- Motor may be noisy
- Sharp objects may damage product
- Proper inflation necessary for optimal effectiveness

MATTRESS OVERLAYS

Air

- Dynamic overlays use alternating inflation and deflation to prevent constant pressure against skin and enhance blood flow
- Interconnected cells inflated with a pump
- Recommended cell depth not less than 3" (7.5 cm)
- Cells with larger diameter and depth produce greater pressure relief over the body

- Assembly required
- Sensation of inflation and deflation may bother patient
- Electricity required
- Sharp objects may damage product
- Slippery surface; patient may slide down or out of bed during transfers
- Proper inflation necessary for optimal effectiveness

Foam

- For contoured foam, base height and height from bottom of foam to start of contour shouldn't be less than 2" (5 cm); overall height shouldn't be less than 3½" (8.8 cm)
- Foam density should range from 1.35 to 1.8 lb/ft³
- 25% indentation load deflection should be about 30 lb

- Types of foam vary considerably
- Effectiveness of foam needs monitoring
- Plastic protective sheet is usually necessary for incontinent patients
- Foam may trap perspiration and be hot
- Cleaning may remove flame-retardant coating

Tissue load management surfaces *(continued)*

Description	**Considerations**

Gel
- Provides flotation with pressure re-duction
- May be manufactured in combina-tion with foam
- Recommended depth not less than 2″

- Product heavy
- Research to prove effectiveness limited
- Sharp objects may damage product
- Some surfaces may be slippery; pa-tient may slide down or out of bed during transfers
- Proper inflation necessary for opti-mal effectiveness

Water
- Provides lower interface pressures than standard hospital mattresses
- Recommended depth not less than 3″

- Water heater required to maintain comfortable temperature
- Fluid motions can make procedures and patient transfers difficult
- Precautions needed to prevent mi-croorganism growth
- Product is heavy
- Sharp objects may damage product

MATTRESS REPLACEMENTS

Air
- Reduces interface pressures and re-places the standard hospital mat-tress
- May be manufactured in combina-tion with other materials, such as foam
- May have removable shapes within the mattress
- Recommended height not less than 5″
- Waterproof cover should be applied to reduce shear and friction
- 2-year warranty recommended

- Moisture not always controlled
- Need for overlays reduced
- No therapeutic benefit when used with overlays
- Initial cost is high
- Low-maintenance product that's easy to clean
- Sharp objects may damage product
- Slippery surface; patient mayslide down or out of bed during transfers
- Proper inflation necessary for opti-mal effectiveness

(continued)

Tissue load management surfaces *(continued)*

Description	**Considerations**

Foam

- Reduces interface pressures and replaces the standard hospital mattress
- May be manufactured in combination with other materials, such as gel
- May have removable shapes within the mattress
- For contoured foam, base height and height from bottom of foam to start of contour shouldn't be less than 2"; overall height shouldn't be less than 3½"
- Foam density should range from 1.35 to 1.8 lb/ft^3
- 25% indentation load deflection should be about 30 lb
- Waterproof cover that reduces friction and shear is recommended.

  - Moisture not always controlled
  - Need for overlays reduced
  - No therapeutic benefit when used with overlays
  - Initial cost is high
  - Low-maintenance product that's easy to clean

Gel

- Reduces interface pressures and replaces the standard hospital mattress
- May be manufactured in combination with other materials, such as foam
- May have removable shapes within the mattress
- Recommended height not less than 5"
- Waterproof cover should be applied to reduce shear and friction
- 2-year warranty is recommended

  - Product is heavy
  - Moisture not always controlled
  - Need for overlays reduced
  - No therapeutic benefit when used with overlays
  - Initial cost is high
  - Low-maintenance product that's easy to clean
  - Sharp objects may damage product
  - Some surfaces may be slippery; patient may slide down or out of bed during transfers

Water

- Reduces interface pressures and replaces the standard hospital mattress
- May be manufactured in combination with other materials, such as gel

  - Moisture is not always controlled
  - Reduces the need for overlays
  - No therapeutic benefit when used with overlays
  - Initial cost is high

Tissue load management surfaces *(continued)*

Description	**Considerations**

Water (continued)

- May have removable shapes within the mattress
- Recommended height not less than 5″
- Waterproof cover should be applied to reduce shear and friction
- 2-year warranty recommended

- Low maintenance and easy to clean
- Sharp objects may damage product

ENHANCED OVERLAYS AND MATTRESSES

Alternating-pressure mattress

- Recommended depth not less than 5″
- Configuration of the system's chambers allows for cyclical changes in pressures in different chambers, creating a low- and high-pressure area
- Fabric covering generally air-permeable, bacteria-impermeable, and waterproof; cover should also reduce friction and shear

- Sensation of inflation and deflation may bother patient
- Motor may be noisy
- Moisture buildup may occur
- Sharp objects may damage product
- Slippery surface; patient may slide down or out of bed during transfers
- Proper inflation necessary for optimal effectiveness

Low-air-loss overlay

- Overlay connected to system of air cells with a minimum cell depth of 3″
- System allows for air to escape from the surface
- Fabric covering generally air-permeable, bacteria-impermeable, and waterproof; cover should also reduce friction and shear

- Motor may be noisy
- Sharp objects may damage product
- Some surfaces may be slippery; patient may slide down or out of bed during transfers
- Moisture buildup controlled
- Proper inflation necessary for optimal effectiveness

Nonpowered adjustable zone overlay

- Must have at least three independent adjustable zones
- Manifold system should provide constant force equalization within each section
- Cover material should have a low coefficient of friction

- Motor may be noisy
- Sharp objects may damage product
- Some surfaces may be slippery; patient may slide down or out of bed during transfers
- Proper inflation necessary for optimal effectiveness

(continued)

Tissue load management surfaces *(continued)*

Description	Considerations
Low-air-loss mattress	
■ Interconnected air cells with a minimum depth of 5″ ■ System allows air to escape from the surface ■ Dedicated power supply unit integrated into the system	■ Motor may be noisy ■ Sharp objects may damage product ■ Some surfaces may be slippery; patient may slide down or out of bed during transfers ■ Not recommended for patients who have cervical or skeletal traction ■ Proper inflation necessary for optimal effectiveness
Low-air-loss mattress with adjuvant therapies	
■ Interconnected air cells with a minimum depth of 5″ ■ System allows for air to escape from the surface ■ System has a dedicated power supply unit ■ System may provide other therapies, such as pulsation, percussion, and kinetic therapy	■ Not recommended for patients who have cervical or skeletal traction ■ Slippery surface: patient may slide down or out of bed during transfers ■ Motor may be noisy ■ Sharp objects may damage product ■ Proper inflation needed for optimal effectiveness
Seating devices	
■ Cushions or other seating surfaces used for patients at risk for skin breakdown ■ Generally used in conjunction with a pressure-reducing or pressure-relieving device for the bed ■ May be static or dynamic and constructed of air, fluid, foam, or gel ■ May be powered or nonpowered	■ Each patient must be evaluated for correct product based on his needs ■ Products should be reevaluated routinely for effectiveness

refers to the height of the overlay from the base to where the convolution begins. Indentation load deflection (ILD) indicates the firmness of the foam, and modulus is the ratio of 60 percent ILD to 25 percent ILD. The support surface should have enough compression resistance to support the weight (or load) of the patient.

The height of a 2-inch convoluted foam mattress overlay does not significantly reduce pressures below the standard hospital mattress level and should be used only as a comfort measure. As opposed to 2-inch convoluted foam, 3-inch or 4-inch foam may be an effective device to reduce pressures. These products should be evaluated for effectiveness on an individual basis. This can be accomplished by observing the patient for signs of improvement or deterioration, or by measuring the tissue interface pressures (TIP) if the equipment is available. TIP can be defined as the pressure between the patient's body and the support surface and can be measured using an electropneumatic sensor. Considerations for this product include the need to monitor moisture, as it isn't always controlled on a foam surface and there is no therapeutic benefit when used in conjunction with overlays.

Static air mattress overlays and mattress replacements

The static air mattress overlays are filled with air using an inflating device, such as a handheld pump. It is critical that the mattress overlay be monitored for inflation using a hand check. To perform this task, the practitioner places a hand (palm up) under the overlay and directly below the patient's bony prominence. In accordance with the AHRQ guidelines, if the practitioner feels less than an inch of support material, the patient has bottomed out and the support surface is inadequate. The air mattress replacements reduce interface pressure and replace the standard hospital mattress. These products can be manufactured in combination with other materials, such as foam. They may have removable shapes with the mattress. The recommended height is no less than 5 inches. The products generally have a waterproof cover to reduce shear and friction. Considerations include proper inflation for optimal effectiveness, and understanding that a slippery surface may cause a patient to slide down or out of the bed, and that sharp objects may damage the surface.

Alternating air mattress overlays and mattress replacements

Dynamic motion of an alternating air mattress overlay and mattress, alternating inflation and deflation of the tubules, is used to prevent constant pressure against skin and enhance blood flow. These interconnected cells or tubules are inflated with an electric pump. Configuration of the system's chambers allow for cyclical changes in pressure within different chamber, creating a low- and high-pressure area. The cell depth of the overlay is recommended at more than 3 inches. Alternating air pressure mattresses' recommended depth is no less than 5 inches. A consideration for both products is its dependence on electricity. Proper inflation is also necessary for optimal effectiveness. Additionally, sharp objects may damage the product, and the sensation of inflation and deflation may bother the patient.

Gel and water products as overlays and mattress replacements

These products are filled with either gel or water. Though heavy in weight, they require little maintenance and are easy to clean. Gel products provide flotation with pressure reduction and may be manufactured in combination with foam. The recommended depth is no less than 2 inches. The considerations of gel mattresses are that some surfaces may be slippery, and proper inflation is necessary for optimal effectiveness. Additionally, limited clinical research has been done to evaluate their effectiveness. Water products provide lower interface pressure than standard hospital mattresses, and the recommended depth is no less than 3 inches. The disadvantages of water mattresses are that fluid motions can make procedures and patient transfers difficult, precautions are needed to prevent microorganism growth, and a water heater is required to maintain a comfortable temperature for the patient. Gel and water products both are prone to damage in the presence of sharp objects.

Low-air-loss mattress overlays and mattress replacements

J.T. Scales first reported clinical studies of low-air-loss therapy in the early 1970s. These products prevent capillary occlusion by even distribution of weight over a number of cells or pillows, which are usually grouped by zones. Each zone of pillows is inflated with air, based primarily on the patient's height, weight, and body distribution. The flotation depth of each pillow should have a minimum depth of 5 inches. This allows the patient to float or immerse his body in any position on the product and maintain pressure relief. These products provide a generous amount of dry airflow between the patient and the support surface that controls moisture and heat buildup, defraying maceration and friction. Low-air-loss settings are adjustable. Low-air-loss mattress replacements are manufactured with interconnected air cells with a minimum depth of at least 5 inches. They provide the same benefits as the mattress overlay, although some products have adjuvant therapies incorporated in the product. These features include percussion, pulsation, and kinetic therapy. The considerations of either product include recognizing that the slippery surface may cause a patient to slide down or out of the bed. Additionally, the motor may be noisy. The low-air-loss product with adjuvant therapy isn't recommended for patients who have cervical or skeletal traction. Both products need proper inflation for optimal effectiveness and electricity to maintain inflation; sharp objects may damage the products.

Total bed replacement: Low-air-loss therapy

These products are integrated support surfaces attached to a bed frame. They distribute the patient's body weight evenly over a sequence of pillows inflated with air by a motor. They have interconnected air cells that have a minimum depth of five inches. Low-air-loss therapy provides a generous amount of dry airflow between the patient and the surface, which controls moisture and heat buildup and prevents maceration and friction. These systems have a dedicated power supply unit. The low-air-loss beds with adjuvant features combine other therapies such as pulsation, percussion, and kinetic therapy. One consideration of these products is that their slippery surfaces may make patient transfers difficult. The slippery surface may also cause the patient to slide down in bed. The low-air-loss therapy with adjuvant features isn't recommended for patients who have cervical or skeletal traction.

Total bed replacement: Air-fluidized or high-air-loss therapy

Air-fluidized therapy products, originally developed for burn patients in the 1960s, are an integrated system of a support surface attached to a bed frame. This therapy provides a medium on which patients float that is denser than water by pumping air through silicon-coated microspheres, separated from the patient by a monofilament sheet. Patients float on this surface with capillary readings less than capillary closure. Air-fluidized therapy also has the capability to control large amounts bodily fluids, exudate, or drainage from the wound and is an excellent product for postoperative flap and burn patients. This product, like all other support surfaces, has considerations for use. It isn't recommended for mobile patients, patients with pulmonary disease, or patients with an unstable spine. The continuous circulation of warm, dry air may dehydrate the patient or desiccate the wound bed. The head of the bed can't be raised. Finally, the weight of the product needs to be taken into consideration when placed in any site of service.

Seating devices

If a patient is deemed at risk for skin breakdown, and the patient will be transferred to a chair or wheelchair during his course of care, the patient should be evaluated for a seating device to prevent skin breakdown or to assist in offloading pressures to a wound or wounds. These products are generally used in conjunction with a pressure-reducing or pressure-relieving device for the bed. The products may be static or dynamic, powered or nonpowered, and constructed of air, a fluid medium, foam, or gel. Considerations for use of these products include evaluation of each patient for correct product choice, based on the patient's clinical presentation, and reevaluating these products routinely for effectiveness.

Modifying wheelchairs for pressure relief and reduction

Effective November 12, 2004, significant revisions were released by Centers for Medicare and Medicaid Services (CMS) directing surveyors for long-term care facilities in the assessment of Tag F314 (pressure sores) and Tag F309 (quality of care). (See chapter 7, Wound care and the regulatory process.) The revision to Appendix PP Tag F314 has been entirely replaced and permits surveyors to focus heavily on the prevention and treatment of pressure ulcers. The purpose of these revisions is to ensure that a resident who enters a facility without pressure sores does not develop them, unless that resident's clinical condition demonstrates that they were unavoidable. While these documents were written clearly for long-term care, the information in the documents provides direction for all health care settings to follow.

CMS guidelines clearly state: "An at-risk resident who sits too long on a static surface may be more prone to get ischial ulceration." CMS goes on to say that "Slouching in a wheelchair may predispose an at-risk resident to pressure ulcers of the spine, scapula, or elbow." CMS further notes that "Friction and shearing are also important factors in tissue ischemia, necrosis, and pressure ulceration." The problem, the CMS guidelines tell us, is that wheelchairs "limit repositioning options and increase the risk of pressure development." However, the guidelines explain that "available modification to the seating can provide a more stable surface and provide better pressure reduction."

According to CMS, these wheelchair modification devices must provide:
- postural alignment
- pressure redistribution
- sitting balance and stability
- weight distribution.

Consider the following interventions to improve upper-body positioning and pressure reduction and relief for the resident in a wheelchair:

1. *Correct lateral leaning.* Lateral leaning increases pressure on the ischials. Many types of interventions are available for residents who lean predominantly to the left or right and for those who lean bilaterally.

2. *Control forward leaning.* Forward leaning causes improper weight distribution. Padded lap trays permit residents to use their arms and elbows to achieve proper positioning. Reclining wheelchairs and add-on reclining backrests for standard wheelchairs are recommended for residents who can't brace themselves on a tray. Always use a wedge cushion when reclining a resident.

3. *Control forward sliding.* Forward sliding places increased pressure on the scapula, ischials, and coccyx. Cushions with low-rise front barriers prevent the pelvic thrust which causes forward sliding. Remember that proper support and positioning for the feet is the first step in controlling forward sliding.

4. *Protect elbows.* F314 guidelines tell us that "elbow ulceration is often related to arm rests or lap boards." Vulnerable elbows are easily protected against armrests by means of padded armrest cushions and various types of elbow protectors. Using padded lap trays instead of hard surface lap trays reduces pressure on elbows.

5. *Provide proper head positioning.* Improper positioning of the head may cause pressure ulcers to develop on the ear lobes. Provide residents in reclining wheelchairs, geri-chairs, and other high-back chairs with head positioners or head rests that prevent extreme left-right head rotation. This will reduce pressure on the ear lobes.

6. *Teach weight shifting in chair.* The F314 guidelines say that "a teachable resident should be taught to shift his or her weight approximately every 15 minutes while sitting in a chair." A regular schedule of ambulation is an effective way to offload pressure and provide valuable exercise. Be certain to incorporate regularly scheduled repositioning and pressure offloading into each resident's care plan.

Additional interventions include:

1. *Provide foot support for the wheelchair.* Foot support is the foundation for proper positioning and weight distribution. Your resident must be able to reach the footrests and be provided with a device that prevents his feet from slipping off the sides or back of the footrests.
2. *Eliminate sling-seat hammocking.* Sling-seat hammocking increases interface pressure and contributes to sliding. A leveling pad or a cushion with an integral contoured firm foundation will eliminate sling-seat hammocking.
3. *Eliminate interface heat buildup.* Interface heat buildup promotes skin breakdown and pressure sore formation by causing perspiration and increasing the skin's metabolic demand for oxygen. Water-based gel seating devices prevent these problems by providing protective cooling.
4. *Conduct skin asssessments.* It's important that clinical staff conduct skin assessments regularly on each resident who is at risk for developing pressure ulcers.

The F314 guidelines tell us that based on the "assessment and the resident's clinical condition, choices and identified needs, basic or routine care should include interventions to: a) Redistribute pressure (such as repositioning, protecting heels, etc); b) Minimize exposure to moisture and keep skin clean, especially of fecal contamination; c) Provide appropriate, pressure redistributing, support surfaces; d) Provide non-irritating surfaces; and e) Maintain or improve nutrition and hydration status, where feasible."

When creating a support surface formulary, be sure to include wheelchair modifications and interventions, which are important components of an overall strategy for reducing and relieving pressure.

Preventing pressure ulcers and healing existing ones are top-of-the-list objectives for health care professionals.

SELECTING THE PROPER SURFACE

There are many factors to consider when selecting a support surface for a patient. The first course of action is to work with a multidisciplinary team to review the patient's status and special needs. Determine if the product considered is pressure-reducing for prevention of pressure ulcers or pressure-relieving for treatment of pressure ulcers. Determine the cost parameters based on the patient's payer source. Review each product's benefits and considerations. Investigate the rental agreement for the facility as well as the patient's reimbursement sources. If the patient is Medicare Part B, review the medical policy coverage and payment rules for the specific support surface.

Carefully document the ongoing medical necessity for the product. It's essential to document details, because they become the facts for a medical record. The clinician understands that the medical record serves as the vehicle for demonstrating the clinician's planning, evaluating, coordination of patient care, and justification for payment.

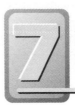

WOUND CARE AND THE REGULATORY PROCESS

Wound care is a business. You're paid for the services you provide to your patients. Some clinicians don't want to look at wound care in these terms. They simply want to march through their day providing the care they were trained to give—and that's OK. On the other hand, some clinicians choose to provide management oversight for wound care programs. Generally these clinicians have provided frontline wound care but now choose to move into a management role for their organization. Their role is to make sure that the care provided in the wound care facility is clinically effective and to verify that the wound care documentation supports the patient's care. No matter which position you choose—hands-on clinician or manager— you must be educated regarding the proper documentation to support history and assessment conducted, examinations completed, work performed, and services provided. This documentation translates into payment for the facility and eventually affects your own paycheck. In order for proper documentation and payment to occur, the facility must practice by a process.

Process is essential

Process is the thread that pulls work, documentation, and payment together. Regulations and guidelines formulated by third-party payers often dictate the actions of these threads. It becomes critical that all personnel associated with the performance of wound care become knowledgeable of stated guidelines and regulations.

Health care expenditures in the United States soon may exceed the $15 billion mark. These expenses most likely will be covered by some form of medical health insurance, which requires providers to file a health insurance claim. The accuracy of this claim reporting, besides supporting medical record documentation, will be imperative to recover all potential revenues and offer substantiation for the payment received. Many issues must be addressed to bring the practice of wound care into compliance with regulations and guidelines set forth by medical health insurance providers. These will include development of a compliance program, knowledge of specific health insurance regulations, and education and training.

The development of a compliance program will provide a structure within the organization to monitor and to know and comply with the laws and regulations and policies and procedures related to the performance of each individual's job. Benefits of the establishment of a compliance program, according to the Office of Inspector General (OIG), are:

- avoidance of potential liability arising from noncompliance
- better communication and more comprehensive policies
- effective internal procedures to ensure compliance with regulations, payment policies, and coding rules
- improved education for all personnel
- improved medical record documentation
- reduced exposure to penalties
- reduction in the denial of submitted claims.

With the initiation of a compliance program, the practice should be committed to addressing the applicable elements set forth in the Federal Sentencing Guidelines and defined by the OIG in their publications addressing the seven basic compliance elements:

- Establish compliance standards through the development of a code of conduct and written policies and procedures.
- Assign compliance monitoring efforts to a designated compliance officer or contact.
- Conduct comprehensive training and education on practice ethics and policies and procedures.
- Conduct internal monitoring and auditing focusing on high-risk billing and coding issues through performance of periodic audits.
- Develop accessible lines of communication, such as discussions at staff meetings regarding fraudulent or erroneous conduct issues and community bulletin boards, to keep employees updated regarding compliance activities.
- Enforce disciplinary standards by making sure that employees are aware that compliance is treated seriously and that violations will be dealt with consistently and uniformly.
- Respond appropriately to detected violations through the investigation of allegations and the disclosure of incidents to appropriate government entities.

Additional information for the establishment of a compliance program can be found on the OIG Web site: *www.oig.hhs.gov*

The objective for a facility-, practice-, or department-specific compliance plan is to create a process for identifying and reducing risk and improving internal controls specific to the facility, practice, or department. The plan shouldn't contradict or conflict with the corporate compliance plan in any way.

Policies and procedures

These written standards communicate departmental values and expectations regarding employee behaviors and establish standards for compliance with laws and regulations.

IMPLEMENTATION AND MONITORING

- Develop relevant policies and procedures.
- Orient staff members to new and revised policies.
- Periodically review policies and procedures and update to reflect changes in laws, regulations, or processes.
- Monitor departmental adherence to policies and procedures.
- Develop a disciplinary plan regarding nonadherence to policies and procedures.
- Provide appropriate resources and educational opportunities to staff members.
- Define risk areas and establish need for self-audit.
- Consider your departmental resources for practicable auditing.
- Determine subject, method, and frequency of audits.
- Review records such as medical and financial records that support claims for reimbursement.
- Prepare the internal audit report.
- Present findings to applicable parties.
- Develop corrective action plan.
- Continue ongoing monitoring.

Ongoing education and training

Training should be designed to promote the understanding of internal standards and the requirements of external laws and regulations.

IMPLEMENTATION AND MONITORING

- Develop departmental-specific educational sessions. These could include admitting and registration requirements, documentation requirements, privacy and confidentiality issues, coverage and billing rules, medical necessity, charge entry risks, and coding requirements. This isn't an exhaustive list, and issues specific to the department should be addressed.
- Provide sufficient time and resources to staff to attend educational sessions.
- Document that training and education of staff has occurred.

Internal auditing

Proactive monitoring and auditing are designed to test and confirm compliance with legal requirements. Auditing is done to assess the completeness of a medical record, determine the accuracy of documentation, and discover lost revenues. During a medical record audit, the documentation is examined to determine if it adequately substantiates the services billed and identifies medical necessity for the services rendered. If this process isn't conducted on an ongoing basis, incorrect or inappropriate documentation and coding practices, potential risks to the organization, compliance with the organizations policies and procedures, and compliance with payer regulations may not be identified.

As a health care provider and a recipient of health insurance dollars, it's important for your organization to conduct internal auditing to prevent improper payments. Effective compliance auditing includes proactive monitoring and auditing, which will confirm the provider's compliance with any legal requirements. The auditing function is the check and balance for your documentation.

IMPLEMENTATION AND MONITORING

- Establish and identify the need for an internal audit.
- Define the specific issues of the audit.
- Determine an appropriate sample size.
- Establish an audit schedule.
- Perform the audit.
- Prepare concise audit report.
- Present audit results to applicable personnel.
- Develop action plan.
- Perform ongoing monitoring.

External auditing

Periodic external audits should be conducted as part of your organizational compliance auditing. This outside audit would confirm your internal audit findings and provide your establishment with any needed corrective actions, should inaccuracies be found.

When an entity chooses an outside auditor or consultant there are many factors to consider. The audit organization must make sure that each audit is conducted by staff that collectively has the knowledge and skills necessary for that audit. The chosen auditor or consultant must have expanded knowledge of medical records and documentation, based on his education, skills, and experience. At a time in the industry when quality of documentation for survey and litigation, coding, confidentiality, and security are emerging as critical issues, it's critical that those chosen to direct your facility have the appropriate credentials.

The audit results should be reported in a professional report that is delivered in a timely manner after the audit or consultation visit. The report should summarize the activities, findings, and recommendations and include concise information to support the determinations made during the audit. When developing an action plan based on an external audit, the provider must identify the regulation or guideline from which the plan was created.

Education

Education also should be a focus for all of your staff. When your entire staff understands the concepts required for the billing and payment of services rendered, it becomes much easier for the organization to meet its compliance standards. Remember, the culture of the medical community in each facility is different. In order to blend the skill sets of the clinicians and physicians, a solid, ongoing wound care education program needs to be implemented. A solid program should be coupled with a multidisciplinary team to lead the charge. A strong wound care team strengthens the problem-solving ability of the program.

Educational process is essential to capitalizing on the strengths of your staff. The following list of solutions may assist you in supporting your program:

- Educate your staff on the standards of care approved by your organization. Not all clinicians are able to learn in the same way.
- Investigate the best method of teaching your staff, just as you would your patient. For example, some physicians and clinicians are visual learners, as opposed to learning by listening to a presentation.
- Provide the targeted learning experience in creative ways. Many educational tools exist, including videotapes, cassette tapes, reading material, verbal presentations, and World Wide Web-architected learning products.
- Mentor your staff. Discuss realistic goals to achieve after the educational process is complete.
- Educate, re-educate, and support the staff of the facility.

Determining which items and services are covered and how often they are covered can be confusing to all entities asking for reimbursement from health care insurers, due to the fact there's inconsistent coverage among insurers. All providers must understand the coverage policies from insurers.

Medicare, Medicaid, and third-party payer standards

Medicare is a federal health insurance program that provides medical coverage for people 65 or older, certain disabled individuals, and some individuals with end-stage renal disease. The U.S. Department of Health and Human Services manages Medicare through the Centers for Medicare & Medicaid Services (CMS).

CMS provides operational direction and policy guidance for nationwide administration of the program. Contracts are awarded to organizations,

Medicare plans

Medicare	Contractors	Coverage
Medicare A	Fiscal Intermediaries (FI)	■ Inpatient hospital care ■ Inpatient care in skilled nursing facility following a covered hospital stay ■ Some home healthcare ■ Hospice care
Medicare B	Carriers	■ Medically necessary services provided by physicians ■ Home healthcare ■ Ambulance services ■ Clinical laboratory and diagnostic services ■ Surgical supplies ■ Durable medical equipment and supplies ■ Services provided by practitioners with limited licensing
Medicare C	■ Health Maintenance Organization (HMO) ■ Point of Service option (POS) ■ Provider Sponsored Organization (PSO) ■ Preferred Provider Organization (PPO) ■ Medical Savings Account (MSA) ■ Private fee-for-service plan ■ Religious fraternal benefit society plan	The beneficiary is still technically "on Medicare" but has selected a different contractor and is required to receive service according to that contractor's arrangement with the U.S. Department of Health and Human Services
Medicare D	Contracted plans	Prescription drug coverage outside of the Part A and Part B coverage elements.

called contractors, to perform Medicare claims processing and related administrative functions. (See *Medicare plans*.)

Medicare pays for services that are considered medically reasonable and necessary to the overall diagnosis and treatment of a patient's condition.

Providers have many avenues that they should monitor when researching Medicare coverage. These would include:

- National coverage, which is published in CMS regulations and the Federal Register, contained in rulings from CMS, or issued as program instruction in coverage or contracted provider manuals
- Local coverage determination, which is developed by the contracted providers in the absence of national coverage determinations and establishes specific criteria as to the coverage or noncoverage and under which clinical circumstances the services are considered reasonable, necessary, and appropriate
- CMS publications
- CMS manual updates.

Medicaid is a joint federal and state health care plan for beneficiaries who are financially unable to obtain health insurance. Medicare and Medicaid payments represent payment in full for services rendered when the provider accepts Medicaid assignment. Medicaid payment regulations differ from state to state and require the provider to obtain specific state regulations when seeking payment.

Other third-party payers such as health organizations and private insurers also have their own guidelines and regulations for payment. Again, this would require the provider to acquire the appropriate payment regulations for submission of claims.

Focus on skin and wound care

Wound care in any health care setting requires concise assessments, documentation, and specialized care. Many regulating bodies and organizations have developed specific language focusing on skin and wound care. (See *Regulations/Guidelines at-a-glance: Focus on skin and wound care*, pages 144 to 157.) The State Operation Manual published by CMS contains supplemental changes to the "Guidance for Surveyors" (Appendix PP), which delineates specific assessment and treatment guidelines.

Even though all health care facilities aren't held to the standards in the State Operation Manual, the guidance will assist in performing assessments, presenting documentation and identifying the necessary treatment for pressure ulcers and incontinent care. Documentation in any health care setting becomes critical when addressing wound and skin care issues. This guidance also provides documentation guidelines to support the assessments, interventions, and care provided to clients with issues related to skin and wound issues. The following documents identify the areas of clinical instruction when caring for individuals with wound and skin problems.

F-Tag 309 Quality of Care

In the skilled nursing facility arena this tag is one that provides guidance in defining the goals of care that are to be provided to the residents who reside in the facility. Because these regulations are being pursued by the federal payment systems in nursing facilities, one could project that other health care providers will be held to similar standards in the very near future. These guidelines can be utilized by other health care providers when determining the appropriate assessments, interventions, and treatments. Being aware of these guidelines can allow other health care entities to provide better care to their clientele when treating specific wound and skin problems.

Each resident must receive—and the facility must provide—the necessary care and services to attain or maintain the highest practicable physical, mental, and psychosocial well-being, in accordance with the comprehensive assessment and plan of care.

The intent of F-Tag 309 is to make sure that the resident obtains optimal improvement or doesn't deteriorate within the limits of a resident's right to refuse treatment, and within the limits of recognized pathology and the normal aging process.

F-TAG 309 DEFINITION OF TERMS

The following definitions and descriptions can be found within the text of F-Tag 309.

- *Highest practicable* is defined as the highest level of functioning and well-being possible, limited only by the individual's presenting functional status and potential for improvement or reduced rate of functional decline. Highest practicable is determined through the comprehensive resident assessment by competently and thoroughly addressing the physical, mental, or psychological needs of the individual.
- *Skin ulcer/wound:* Skin ulcer definitions are included to clarify clinical terms related to skin ulcers. At the time of the assessment and diagnosis, the clinician is expected to document the clinical basis that permits differentiating the ulcer type, especially if the ulcer has characteristics consistent with a pressure ulcer but is determined not to be one.
- *Arterial ulcer:* This is an ulceration that occurs as the result of arterial occlusive disease when nonpressure-related disruption or blockage of the arterial blood flow to an area causes tissue necrosis.

Inadequate blood supply to the extremity may initially present as intermittent claudication. Arterial or ischemic ulcers may be present in individuals with moderate to severe peripheral vascular disease, generalized arteriosclerosis, inflammatory or autoimmune disorders, or significant vascular disease elsewhere. The arterial ulcer is characteristically painful, usually occurs in the distal portion of the lower extremity, and may be over the ankle or bony areas of the foot. The wound bed is frequently dry and pale with minimal or no exudates. The affected foot may exhibit diminished or absent pedal pulse, coolness to touch, decreased pain when hanging down or increased pain when elevated, blanching upon elevation, delayed capillary fill time, hair loss on top of the foot and toes, or toenail thickening.

(Text continues on page 158.)

Regulations/Guidelines at-a-glance*
Focus on skin and wound care

Regulation/Guideline	Purpose
Quality Improvement Roadmap July 2005 (CMS)	This document was created by the CMS Quality Council, in an effort to delineate and advance a vision for improving of medical care. It provides a summary of CMS's many quality-related initiatives. The goal of the quality roadmap is to ensure the right care for every person every time and to do this by making care safe, effective, efficient, patient-centered, timely and equitable.

Specific points	Clinical importance
CMS is working with broad partnerships to clinically validate and provide reliable measures to improve quality of care. Organizations such as AARP, AFL-CIO, AHRQ, AHA, AHIP, AMA, ANA, and The Joint Commission. 5 Major Strategies are being developed: **1. Work through partnerships, within CMS, with Federal and State agencies, and especially with nongovernmental partners to achieve specific quality goals.** Partnering with the following organizations: - Public and private sector groups in the Institute for Healthcare Improvement Campaign - Surgical care Improvement Partnership - Reduce surgical complications - Fistula First National Renal Coalition - Alliance for Cardiac Care - Implement performance measurement through stakeholders such as Hospital Quality Alliance (HQA) and Ambulatory Care Quality Alliance (AQA) CMS recognizes that to achieve real improvements in quality they will need to work together with other stakeholders from throughout our health care system. **2. Develop and provide quality measures and information, as a basis for supporting more effective quality improvement efforts.** CMS is working with broad partnerships to clinically validate and provide reliable measures to improve quality of care. Organizations such as AARP, AFL-CIO, AHRQ, AHA, AHIP, AMA, ANA, and The Joint Commission. **3. Pay in a way that reinforces our commitment to quality, and that helps providers and patients take steps to improve health and avoid unnecessary costs.** This initiative hopes to reverse the payment process of the rewarding of increased payment for ordering more lab tests or imaging, or having more specialists see a patient or do more procedures in order for the medical office to make ends meet. The best way to help health care providers deliver high-quality, efficient care is to pay for it. CMS is implementing and evaluating payment reforms so that there is payment reward for quality not quantity of care.	- The measures have been expanded to include outcomes such as patient satisfaction and surgical complications. Measures of hospital efficiency have been expanded. - Nursing Home quality is part of the Nursing Home Quality Initiative and it has been recently expanded to improve outcomes and efficiencies to reduce pressure ulcers and avoid hospital admission with preventable complications. - A recent Medicare Coverage Advisory Committee (MCAC) made recommendations that have resulted in the development of a guidance document for the management of chronic, non-healing wounds.

(continued)

Regulations/Guidelines at-a-glance*
Focus on skin and wound care *(continued)*

Regulation/Guideline	Purpose
Quality Improvement Roadmap **July 2005 (CMS)** *(continued)*	
Joint Commission 2007 National Patient Safety Goals: Implementation Expectations	The Joint Commission is committed to improving safety for patients and residents in health care organizations. This commitment is inherent in its mission to continuously improve the safety and quality of care provided to the public through the provision of health care accreditation and related services that support performance improvement in health care organizations. At its heart, accreditation is a risk-reduction activity; compliance with standards is intended to reduce the risk of adverse outcomes. The Joint Commission demonstrates its commitment to patient safety through numerous efforts.

Specific points	**Clinical importance**

4.   Assist practitioners and providers in making care more effective, particularly including the use of effective electronic health systems.

Assisting practices to get electronic health systems at a reasonable cost

5.   Bring effective new treatments to patients more rapidly and help develop better evidence so that doctors and patients can use medical technologies more effectively.

CMS is supporting the availability of better treatments for our beneficiaries, along with better evidence on the benefits, risks, and costs of using medical treatments.

Along with the improvement of guidance documents, CMS is working on a more transparent and opportunity for public input on coverage issues. A recent Medicare Coverage Advisory Committee (MCAC) made recommendations that have resulted in the drafting of a guidance document for the management of chronic, non healing wounds.

There are 14 Goals and Requirements declared by The Joint Commission.

Goal 1: Improve accuracy of patient/resident/client identification.

Goal 2: Improve the effectiveness of communication amongst caregivers.

Goal 3: Improve the safety of using medications.

Goal 4: Eliminate wrong patient, wrong site, wrong surgical procedure surgery.

Goal 5: Improve the safety of using infusion pumps.

Goal 6: Improve the effectiveness of clinical alarm systems.

Goal 7: Reduce the risk of health care associated infections.

Goal 8: Accurately and completely reconcile medications across the continuum of care.

Goal 9: Reduce the risk of harm related to patient/resident/client falls.

Goal 10: Reduce the risk of influenza and pneumococcal disease in older adults.

Goal 11: Reduce the risk of surgical infections.

New Goals:

8B- The complete list of medications is also provided to the resident/patient on discharge from the facility.

13A- Define and communicate the means for patients/residents and their families to report concerns about safety and encourage them to do so.

(continued)

Regulations/Guidelines at-a-glance*
Focus on skin and wound care *(continued)*

Regulation/Guideline	Purpose
Joint Commission 2007 National Patient Safety Goals: Implementation Expectations *(continued)*	
Guideline for prevention and management of pressure ulcers Wound, Ostomy, and Continence Nurses Society (WOCN). Guideline for prevention and management of pressure ulcers. Glenview (IL): Wound, Ostomy, and Continence Nurses Society (WOCN); 2003. 52 p. (WOCN clinical practice guideline; no. 2). [141 references]	To present an evidence-based guideline for pressure ulcer prevention and management; and To improve cost-effective patient outcomes as well as increase wound research in the areas where there are gaps between research and practice.

Specific points	Clinical importance
Goal 12: Implementation of applicable National Patient Safety Goals and associated requirements by components and practitioner site. **NEW Goal 13:** Encourage the active involvement of patients and their families in the patient's own care as a patient safety strategy. **Goal 14:** Prevent health care related pressure ulcers. **NEW Goal 15:** The organization identifies safety risks inherent in its patient/resident population.	

Assessment 1. Assessment of individual risk for developing pressure ulcers using risk assessment tools (e.g., Braden Scale, Norton Scale, Braden Q Scale) 2. Identification of high-risk settings and groups to target prevention efforts and minimize risk 3. Assessment of skin 4. Assessment of cognition, sensation, immobility, friction and shearing, and incontinence 5. Assessment of nutritional status and laboratory parameters for nutrition status 6. Assessment for history of prior ulcer and/or presence of current ulcer, previous treatments, or surgical interventions 7. Assessment and monitoring of pressure ulcers at each dressing change 8. Assessment for factors that impede healing 9. Evaluation of healing 10. Assessment for potential complications associated with pressure ulcers	■ Assessment of skin ■ Management of incontinence (bowel and bladder program; skin cleansing; skin barriers; use of absorbent material next to skin; collection devices for urine and stool)
Prevention/Management/Treatment 1. Measures to minimize friction and shear (keeping skin dry, using lift sheets or turning devices, overhead trapeze bars) 2. Measures to reduce or relieve pressure (turning and repositioning; avoiding foam rings, donuts, sheepskin; proper positioning of chair-bound patients; use of pressure-reducing or -relieving devices 3. Management of incontinence (bowel and bladder program; skin cleansing; skin barriers; use of absorbent material next to skin; collection devices for urine and stool)	

(continued)

Regulations/Guidelines at-a-glance*
Focus on skin and wound care *(continued)*

Regulation/Guideline	Purpose
Guideline for prevention and management of pressure ulcers *(continued)*	
Pressure ulcers in adults: Prediction and prevention. Agency for Health Care Policy and Research (AHCPR). Pressure ulcers in adults: prediction and prevention. Rockville (MD): U.S. Department of Health and Human Services, Public Health Service, AHCPR; 1992 May. 63 p. (Clinical practice guideline; no. 3). [127 references]	

pecific points	Clinical importance

4. Nutritional management (correction of deficiencies)

5. Patient/caregiver education (causes, risk factors, prevention and management of pressure ulcers)

6. Wound management (cleansing, debridement of tissue, topical dressing, managing infection)

7. Adjunctive therapies (growth factors; electrical stimulation; noncontact normothermic radiant heat therapy; topical negative pressure)

8. Note: The guideline developers considered but did not recommend other adjunctive therapies (ultrasound, electromagnetic therapy, hyperbaric oxygen therapy; use of sugar, honey, or skin equivalents; topical phenytoin; topical estrogen; phototherapy)

9. Evaluation of need for operative repair

9. Evaluation and management of pain

**sk Assessment Tools and Risk Factors: Identify at-
sk Individuals needing prevention and the specific
ctors placing them at risk**

ed- and Chair-Bound Individuals

in Care and Early Treatment

aintain and improve tissue tolerance to pressure in order
prevent injury

Skin Inspection

individuals at risk should have a systematic skin inspection at least once a day, paying particular attention to the ny prominences. Results of skin inspection should be cumented. (Strength of Evidence = C.)

Skin Cleansing

in cleansing should occur at the time of soiling and at utine intervals. The frequency of skin cleansing should be dividualized according to need and/or patient preference. oid hot water, and use a mild cleansing agent that minimizes irritation and dryness of the skin. During the cleansing process, care should be utilized to minimize the force d friction applied to the skin. (Strength of Evidence = C.)

Dry Skin

nimize environmental factors leading to skin drying, such low humidity (less than 40 percent) and exposure to cold.

(continued)

Regulations/Guidelines at-a-glance*
Focus on skin and wound care *(continued)*

Regulation/Guideline	Purpose
Pressure ulcers in adults: Prediction and prevention. *(continued)*	

| pecific points | Clinical importance |

y skin should be treated with moisturizers. (Strength of
idence = C.)

Massage

void massage over bony prominences. (Strength of Evi-
nce = B.)

Exposure to Moisture

inimize skin exposure to moisture due to incontinence,
rspiration, or wound drainage. When these sources of
oisture cannot be controlled, underpads or briefs can be
ed that are made of materials that absorb moisture and
esent a quick-drying surface to the skin. Topical agents
at act as barriers to moisture can also be used. (Strength
Evidence = C.)

Friction and Shear Injuries

in injury due to friction and shear forces should be mini-
zed through proper positioning, transferring, and turning
chniques. In addition, friction injuries may be reduced by
e use of lubricants (such as corn starch, and creams), pro-
ctive films (such as transparent film dressings, and skin
alants), protective dressings (such as hydrocolloids), and
otective padding. (Strength of Evidence = C.)

Nutrition

ien apparently well-nourished individuals develop an in-
equate dietary intake of protein or calories, caregivers
ould first attempt to discover the factors compromising
ake and offer support with eating. Other nutritional sup-
ements or support may be needed. If dietary intake re-
ins inadequate and if consistent with overall goals of
erapy, more aggressive nutritional intervention such as
teral or parenteral feedings should be considered.
rength of Evidence = C.)

nutritionally compromised individuals, a plan of nutri-
nal support and/or supplementation should be imple-
nted that meets individual needs and is consistent with
overall goals of therapy. (Strength of Evidence = C.)

Mobility and Activity

otential for improving mobility and activity status exists,
abilitation efforts should be instituted if consistent with
overall goals of therapy. Maintaining current activity

(continued)

Regulations/Guidelines at-a-glance*
Focus on skin and wound care *(continued)*

Regulation/Guideline	Purpose
Pressure ulcers in adults: Prediction and prevention *(continued)*	
F-Tag 314: Pressure Sores	The intent of this requirement is that the resident does not develop pressure ulcers unless clinically unavoidable and that the facility provides care and services.

pecific points	Clinical importance
vel, mobility, and range of motion is an appropriate goal r most individuals. (Strength of Evidence = C.) **Documentation** terventions and outcomes should be monitored and docu-ented. (Strength of Evidence = C.) **echanical Loading and Support Surfaces** otect against the adverse effects of external mechanical rces: pressure, friction, and shear. **ucation** duce the incidence of pressure ulcers through education-programs.	
comprehensive admission assessment should address ose factors that have been identified as having an impact the development, treatment and/or healing of pressure ers, including, at a minimum: risk factors, pressure nts, under-nutrition and hydration deficits, and moisture d the impact of moisture on skin. Assessment upon admission, weekly assessments for e first 4 weeks for residents at risk, then quarterly, or enever there is a change in cognition or functional lity The clinicians responsible for the resident's care should iew each risk factor and potential cause(s) **individually**. Both urine and feces contain substances that may irri-e the epidermis and may make skin more susceptible to akdown. It may be difficult to differentiate dermatitis ated to incontinence from partial thickness skin loss essure ulcer). This differentiation should be based on the ical evidence and review of presenting risk factors. A facility should be able to show that its treatment pro-ols are based upon current standards of practice and are accord with the facility's policies and procedures as de-oped with the medical director's review and approval. Potential changes in skin condition should be monitored east daily. Additionally residents should be monitored condition changes that might increase the risk of break-vn and the defined interventions should be implemented monitored for effectiveness.	Related skin care and pressure ulcer care infor-mation threaded through-out the regulation.

(continued)

Regulations/Guidelines at-a-glance*
Focus on skin and wound care *(continued)*

Regulation/Guideline	Purpose
F-Tag 315: Incontinence and Catheters	A resident who enters the facility without an indwelling catheter is not catheterized unless the resident's clinical condition demonstrates that catheterization was necessary; and a resident who is incontinent of bladder receives appropriate treatment and services to prevent urinary tract infections and to restore as much normal bladder function as possible.
F-Tag 309: Quality of Life	New language is added to include definitions of nonpressure related ulcers.
Quality Improvement Matters	Quality improvement strategies to improve the care in nursing homes

pecific points	Clinical importance
kin-related complications in problems associated with incontinence and moisture range from irritation to increased risk of skin breakwn. Moisture may make the skin more susceptible to mage from friction and shear during repositioning. One m of early skin breakdown is maceration. Lastly, the pertent exposure of perineal skin to urine and/or feces can tate the epidermis and can cause sever dermatitis or skin osion.	1. Keep the perineal skin clean and dry. Research has shown that soap and water regimen alone may be less effective in preventing skin breakdown compared with moisture barriers and no-rinse incontinence cleansers. 2. Because frequent washing with soap and water can dry the skin, the use of a perineal rise may be indicated. 3. Moisturizers help preserve the moisture in the skin by either sealing in existing moisture or adding moisture to the skin. 4. Moisturizers include lotions or pastes. However, moisturizers should be used sparingly, if at all, on already macerated or excessively moist skin.

the time of the assessment and diagnosis, the clinician
expected to document the clinical basis (e.g., underlying
dition contributing to the ulceration, ulcer edges and
und bed, location, shape, condition of surrounding tis-
e), which permits differentiating the ulcer type, especially
he ulcer has characteristics consistent with a pressure
er, but is determined not to be one.
inition of the following are provided: Arterial Ulcer, Di-
tic Neuropathic Ulcer, and Venous Insufficiency Ulcer.

ks at pressure ulcers, pain and infections

- *Diabetic neuropathic ulcer:* This requires that the resident be diagnosed with diabetes mellitus and have peripheral neuropathy. The diabetic ulcer characteristically occurs on the foot, at midfoot, at the ball of the foot over the metatarsal heads, or on top of toes with Charcot deformity.
- *Pressure ulcer:* This is addressed under F-Tag 314.
- *Venous insufficiency ulcer:* This is an open lesion of the skin and subcutaneous tissue of the lower leg usually occurring in the pretibial area of the lower leg or above the medial ankle. Venous ulcers are reported to be the most common vascular ulceration and may be difficult to heal, may occur off and on for several years, and may occur after relatively minor trauma. The ulcer may have a moist, granulating wound bed, may be superficial, and may have minimal to copious serous drainage unless the wound is infected. The resident may experience pain that may be increased when the foot is in a dependent position, such as when the resident is seated with his feet on the floor. Recent literature implicates venous hypertension as a causative factor. Earlier the ulceration was believed to be due to the pooling of blood in the veins.

    Venous hypertension may be caused by one or a combination of factors including loss of valve function in the vein, partial or complete obstruction of the vein, or failure of the calf muscle to pump the blood. Venous insufficiency may result in edema and induration, dilated superficial veins, cellulites in the lower third of the leg, or dermatitis. The pigmentation may appear as darkening skin: tan or purple areas in light-skinned patients and dark purple or black in dark brown-skinned patients.

    In any instance in which there has been a lack of improvement or decline, the facility must determine if the occurrence was unavoidable or avoidable. An unavoidable determination can be made only if the following are present:

- an accurate and complete assessment
- a care plan that is implemented consistently and based on information from the assessment
- evaluation of the results of the interventions and revision of the interventions as necessary.

F-TAG 314 PRESSURE ULCERS

Pressure ulcers aren't treated only in a skilled nursing facility. Inpatient facilities have seen admissions and inhouse development of pressure ulcers within their patient population. Outpatient wound care departments and home health agencies are seeing pressure ulcers in consultation and providing care. The CMS State Operations Manual provides extensive guidance for the identification, assessment, treatment, and prevention of pressure ulcers under F-Tag 314. Currently these regulations are mandated only to skilled nursing facilities, but all other health care providers could benefit from awareness of the information.

"Based on the comprehensive assessment of a resident, the facility must make sure that:

- a resident who enters the facility without pressure ulcers doesn't develop pressure ulcers unless the individual's clinical condition demonstrates that they were unavoidable
- a resident with pressure ulcers receives necessary treatment and services to promote healing, prevent infection, and prevent new sores from developing."

As stated within the text of F-Tag 314, the intent of this guidance is to prevent the resident from developing pressure ulcers unless clinically unavoidable and to make sure that the facility provides care and services to:

- promote prevention of pressure ulcer development
- promote the healing of pressure ulcers that are present (including prevention of infection to the extent possible)
- prevent development of additional pressure ulcers.

The facility should have the following supportive documentation:

- to identify if the pressure ulcer or ulcers were avoidable or unavoidable
- to identify the adequacy of the facility's interventions and efforts to prevent and treat pressure ulcers.

F-TAG 315 INCONTINENCE AND CATHETERS

Many conditions precipitate wound and skin conditions. Incontinence and the occurrence of urinary tract infections historically either have caused skin deterioration or contributed to the worsening of symptoms. Addressing these two issues in any health care setting could lead to the prevention or improvement of any skin breakdown. In the published guidelines of the CMS State Operations Manual for skilled nursing facilities, the issues related to incontinence and catheters are defined, and documentation guidance is provided to support the care provided.

As stated within the text of F-Tag 315, a resident who enters the facility without an indwelling catheter isn't catheterized unless the resident's clinical condition demonstrates that catheterization was necessary. Some residents are admitted to the facility with indwelling catheters already placed. The facility is responsible for the assessment of the resident at risk for urinary catheterization and for the ongoing assessment of the resident who currently has a catheter. This is followed by implementation of appropriate individualized interventions and monitoring for the effectiveness of the interventions.

The guidelines continue to state that a resident who's incontinent of bladder receives appropriate treatment and services to prevent urinary tract infections and to restore as much normal bladder function as possible. Whether the resident is incontinent of urine on admission or develops incontinence after admission, the steps of assessment, monitoring, reviewing, and revising approaches to care are essential to managing urinary incontinence and to restoring as much normal bladder function as possible.

The intent of F-Tag 315 is to make sure that:

- Each resident who's incontinent of bladder is identified, assessed, and provided appropriate treatment and services to achieve or maintain as much normal urinary function as possible.
- An indwelling catheter isn't used unless there's valid medical justification.
- An indwelling catheter for which continuing use isn't medically justified is discontinued as soon as clinically warranted.
- Services are provided to restore or improve normal bladder function, to the extent possible, after removal of the catheter.
- A resident, with or without a catheter, receives the appropriate care and services to prevent infections, to the extent possible.

The facility should have documentation to support:

- whether the initial insertion or continued use of an indwelling catheter is based on clinical indication for use of a urinary catheter
- the adequacy of interventions to prevent, improve, and manage urinary incontinence
- determination of whether appropriate treatment and services to prevent or treat urinary tract infections was provided.

No matter which health care setting provides care to clients for wound and skin treatment, the physician should provide the initial treatment plan and continued periodic followup. Two F-Tag guidance documents for skilled nursing care address the need for physician input into the care for individuals with skin and wound care issues. These two publications can be utilized as guidance tools in any other health care setting when addressing the physician's role in the assessment and treatment of individuals with these types of issues. There should be medical record documentation in any health care setting, identifying that the physician is involved in the assessment, intervention, and treatment of wound and skin problems. Appropriate follow-up also should be documented. Again, even though the guidance of the State Operations Manual is specifically targeted to skilled facilities, the document can be utilized by other health care providers as a guidance tool. The two following F-Tag documents address physician services and the role of a medical director.

F-TAG 385 PHYSICIAN SERVICES

A physician must personally approve, in writing, a recommendation that an individual be admitted to a facility. Each resident must remain under the care of a physician.

The facility must make sure that:

- the medical care of each resident is supervised by a physician
- another physician supervises the medical care of residents when their attending physician is unavailable.

As stated within the text of F-Tag 385, the intent of this regulation is to ensure medical supervision of the care of nursing home residents by a personal physician.

Supervising the medical care of a resident means participating in the resident's assessment and care planning, monitoring changes in a resident's medical status, and providing consultation or treatment when called by the facility. It also includes, but isn't limited to, prescribing new therapy, ordering a resident's transfer to the hospital, conducting required routine visits, or delegating and supervising follow-up visits to nurse practitioners or physician assistants. Each resident should be allowed to designate a personal physician. The facility's responsibility in this situation is to simply assist the resident, when necessary, in his efforts to obtain these services. For example, the facility could put the resident in touch with the county medical society for the purpose of obtaining referrals to practicing physicians in the area.

The guidelines continue to state that the facility should maintain the following in its documentation:

- documentation that supports the supervising physician's involvement in the resident's assessment and care planning
- documentation of a response to staff report of a significant change in medical status to the supervising physician
- documentation that the supervising physician has appropriate coverage when he's unavailable
- documentation to support that residents aren't routinely cared for in the emergency department because of the lack of an on-call physician.

F-Tag 501 MEDICAL DIRECTOR

The medical director has an important leadership role in actively helping long-term care facilities provide quality care. This individual accepts the responsibility for the implementation of resident care policies and the coordination of medical care. The medical director's roles and functions require the physician serving in that capacity to be knowledgeable about current standards of practice in caring for long-term care residents and about how to coordinate and oversee related practitioners. As a clinician, the medical director plays a pivotal role in providing clinical leadership regarding application of current standards of practice for resident care, and new or proposed treatments, practices, and approaches to care. The medical director's input promotes the attainment of optimal resident outcomes, which may also be influenced by many factors, such as resident characteristics and preferences, individual attending physician actions, and facility support.

As stated within the text of F-Tag 501, the intent of this guidance is to make sure that:

- The facility has a licensed physician who serves as the medical director to coordinate medical care in the facility and provide clinical guidance and oversight regarding the implementation of resident care policies.

- The medical director collaborates with the facility leadership, staff, and other practitioners and consultants to help develop, implement, and evaluate resident care policies and procedures that reflect current standards of practice.
- The medical director helps the facility to identify, evaluate, and address or resolve medical and clinical concerns and issues that:
  –affect resident care, medical care, or quality of life
  –are related to the provision of services by physicians and other health care practitioners.

The facility should be able to provide documentation to support the following:

- It has a designated medical director who is a licensed physician.
- The physician is performing the functions of the position.
- The medical director provides input and helps the facility develop, review, and implement resident care policies, based on current clinical standards.
- The medical director assists the facility in the coordination of medical care and services in the facility.

The medical record

As health care providers, we believe that the most critical function of the medical record's multiple purposes is to plan and provide continuity of care for a patient's medical treatment. The documentation in the medical record does provide this function, but in many instances we, as health care providers, forget that the additional functions of the medical record include:

- providing information for the financial reimbursement to hospitals, health care providers, skilled nursing facilities, and patients
- providing legal documentation in cases of injury or other legal proceedings
- providing information for quality assurance and peer review committees, state licensing agencies, and state regulatory agencies when assessing the quality of care provided
- providing the critical information in an accreditation process such as The Joint Commission.

Throughout this chapter we have discussed compliance, reimbursement, guidelines, and regulations. These elements can be met only through the appropriate documentation in the medical record. (See chapter 5, Developing a skin and wound care formulary.) No matter the health care setting in which one provides care for wound and skin issues, the critical element becomes the documentation in the medical record.

Wound care in any health care setting requires concise assessments, documentation, and specialized care. The following documents identify the areas of clinical instruction when caring for individuals with wound and

Audit tool for outpatient wound care department

HOSPITAL-OWNED OUTPATIENT WOUND CARE DEPARTMENT

Review Audit Checklist for Medical Necessity of Provided Services

In the hospital outpatient setting, both the facility and the professional receive payment from Medicare for the services rendered. Each entity must maintain their documentation standards to allow for payment of their services. This checklist is provided as the first step in the review audit process to identify obvious discrepancies and prompt a more intense compliance review.

Facility Review Audit Checklist

Task	Met	Not Met	Specific Follow-up Required (Identify type of follow-up)
1. Has your facility developed a requirement crosswalk between the E/M level and the APC level?			
2. Does the medical record documentation support the requirements from the facility developed crosswalk?			
3. Does the departmental staff understand the requirements for medical record documentation to support the facility developed crosswalk?			
4. Has the department staff received the appropriate education and training in the utilization of the crosswalk?			
5. Are the appropriate modifiers being utilized in the department?			
6. Has the departmental staff been trained in the use of modifiers?			
7. Does the medical record documentation support the utilization of a modifier?			
8. Does the wound care department have a tool which provides the facility billing entity with a listing of the services rendered?			
9. Is there appropriate communication between the departmental staff and the billing entity of the facility (i.e. coding/billing updates, revisions to facility crosswalk, etc.)?			
10. Does the facility billing entity audit the wound care departments documentation in order to support the APC levels billed?			

Professional Review Audit Checklist

Task	Met	Not Met	Specific Follow-up Required (Identify type of follow-up)
1. Is there an appropriate tool to correspond the services rendered to the professional billing entity?			
2. Does the professional billing entity audit the medical record documentation to assure that the appropriate E/M level has been billed?			
3. Does the professional billing entity provide the practicing professional with necessary updates to determine service codes?			
4. When modifiers are appended, is there supporting medical record documentation?			
5. Does the practicing professional provide supporting medical record documentation to correspond with the level of E/M billed for his/her professional service?			
6. If templates are utilized, does the practicing professional document utilizing the guidelines for the template?			
7. Does the documentation require the date and the signature of the practicing professional providing the service?			
8. Has the practicing professional identified the appropriate diagnosis code for the services rendered?			
9. Has the practicing professional identified the appropriate diagnosis coding for ancillary services ordered?			
10. Does the medical record documentation for the wound assessment and description support the dressing ordered? (following appropriate Medicare Part B Surgical Dressing Policy for specific region)			
11. Are procedures appropriately documented in the medical record to support the service code identified and billed?			
12. Are the services being rendered by the professional appropriate for the Wound Care Department setting?			

skin problems. (See *Audit tool for outpatient wound care department.* See also *Positioning and support services assessment audit form,* page 164.)

Positioning and support services assessment audit form

we bring it all together™

POSITIONING AND SUPPORT SURFACES ASSESSMENT AUDIT*

Directions:
Complete all sections of this form. If the answer to any question is No or N/A, explain responses on the back of this form.
Complete the entire audit process per facility protocol.

Positioning and Support Surfaces Assessment

1. Were the appropriate risk assessments performed to determine the level of risk for skin breakdown? θ YES θ NO θ N/A

2. Were the appropriate skin care measures instituted? θ YES θ NO θ N/A

3. Were the appropriate interdisciplinary team members consulted to evaluate at risk residents? θ YES θ NO θ N/A

4. Were resident/patients with existing pressure ulcers assessed appropriately for preventive support surfaces? θ YES θ NO θ N/A

5. Was the resident/patient's activity level and mobility assessed appropriately? θ YES θ NO θ N/A

6. Does the medical record documentation by the staff caring for resident/patient indicate that preventative care was given to the resident (repositioning, skin care, utilization of lifting devices when indicated) ? θ YES θ NO θ N/A

7. Were the resident/patient's nutritional needs assessed appropriately? θ YES θ NO θ N/A

8. Was the resident/patient's continence assessed appropriately? θ YES θ NO θ N/A

9. Were the appropriate support surfaces provided to the resident/patient (static vs. dynamic)? θ YES θ NO θ N/A

10. Did the care plan reflect the need for support surface? θ YES θ NO θ N/A

11. Did the care plan indicate the care needed in providing a support surface? θ YES θ NO θ N/A

12. Was the appropriate maintenance provided for the indicated support surface? θ YES θ NO θ N/A

13. Was the appropriate infection control issues addressed related to the support surface being utilized? θ YES θ NO θ N/A

14. Were residents/patients re-evaluated at intervals to assess the success of the support surface and to determine necessary changes? θ YES θ NO θ N/A

15. Does medical record documentation support timely re-evaluations and documentation of anticipated plan? θ YES θ NO θ N/A

_____   Date of audit
Chart/Medical Record Number audited

_____   Date
Signature of Clinician completing audit

*An audit should be differentiated from a review. An audit should have measurable criteria, formal identification of action to resolve discrepancies and a recording process to retain information and make recommendations. This audit tool provides the components for needed follow-up identification.

PART TWO

SKIN AND WOUND CARE PRODUCTS

OVERVIEW

For centuries, humans have been combining substances for use in topical skin and wound care. Early Egyptians mixed concoctions of naturally occurring products, such as honey, animal fat, and vegetable fibers. Shamans and witch doctors created poultices of plant extracts and animal products. As the culture progressed, mixtures became more complex, and the relative amounts of various ingredients became more important for a successful mixture, so the compounders began keeping records of specific compositions and preparation methods.

In the 19th and 20th centuries, synthetic ingredients such as polymers joined the list of naturally occurring ingredients in various products. The complexity of products soared along with the explosion of new products. And with this explosion has come confusion over dressing selection.

Clinical Guide: Skin and Wound Care can help you, the practitioner, choose the proper skin and wound care products to facilitate skin health and wound healing based on the classification of the wound and skin condition. To use this tool properly, remember that the composition of a product is often key to its success and may be kept a trade secret. However, for fundamental safety reasons, the U.S. Food and Drug Administration requires a basic level of disclosure about the ingredients in products. Some products may contain ingredients that cause an allergic reaction in certain people or ingredients that shouldn't be mixed with certain other ingredients. For example, many people are allergic to latex and need to know if it's a component of a certain product. Labels of most food and household products contain information about their ingredients, which are listed in order of abundance in the mixture. In addition to the label, a Material Safety Data Sheet (MSDS) is available upon request from any manufacturer for any of its products. An MSDS contains health and safety information on the product and its ingredients. Practitioners should be careful when mixing products and should always read the product label and package insert before use.

Practitioners must provide comprehensive product choices for skin and wound care management, including products for skin health, topical wound care products, support surfaces, nutritional products, and adjunctive therapies that promote healing.

166

Part Two provides quick-reference descriptions of skin and wound care products grouped under generic categories. The skin care product categories include antifungals and antimicrobials, liquid skin protectants, moisture barriers, skin cleansers, therapeutic moisturizers, and other skin care products. Included in the wound care product section are alginates, antimicrobials, collagens, composites, contact layers, drugs, foams, hydrocolloids, hydrogels, specialty absorptives, surgical dressings, transparent films, and more. For specific packaging information, you may want to contact the manufacturer. (See *Manufacturer resource guide,* pages 582 to 583.)

No single skin or wound care product provides an optimum environment for skin health or healing of all wounds. It's your responsibility to understand the characteristics, function, and appropriateness for each patient of the skin care products, dressings, drugs, and devices.

Skin care products

Overview

The fundamental building blocks addressing prevention of skin breakdown are generally overshadowed by the deluge of intervention strategies touted for patients with chronic wounds. It's paramount that providers take these proactive steps in clinical practice to develop sound skin care prevention and intervention pathways. To that end, the clinician must understand the anatomy and physiology of the skin, current practice guidelines, and indications and contraindications of skin care products used in clinical practice.

Use the skin care products section to help you develop a skin care formulary for your facility. When creating the skin care formulary, be sure to include products under categories such as:

- Antifungals and antimicrobials (topical): products that inhibit the growth of organisms that cause superficial skin infections, such as yeast
- Liquid skin protectants (also called *skin sealants*): products that protect the skin by forming a transparent protective barrier
- Moisture barriers (also called *skin protectants*): ointments, creams, or pastes that protect the skin from urinary and fecal incontinence by shielding the skin from irritants or moisture (for example, dimethicone, petrolatum, and zinc oxide).
- Skin cleansers: pH-balanced products used to provide moisture and to effectively remove urine, feces, or both without patient discomfort
- Therapeutic moisturizing products: lotions and creams used to replace lost lipids in skin

HCPCS code overview

Health Care Financing Administration Common Procedure Coding System (HCPCS) is a standardized coding system that is used for describing and identifying health care equipment and supplies in health care transactions not included in the current procedural terminology (CPT) codes. Because Medicare and other insurers cover a variety of services, supplies, and equipment that aren't identified by CPT codes, the level II HCPCS codes were established for submitting claims for these items.

The Statistical Analysis Durable Medical Equipment Regional Contractor (SADMERC) is responsible for providing suppliers and manufacturers with assistance in determining which HCPCS code should be used to describe health care equipment and supplies for the purpose of billing Medicare. This standardized process to request a code for a particular supply or a request for a modification to the alpha-numeric coding system for a particular product has been defined and is accessible to all suppliers and manufacturers.

You may find that many skin care products are considered routine supply items and are included in the general cost of an inpatient stay, whether the stay is for acute or long-term care. It's the clinician's responsibility to verify whether a product has been assigned a HCPCS code. The ultimate responsibility for correct HCPCS coding lies with the provider or supplier who is submitting a claim to a third-party payer.

Antifungals and antimicrobials

The pH of the skin is in the acidic range but varies in different areas of the body. The pH is important because it regulates some of the functions of the stratum corneum including its permeability function; the integrity and cohesion of skin cells, or what holds the cells together; and the defense against bacteria and fungi. Skin flora, or the microorganisms that live on or infect the skin, grow differently based on the skin pH. Antifungal and antimicrobial products inhibit the growth of organisms that cause superficial skin infections, such as yeast. These products are formulated as creams, ointments, lotions, or powders and may be found in select moisture barriers.

Because of the variation in coding for antifungals and antimicrobials, it's the clinician's responsibility to verify coding and payment of each product with the manufacturer.

Product name	Manufacturer/Distributor
Aloe Vesta Antifungal Ointment	ConvaTec
Baza Antifungal Cream	Coloplast Corporation
Carrington Antifungal Cream	Carrington Laboratories, Inc.
Micro-Guard	Coloplast Corporation
Remedy Antifungal powder & cream	Medline Industries, Inc.
SECURA Antifungal Extra Thick	Smith & Nephew, Inc. Wound Management
SECURA Antifungal Greaseless	Smith & Nephew, Inc. Wound Management
Soothe & Cool INZO Antifungal Cream	Medline Industries, Inc.

Liquid skin protectants

Liquid skin protectants, or skin sealants, are formulated with a polymer and solvent. When the product is applied to the skin, the solvent evaporates, and the polymer dries to form a transparent, protective barrier. Select liquid skin protectants may irritate denuded or compromised skin. The clinician should be aware that liquid skin protectants can be formulated with or without alcohol. Liquid skin protectants are manufactured in wipes, swabs, sprays, and foam applicators.

Because of the variation in coding for liquid skin protectants, it's the clinician's responsibility to verify coding and payment of each product with the manufacturer.

Product name	Manufacturer/Distributor
Sureprep No-Sting Skin Prep Wipes	Medline Industries, Inc.

Moisture barriers

Moisture barriers, sometimes called skin protectants, are ointments, creams, or pastes that shield the skin from exposure to irritants or moisture from sources such as incontinence, perspiration, and enzymatic and wound drainage. Three common ingredients found in moisture barriers include dimethicone, petrolatum, and zinc oxide or a combination thereof. Some products are formulated with additional properties such as antibacterial, antiyeast, or antifungal ingredients. A moisture barrier may be formulated with a skin cleanser or as a stand-alone paste, cream, powder, or ointment. Once the moisture barrier is applied to the skin, it may appear clear, translucent, or opaque depending on the formulation.

Because of the variation in coding for moisture barriers, it's the clinician's responsibility to verify coding and payment of each product with the manufacturer.

Product name	Manufacturer/Distributor
AlexaCare Barrier Lotion	Acies Health, Inc.
Aloe Vesta Protective Barrier Spray	ConvaTec
Aloe Vesta Protective Ointment	ConvaTec
Amerigel Barrier Lotion	Amerx Health Care Corporation
Baza Cleanse Protect Cloth	Coloplast Corporation
Baza Clear	Coloplast Corporation
Baza Protect	Coloplast Corporation
Carrington Moisture Barrier Cream and Moisture Barrier with Zinc and Acemannan Hydrogel	Carrington Laboratories, Inc.
Carrington Moisture Guard with Dimethicone and Acemannan Hydrogel	Carrington Laboratories, Inc.

Product name	Manufacturer/Distributor
Critic-Aid Clear	Coloplast Corporation
Critic-Aid Clear AF	Coloplast Corporation
Critic-Aid Skin Paste	Coloplast Corporation
Fordustin' Body Powder	Coloplast Corporation
Remedy Calazime Protectant Paste	Medline Industries, Inc.
Remedy Dimethicone Moisture Barrier	Medline Industries, Inc.
Remedy Nutrashield	Medline Industries, Inc.
SECURA Dimethicone Protectant	Smith & Nephew, Inc. Wound Management
SECURA Extra Protective Cream	Smith & Nephew, Inc. Wound Management
SECURA Protective Cream	Smith & Nephew, Inc. Wound Management
SECURA Protective Ointment	Smith & Nephew, Inc. Wound Management
Sensi-Care Protective Barrier	ConvaTec
Shield & Protect	GENTELL, Inc.
Soothe & Cool Body Powder	Medline Industries, Inc.
Soothe & Cool INZO Invisible Zinc Oxide Barrier Cream	Medline Industries, Inc.
Soothe & Cool Moisture Barrier Ointment	Medline Industries, Inc.
Soothe & Cool Skin Paste	Medline Industries, Inc.

Skin cleansers

Skin cleansing removes unwanted microorganisms while maintaining the skin's barrier function. The characteristics of skin cleansers vary according to the needs of those using the product. For example, skin cleaners are available as a rinse or no-rinse formulation, an all-in-one product that cleanses, moisturizes, and protects or a variation thereof. Additionally, some products are manufactured for cleansing the entire body or only the perineal area. Therefore, when choosing a skin cleanser, it's important to understand the ingredients and total formulation and match the product to the patient's clinical goals.

Because of the variation in coding for skin cleansers, it's the clinician's responsibility to verify coding and payment of each product with the manufacturer.

Product name	Manufacturer/Distributor
Aloe Vesta Bathing Cloths	ConvaTec
Aloe Vesta Body Wash & Shampoo	ConvaTec
Aloe Vesta Cleansing Foam	ConvaTec
Baza Cleanse & Protect	Coloplast Corporation
Bedside Care EasiCleanse Bath	Coloplast Corporation

Product name	Manufacturer/Distributor
Bedside-Care Foam No-Rinse Foaming Body Wash, Shampoo and Incontinent Cleanser	Coloplast Corporation
Bedside-Care No-Rinse All Body Wash and Incontinent Cleanser	Coloplast Corporation
Bedside-Care Perineal Wash No-Rinse Incontinent Cleanser	Coloplast Corporation
CarraFoam Skin & Perineal Cleanser with Acemannan Hydrogel	Carrington Laboratories, Inc.
CarraWash Liquid Skin & Perineal No-Rinse Cleanser with Acemannan Hydrogel	Carrington Laboratories, Inc.
Carrington Shampoo & Body Wash with Acemannan Hydrogel	Carrington Laboratories, Inc.
Gentell Liquid Clean	GENTELL, Inc.
Gentle Rain Antibacterial Moisturizing Body Wash & Shampoo	Coloplast Corporation
Gentle Rain Extra Mild Sensitive Skin Moisturizing Body Wash & Shampoo	Coloplast Corporation
Remedy 4-in-1 Antimicrobial Cleanser	Medline Industries, Inc.
Remedy 4-in-1 Body Cleanser	Medline Industries, Inc.
Remedy 4-in-1 Cleansing Lotion	Medline Industries, Inc.
SECURA Moisturizing Cleanser	Smith & Nephew, Inc. Wound Management
SECURA Personal Cleanser	Smith & Nephew, Inc. Wound Management
SECURA Total Body Foam Cleanser	Smith & Nephew, Inc. Wound Management
Septi-Soft Concentrate	ConvaTec
Soothe & Cool Bath Oil	Medline Industries, Inc.
Soothe & Cool Foaming Perineal Wash	Medline Industries, Inc.
Soothe & Cool No-Rinse Shampoo & Body Wash	Medline Industries, Inc.
Soothe & Cool Perineal Wash	Medline Industries, Inc.
Soothe & Cool Perineal Wash, No Rinse	Medline Industries, Inc.
Soothe & Cool Shampoo & Body Wash	Medline Industries, Inc.

Therapeutic moisturizers

One of the skin's main functions is to hold in moisture. The epidermis produces lipids, oily substances that limit the passage of water into or out of the skin. If the skin is deficient in lipids, moisture can escape. The loss of moisture causes dry, flaky, itchy skin. Therapeutic moisturizers replace skin lipids and maintain skin hydration. These products can be found as creams, lotions, or ointments with or without an antimicrobial ingredient. Common ingredients found in therapeutic moisturizers include emollients and humectants. Some products are applied daily while other products are indicated to be applied more frequently.

Because of the variation in coding for therapeutic moisturizers, it's the clinician's responsibility to verify coding and payment of each product with the manufacturer.

Product name	Manufacturer/Distributor
AlexaCare Therapeutic Moisturizer	Acies Health, Inc.
Aloe Vesta Skin Conditioner	ConvaTec
Atrac-Tain Lotion	Coloplast Corporation
CarraDerm Moisturizing Cream with Acemannan Hydrogel	Carrington Laboratories, Inc.
DiaB Cream with Acemannan Hydrogel	Carrington Laboratories, Inc.
RadiaCream with Acemannan Hydrogel	Carrington Laboratories, Inc.
Remedy Skin Repair Cream	Medline Industries, Inc.
SECURA Moisturizing Cream	Smith & Nephew, Inc. Wound Management
SECURA Moisturizing Lotion	Smith & Nephew, Inc. Wound Management
Sensi-Care Moisturizing Body Cream	ConvaTec
Soothe & Cool Extra-Thick Cream	Medline Industries, Inc.
Soothe & Cool Moisture Body Lotion	Medline Industries, Inc.
Soothe & Cool Skin Cream	Medline Industries, Inc.
Sween 24	Coloplast Corporation
Sween Cream	Coloplast Corporation
UNICARE Moisturizing Lotion	Smith & Nephew, Inc. Wound Management
UNIDERM Moisturizing Cream	Smith & Nephew, Inc. Wound Management
WHIRL-SOL	Coloplast Corporation
Xtra-Care Lotion	Coloplast Corporation

DRESSINGS AND DEVICES

Overview

With more than 2,000 wound care products on the market, choosing the correct dressing or device may be difficult. In developing a management pathway and planning wound care, the health care professional must consider:

- wound- and skin-related factors, such as cause, severity, environment, condition of periwound skin, size and depth, anatomic location, volume of exudate, and the risk or presence of infection
- patient-related factors, such as vascular, nutritional, and medical status; odor-control requirements; comfort and preferences; and cost-benefit ratio
- dressing-related factors, such as availability, durability, adaptability, and uses.

Familiarizing yourself with the major categories of wound care products and their actions, indications, contraindications, advantages, and disadvantages will help you choose the most appropriate dressing. Also consider the product's availability and its application and removal procedures. In many cases, one product can help you meet more than one therapeutic goal.

The wound care products in this section include alginates, antimicrobials, collagens, composites, contact layers, drugs, foams, hydrocolloids, hydrogels, specialty absorptives, surgical dressings, transparent films, and more. For each product, you'll find the size and configuration of the product, the action, indications, contraindications, and instructions for application and removal, as well as the product's code, as assigned by the Health Care Financing Administration Common Procedure Coding System (HCPCS). Product names may be copyrighted or trademarked even when unaccompanied by copyright or trademark characters.

HCPCS code overview

To ensure uniform Medicare claim coding by all suppliers of wound care dressings, the Statistical Analysis Durable Medical Equipment Regional Carrier (SADMERC) performs a coding verification review. If manufacturers wish to have an HCPCS code assigned to their products, they must submit a formal application to SADMERC.

SADMERC and the four Durable Medical Equipment Regional Carriers conduct reviews of products to determine the correct HCPCS codes for Medicare billing. These reviews result in a consensus coding decision. The assignment of a HCPCS code to a product shouldn't be construed as an approval or endorsement of the product by SADMERC or Medicare and doesn't imply or guarantee reimbursement or coverage. Many other payers also require the assigned HCPCS codes on their claim forms.

If a manufacturer has provided the SADMERC-assigned HCPCS codes for its products, the five-digit alphanumeric code is listed beside the size of each product. Conversely, if a manufacturer hasn't provided an HCPCS code for a particular product, it's the provider's responsibility to verify proper coding. The provider and supplier are ultimately responsible for verifying the correct HCPCS codes before submitting claims to a payer.

Alginates

Action

Alginates are derived from brown seaweed. The products are composed of soft, nonwoven fibers shaped as ropes (twisted fibers) or pads (fibrous mats). Alginates are absorbent and conform to the shape of a wound. When packed, an alginate interacts with wound exudate to form a soft gel that maintains a moist healing environment. An alginate can absorb up to 20 times its weight.

Indications

To manage partial- and full-thickness, draining wounds; wounds with moderate to heavy exudate; tunneling wounds; infected and noninfected wounds; and "moist" red and yellow wounds

Advantages

- Absorb up to 20 times their weight
- Form a gel within the wound to maintain a moist healing environment
- Facilitate autolytic debridement
- Fill in dead space
- Are easy to apply and remove

Disadvantages

- Aren't recommended for wounds with light exudate or dry eschar
- Can dehydrate the wound bed
- Require a secondary dressing

HCPCS code overview

The HCPCS codes normally assigned to alginate wound covers or other gelling fiber dressings are:

A6196—pad size < 16 in^2

A6197—pad size > 16 in^2 but < 48 in^2

A6198—pad size > 48 in^2.

The HCPCS code normally assigned to alginate wound fillers or other gelling fiber dressings is:

A6199—wound filler, per 6" (15 cm).

AlgiCell Calcium Alginate
Derma Sciences, Inc.

How supplied
Disk: 1", 2", 4"
Pad: 2" × 2", 4" × 4", 4" × 8"
Rope: ³⁄₄" × 12", ³⁄₄" × 36"

Action

AlgiCell Calcium Alginate dressings
are highly absorptive, soft, white, and sterile. They form a soft gel in contact with wound fluids to maintain a moist healing environment.

Indications
To manage moderately to highly exuding partial- and full-thickness wounds; may be used for smaller wounds, such as biopsy sites (disks) or to pack deep wounds (rope)

Contraindications
- Contraindicated for third-degree burns
- Contraindicated for surgical implantation

Application
- Clean wound with PrimaDerm Dermal Cleanser or saline solution, according to facility policy.
- Apply AlgiCell to the wound bed.
- Loosely pack deeper wounds.
- Cover the dressing with an appropriate secondary dressing.

Removal
- Remove the secondary dressing.
- Gently rinse the affected area to remove remaining gel.
- Reapply a new dressing daily or as indicated by amount of exudate and facility policy.

ALGINATES

AlgiSite M Calcium Alginate Dressing
Smith & Nephew, Inc.
Wound Management

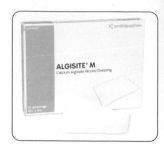

How supplied
Pad: 2" × 2", 4" × 4"; A6196
6" × 8"; A6197
Rope: ³/₄" × 12"; A6199

Action
AlgiSite M is a calcium-alginate dressing that forms a soft gel that absorbs wound exudate. AlgiSite M uses the proven benefits of moist wound management. The exudate produces a gel upon contact with the alginate fibers to create a moist wound surface environment. This helps prevent eschar formation and promotes an optimal moist wound environment. The dressing allows wound contraction to occur, which may help reduce scarring, and also allows the gaseous exchange necessary for a healthy wound bed.

Indications
Under the care of a health care professional, to manage full- and partial-thickness leg ulcers, pressure ulcers, diabetic foot ulcers, and surgical wounds; for over-the-counter applications, to manage lacerations, abrasions, skin tears, and minor burns

Contraindications
- Not for use until the packing in cavities and sinuses has been removed
- Not for use on very lightly exuding wounds
- Not for use on patients allergic to alginates

Application
- Cleanse the wound in accordance with normal procedures.
- Choose a dressing that's slightly larger than the wound and place it in intimate contact with the wound base, making sure that the entire surface is covered. It may be best to use the alginate strip if the wound is deep or undermined. To avoid maceration of the surrounding skin, cut the AlgiSite M to the size of the wound, or fold any dressing material overlying the wound into the wound.
- Apply using an appropriate dressing technique.
- Cover with an appropriate retention dressing. Wound exudate will evaporate from the gel surface; the secondary dressing shouldn't hinder this evaporative process where exudate is heavy.

Removal
- Generally, dressings should be changed daily in heavily draining wounds, reducing to twice weekly (or weekly) as healing proceeds.
- If the dressing isn't easily removed, moisten it with saline, then remove.

ALGINATES

- To remove AlgiSite M, use tweezers, forceps, or a gloved hand to gently lift the dressing away—the high wet strength generally allows it to remain in one piece. The dressing may adhere if used on a very lightly exuding wound. Removal of the dressing is facilitated by saturating the wound with saline.

AQUACEL Ag Hydrofiber Dressing with Silver*

ConvaTec

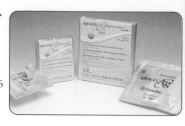

How supplied

Dressing: 2" × 2", 4" × 4"; A6196
6" × 6"; A6197
8" × 12"; A6198

Rope: ³/₄" × 18"; A6199

Action

AQUACEL Ag Hydrofiber Dressing with silver is an advanced technology, sterile, single use, wound dressing comprised of sodium carboxymethyl-cellulose and ionic silver (Ag+). It is a soft and conformable dressing that remains integral when wet or dry. This highly absorbent dressing interacts with wound exudate and forms a soft gel that maintains a moist environment for optimal wound healing and easy removal with little or no damage to healing wounds. The ionic silver gives AQUACEL Ag dressing its silver-gray appearance and broad-spectrum antimicrobial properties.

Indications

To manage wounds at risk of infection; partial-thickness (second-degree) burns; diabetic foot ulcers; venous stasis ulcers, arterial ulcers, and other leg ulcers; pressure ulcers (partial- and full-thickness); surgical wounds left to heal by secondary intent; traumatic wounds prone to bleeding, such as those that have been mechanically or surgically debrided; oncology wounds with exudate, such as fungoides-cutaneous tumors, fungating carcinoma, cutaneous metastasis, Kaposi's sarcoma, and angiosarcoma

Contraindications

- Not for use on patients who are sensitive to or who have had an allergic reaction to the dressing or its components

Application

- Clean the wound with water or saline. Apply the dressing to shallow wounds with an adequate overlap (at least ³/₈" [1 cm]) overlap of the wound edges. For deep wounds, loosely pack ribbon or sheet into wound to about 80% of the depth of the wound to accommodate swelling of the dressing, leaving a small overhang (at least 1" [2.5 cm]) to facilitate removal.
- For dry wounds, place the AQUACEL Ag dressing in the wound and then wet with sterile saline over the wound area only. The vertical absorption properties of the dressing will help to maintain the moist area over the wound only and reduce the risk of maceration. Cover the dressing with a moisture retentive dressing to avoid drying out the dressing and subsequent dressing adherence to the wound.
- Cover and secure with an appropriate dressing.

ALGINATES

Removal

- AQUACEL Ag dressing is designed to be easy to remove without leaving residue or causing trauma to the wound bed. In the unlikely event of adhesion to the wound bed, the dressing can be easily removed by soaking.

*See package insert for complete instructions for use.

ALGINATES

AQUACEL Hydrofiber Wound Dressing*
ConvaTec

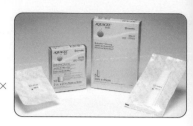

How supplied
Dressing: 2″ × 2″, 4″ × 4″, 6″ ×
             6″; A6251
Ribbon: ³/₄″ × 18″; A6251

Action
AQUACEL Hydrofiber Wound Dressing is a soft, sterile, nonwoven pad or ribbon dressing made from sodium carboxymethylcellulose fibers. This conformable and absorbent dressing forms a soft gel that creates a moist wound environment that supports the healing process and autolytic debridement and allows for nontraumatic removal.

Indications
To manage exuding wounds, pressure ulcers, leg ulcers, abrasions, lacerations, incisions, donor sites, oncology wounds, first- and second-degree burns, and surgical or traumatic wounds that have been left to heal by secondary intent; may be used for wounds that are prone to bleeding, such as mechanically or surgically debrided wounds, donor sites, and traumatic wounds; may also be used to facilitate the control of minor bleeding

Contraindications
- Contraindicated for use in patients with sensitivity to this dressing or its components
- Not intended for use as a surgical sponge

Application
- AQUACEL Hydrofiber Wound Dressings are sterile and should be handled appropriately.
- If necessary, debride the wound prior to application, then cleanse it with an effective cleansing agent such as SAF–Clens AF dermal wound cleanser or normal saline solution.
- Apply AQUACEL Hydrofiber Wound Dressing to the wound site, and cover with an appropriate secondary dressing, such as a moisture-retentive dressing.
- Change the dressing when it becomes saturated with exudate or when good clinical practice dictates.
- Dressing may remain in place for up to 7 days.

Removal
- Remove the secondary dressing gently, according to the product's package insert.
- Remove the AQUACEL Hydrofiber Wound Dressing and discard.

ALGINATES

- Without disrupting the delicate granulation tissue, irrigate the wound with SAF–Clens AF dermal wound cleanser or normal saline solution to remove any residual gel.
- Redress the wound with a new dressing, and cover with a secondary dressing as previously described.

*See package insert for complete instructions for use.

ALGINATES

CarboFlex Odor Control Dressing*

ConvaTec

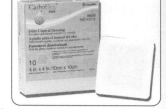

How supplied

Pad: 4" × 4"; A6196
        3" × 6" oval, 6" × 8"; A6197

Action

CarboFlex is a sterile nonadhesive dressing with an absorbent wound-contact layer (containing alginate and hydrocolloid), an activated charcoal central pad, and a smooth, water-resistant top layer.

Indications

To manage acute and chronic wounds; may be used as a primary dressing for shallow wounds or as a secondary dressing over wound fillers for deeper wounds; may also be used on infected malodorous wounds along with appropriate therapy and frequent monitoring of the wound

Contraindications

- Contraindicated in patients with a sensitivity to the dressing or its components

Application

- If required, debride the wound and remove necrotic tissue. Cleanse the wound site, rinse well, and dry the surrounding skin.
- Don't cut the dressing.
- Choose a dressing that is larger than the wound area to ensure that the dressing overlaps the wound edge by at least 1 1/4" (3 cm). For shallow wounds, the dressing may be placed directly onto the wound as a primary dressing; for cavity wounds, CarboFlex can be laid over a wound filler or gel as a secondary dressing.
- Place the fibrous (nonshiny) surface on the wound or cavity filler.
- Secure CarboFlex in place with tape or other appropriate material. The wound contact layer absorbs exudate and forms a soft gel.

Removal

- Change the dressing when clinically indicated, when exudate strikethrough to the top layer occurs, or when the odor is no longer being absorbed. With noninfected malodorous wounds, CarboFlex may be left undisturbed for up to 3 days. If the wound is infected, CarboFlex should be changed more frequently.
- Carefully lift the dressing away from the wound by grasping it at one corner.

*See package insert for complete instructions for use.

ALGINATES

CarraGinate High G Calcium Alginate Wound Dressing with Acemannan Hydrogel

Carrington Laboratories, Inc.

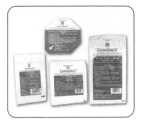

How supplied
Pad: 2" × 2", 4" × 4"; A6196
4" × 8"; A6197
Rope: 14"; A6199

Action
CarraGinate is a nonwoven, preservative-free, nontoxic absorptive dressing with Acemannan Hydrogel manufactured from seaweed.

Indications
To manage pressure ulcers, diabetic ulcers, venous ulcers, arterial ulcers, traumatic wounds, dermal lesions, donor sites, and partial- and full-thickness wounds with moderate to heavy wound exudate

Contraindications
- Contraindicated for surgical implantation
- Contraindicated for third degree burns

Application
- Flush the wound with a suitable wound cleanser, such as CarraKlenz, UltraKlenz, or MicroKlenz.
- Apply the dressing and cover it with a secondary dressing, such as CarraFilm or CarraSmart Film.

Removal
- When changing the dressing, rinse away the remaining gel with a suitable wound cleanser, such as CarraKlenz, UltraKlenz, or MicroKlenz.

ALGINATES

CarraSorb H Calcium Alginate Wound Dressing

Carrington Laboratories, Inc.

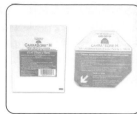

How supplied

Pad: 2″ × 2″, 4″ × 4″; A6196
Rope: 12″ (30 cm); A6199

Action

CarraSorb H is a nonwoven, preservative-free, nontoxic, absorptive dressing manufactured from seaweed. A soft gel forms as calcium in the alginate exchanges with sodium in the exudate. This sterile primary wound dressing insulates, absorbs, and fills dead space.

Indications

To manage pressure ulcers (stages 3 and 4); arterial, venous, and diabetic ulcers; donor sites; traumatic wounds; and dermal lesions; may also be used on tunneling wounds, infected and noninfected wounds, red or yellow wounds; and wounds with undermining or sinus tracts, necrotic tissue and exudate, moderate to heavy exudate, or serosanguineous drainage

Contraindications

- Contraindicated for surgical implantation
- Contraindicated for third-degree burns

Application

- Flush the wound with a suitable wound cleanser, such as CarraKlenz Wound Cleanser, UltraKlenz Wound Cleanser, or MicroKlenz Antimicrobial, Deodorizing Wound Cleanser.
- Apply the dressing to a moist wound bed; loosely pack it into deep wounds to allow room for expansion as it absorbs drainage. Use rope packing in undermined or tunneled areas.
- Cover the dressing with a secondary dressing, such as gauze, CarraFilm, or CarraSmart Film.

Removal

- Change the dressing according to the wound condition and amount of exudate or as directed by the physician. In general, a heavily draining wound may require one or two changes per day. As drainage decreases, gradually reduce the number of changes to once every 2 to 3 days.
- Remove the secondary dressing and nongelled CarraSorb H.
- Rinse away any remaining gel residue with gentle irrigation.

ALGINATES

CarraSorb M Freeze-Dried Gel Wound Dressing with Acemannan Hydrogel
Carrington Laboratories, Inc.

How supplied
Wafer: 4" diameter; A4649

Action
CarraSorb M Freeze-Dried Gel Wound Dressing is pure aloe vera gel containing Acemannan Hydrogel with all water extracted in freeze-drying. It's a sterile, preservative-free primary dressing that's nonirritating and nontoxic. It returns to a moldable hydrogel as it absorbs exudate (up to 20 times its weight) without fiber residue. The gel maintains a moist healing environment.

Indications
To manage and dress pressure ulcers (stages 1, 2, 3, and 4), venous stasis ulcers, first- and second-degree burns, cuts, abrasions, skin irritations, radiation dermatitis, diabetic ulcers, foot ulcers, postsurgical incisions, and skin conditions associated with peristomal care; may also be used on partial- and full-thickness wounds, tunneling wounds, infected and noninfected wounds, wounds with moderate exudate, wounds with serosanguineous drainage, and red, yellow, or black wounds

Contraindications
- Contraindicated in patients with a sensitivity to Acemannan Hydrogel or any other component of the dressing

Application
- Flush wound with a suitable cleanser, such as CarraKlenz, UltraKlenz, or MicroKlenz.
- Apply the dressing to the wound bed by folding it into the wound or tearing it to pack into undermined areas.
- Cover the dressing with a secondary dressing, such as CarraFilm or CarraSmart Film.

Removal
- Change the dressing as needed, according to wound condition and amount of exudate or as directed by the physician. Generally, a daily change is indicated.
- Rinse away any remaining gel residue with gentle irrigation.

ALGINATES

Curasorb

Curasorb Zinc

Tyco Healthcare/Kendall

How supplied

Pad: 2″ × 2″, 4″ × 4″, 4″ × 4″ plus (extra ab-
            sorptive), 2″ × 2″ with zinc, 4″ × 4″
            with zinc; A6196

       4″ × 4″, 4″ × 4″ plus (extra absorptive), 4″ × 5½″, 4″ × 4″ with
zinc, 4″ × 8″, 4″ × 8″ with zinc; A6197

       6″ × 10″, 12″ × 24″; A6198

Rope: 12″, 24″, 36″, 12″ with zinc; A6199

Action

Curasorb and Curasorb Zinc absorb large volumes of exudate and maintain a moist healing environment.

Indications

To manage wounds with moderate to large amounts of exudate; may also
be used on pressure ulcers (stages 2, 3, and 4), tunneling wounds, infected and noninfected wounds, full-thickness wounds, and red or yellow
wounds

Contraindications

- Contraindicated for wounds with dry eschar
- Contraindicated for wounds with minimal exudate

Application

- Apply the dressing dry.
- Cover the dressing with a secondary dressing.

Removal

- Remove the dressing when strike-through to the secondary dressing occurs.

DermaGinate
DermaRite Industries, LLC

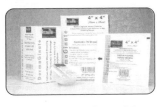

How supplied
Pad: 2″ × 2″; 4″ × 4″; A6196
Rope: 12″; A6199

Action
DermaGinate is a sterile, nonwoven dressing of calcium-sodium alginate fiber designed to promote and maintain a moist healing environment. The fibers absorb wound exudate to form a firm, viscous gel-fiber material.

Indications
To manage infected and noninfected wounds, pressure ulcers, venous ulcers, and diabetic ulcers; may be used for partial- and full-thickness wounds, dermal lesions, tunneling wounds, and wounds with moderate to heavy drainage

Contraindications
- Contraindicated for dry to lightly exuding wounds
- Contraindicated for third-degree burns
- Contraindicated in patients with sensitivity to calcium alginate materials

Application
- Clean the wound by irrigating with DermaKlenz solution
- Pat dry surrounding areas.
- Apply dressing to the wound surface or wound bed; if wound is deep, pack DermaGinate rope gently at site.
- Cover the dressing with a secondary dressing, and secure it.

Removal
- Remove the secondary dressing.
- For wounds with minimal exudate, dampen the dressing with normal saline solution to loosen, then lift.
- If necessary, gently rinse away the remaining gel or dressing fibers.

ALGINATES

GENTELL Calcium Alginate
GENTELL, Inc.

How supplied
Dressing: 2″ × 2″, 4″ × 4″; A6196
Rope: 12″; A6199

Action
GENTELL Alginate dressings are designed
to absorb wound exudate to form a firm gel-fiber material.

Indications
For partial- and full-thickness wounds with moderate to heavy exudate

Contraindications
■ Not recommended for dry wounds or wounds with minimal exudate

Application
■ Apply dressing dry, and cover with a secondary dressing.

Removal
■ Carefully remove the dressing from the wound bed.

KALGINATE Calcium Alginate Wound Dressing
DeRoyal

How supplied
Pad: 2″ × 2″, 4″ × 4″; A6196
        4″ × 8″; A6197
Rope: 6″, 12″; A6199

Action
KALGINATE is a sterile, nonwoven, calcium alginate dressing of heavy fiber. Thick and substantial, it provides maximum absorption of exudate with minimal dressing changes. It allows for gaseous exchange, can be layered or packed for absorbency, and maintains its shape and integrity during removal.

Indications
To manage pressure ulcers (stages 3 and 4); full-thickness wounds; tunneling, infected, and draining wounds; and wounds with moderate to heavy exudate

Contraindications
- Contraindicated for third-degree burns

Application
- Clean the wound area with normal saline solution.
- Place KALGINATE pad or rope into the wound, packing deep wounds loosely.
- Cover the dressing with an absorptive cover dressing, and secure in place.

Removal
- Change the dressing when the outer dressing is saturated with drainage.
- Remove the outer dressing.
- Irrigate the wound with normal saline solution, and lift the dressing from the wound bed.

KALTOSTAT Wound Dressing*

ConvaTec

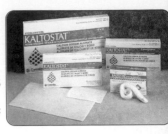

How supplied

Dressing: 2″ × 2″, 3″ × 4³/₄″; A6196
           4″ × 8″; A6197
           6″ × 9¹/₂″, 12″ × 24″;
           A6198
Rope: 2 g; A6199

Action

KALTOSTAT Wound Dressing is a soft, sterile, nonwoven dressing of calcium-sodium alginate fiber. The alginate fibers absorb wound exudate or normal saline solution and form a firm gel-fiber mat. The mat maintains a moist, warm environment at the wound-dressing interface and allows removal of the dressing with little or no damage to newly formed tissue.

Indications

To manage pressure ulcers, venous stasis ulcers, arterial ulcers, diabetic ulcers, donor sites, abrasions, lacerations, superficial burns, postoperative incisions, and other external wounds inflicted by trauma. May also be used as a nasal packing for nosebleeds, dental extraction sites, and postoperative wound debridement

Contraindications

- Contraindicated for third-degree burns
- Not intended to control heavy bleeding
- Not intended for use as a surgical sponge

Application

- Debride the wound of excessive necrotic tissue and eschar, and irrigate with an appropriate nontoxic cleansing solution.
- Trim the dressing to the exact size of the wound.
- For heavily exuding wounds, apply the dry dressing to the wound.
- For lightly exuding wounds or nonexuding wounds, place the dressing on the wound, and moisten it with normal saline solution. Reapply normal saline solution, as necessary, to maintain the gel.
- Apply an appropriate secondary dressing to secure the dressing.
- To effect hemostasis on bleeding wounds, apply the dressing to the bleeding area. Remove the dressing after bleeding has stopped, and then apply a new dressing.

Removal

- To remove a dressing from a nonexuding or lightly exuding wound, saturate the dressing with normal saline solution. If the gel has dried, rehydrate it by saturating it with normal saline solution; softening may take several hours if severe drying has occurred.

- Change the dressing on heavily exuding wounds when strike-through to the secondary dressing occurs, or whenever clinical practice dictates. Removal is easy because the dressing forms a gel at the wound-dressing interface.
- Leave the dressing in place for up to 7 days, depending on the wound.
- Cleanse the wound site before applying a new dressing; any alginate fibers and gels inadvertently left in the wound will be absorbed by the body.

*See package insert for complete instructions for use.

ALGINATES

New Product

Maxorb Extra Ag Antimicrobial Silver CMC/Alginate Dressing

Medline Industries, Inc.

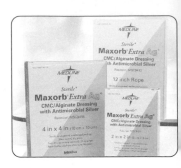

How supplied
Pad: 2″ × 2″; A6196
         4″ × 8″; 4″ × 4.75″; A6197
Rope: 12″ × 1″ (2 g); A6199

Action
Maxorb Extra Ag CMC/Alginate Dressing's nonwoven alginate and carboxymethylcellulose fiber combination reacts with wound exudate to form a gel, providing a moist healing environment. The added presence of carboxymethylcellulose in Maxorb improves the wicking and fluid-handling ability of this dressing and increases wet strength. Because the product doesn't wick exudate laterally, it reduces the potential for damage to delicate periwound tissue. Exposure to wound exudate dissolves the silver and stimulates the release of silver ions. As more fluid is absorbed over time, more silver ions are released, creating a controlled-release antimicrobial effect. Maxorb Extra Ag is biocompatible, nonirritating, nonsensitizing, nonstaining, and will not harm new granulation tissue.

Indications
To manage partial- and full-thickness wounds with moderate to heavy exudate, including venous stasis ulcers, pressure ulcers (stages 2, 3, and 4), arterial ulcers, diabetic ulcers, donor sites, lacerations, abrasions, postsurgical incisions, and second-degree burns; may also be used for infected and noninfected wounds, tunneling wounds, and wounds with serosanguineous or purulent drainage

Contraindications
- Contraindicated for third-degree burns
- Not intended for use as a surgical sponge

Application
- Clean the wound with normal saline solution or an appropriate wound cleanser, such as Skintegrity Wound Cleanser.
- Apply the dressing to a moist wound bed. The dressing doesn't need to be trimmed to fit the wound bed because it won't wick fluid laterally. Loosely pack deep or tunneling wounds.
- Cover the dressing with an appropriate secondary dressing, such as Stratasorb Composite Dressing.

ALGINATES

Removal

- Change the dressing when strike-through to the secondary dressing occurs, at least every 7 days or as directed by the physician.
- The gelatinous pad may be easily lifted away in one piece from the wound bed, making dressing changes easier.
- Remove the secondary dressing as well as gelled and nongelled Maxorb dressing.
- Irrigate the wound with normal saline solution or another appropriate solution, such as Skintegrity Wound Cleanser, to remove any remaining gel.
- If the dressing is dry at the time of removal, moisten it with saline or wound cleanser before removing it. This may indicate the need to consider replacing this type dressing with a moistening, hydrogel product instead.

ALGINATES

Maxorb Extra CMC/Alginate Dressing

Medline Industries, Inc.

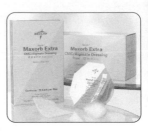

How supplied

Pad: 1″ × 12″, 2″ × 2″, 4″ × 4″; A6196
          4″ × 8″; A6197
Rope: 12″ (2 g); A6199

Dressings are supplied in sterile form in single pouches or a lidded tray. The lidded tray package on the rope is important because it keeps the fibers from compressing. As a result, fluid-handling capacity is increased.

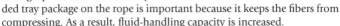

Action

Maxorb Extra CMC/Alginate Dressing's nonwoven alginate and carboxymethylcellulose fiber combination reacts with wound exudate to form a gel, providing a moist healing environment. The added presence of carboxymethylcellulose in Maxorb improves the wicking and fluid-handling ability of this dressing and increases wet strength. Because the product doesn't wick exudate laterally, it reduces the potential for damage to delicate periwound tissue. New "Extra" formulation has more loft and alginate fibers to provide 25% greater fluid handling.

Indications

To manage partial- and full-thickness wounds with moderate to heavy exudate, including venous stasis ulcers, pressure ulcers (stages 2, 3, and 4), arterial ulcers, diabetic ulcers, donor sites, lacerations, abrasions, postsurgical incisions, and second-degree burns; may also be used for infected and noninfected wounds, tunneling wounds, and wounds with serosanguineous or purulent drainage

Contraindications

- Contraindicated for third-degree burns
- Not intended for use as a surgical sponge

Application

- Clean the wound with normal saline solution or an appropriate wound cleanser, such as Skintegrity Wound Cleanser.
- Apply the dressing to a moist wound bed. The dressing doesn't need to be trimmed to fit the wound bed because it won't wick fluid laterally. Loosely pack deep or tunneling wounds.
- Cover the dressing with an appropriate secondary dressing, such as Stratasorb Composite Dressing.

Removal

- Change the dressing when strike-through to the secondary dressing occurs, every 2 to 5 days or as directed by the physician.

- The gelatinous pad may be easily lifted away in one piece from the wound bed, making dressing changes easier.
- Remove the secondary dressing as well as gelled and nongelled Maxorb dressing.
- Irrigate the wound with normal saline solution or another appropriate solution, such as Skintegrity Wound Cleanser, to remove any remaining gel.
- If the dressing is dry at the time of removal, moisten it with saline or wound cleanser before removing it. This may indicate the need to consider replacing this type dressing with a moistening, hydrogel product instead.

ALGINATES

Melgisorb
Mölnlycke Health Care

How supplied
Pad: 2″ × 2″, 4″ × 4″; A6196
         4″ × 8″; A6197
Rope: 12.5″; A6199

Action
Melgisorb is a hydrophilic calcium alginate dressing that absorbs wound exudate. As the alginate fibers absorb exudate, they form a moist gel that provides a moist environment conducive to wound healing.

Indications
To manage infected and noninfected wounds with moderate to heavy exudate, such as pressure ulcers, venous ulcers, arterial ulcers, diabetic ulcers, donor sites, postoperative wounds, and dermal lesions

Contraindications
- Contraindicated for dry wounds
- Contraindicated on third-degree burns
- Not recommended for surgical implantation

Application
- Clean and flush the wound with normal saline solution, then dry the healthy surrounding skin.
- Apply Melgisorb dry to a moist wound bed. For shallow wounds, choose the correct size of the flat dressing to cover the entire wound. For deep or tunneling wounds, choose and cut an appropriate length of rope and pack loosely.
- Cover the dressing with an appropriate secondary dressing.

Removal
- Gently flush the wound with normal saline solution or another appropriate solution. Any nongelled Melgisorb can be moistened with saline and removed.

Restore CalciCare Wound Care Dressing

Hollister Incorporated

How supplied

Pad: 2″ × 2″, 4″ × 4″; A6196
4″ × 8″; A6197
Rope: 12″ (2 g); A6199

Action

Restore CalciCare Wound Care Dressings are absorptive and made from calcium and sodium alginate. They conform to the wound and form a gel when in contact with exudate, creating a moist interface with the wound, which provides a moist healing environment.

Indications

To manage partial- and full-thickness wounds with moderate to heavy exudate, including pressure ulcers (stages 1, 2, 3, and 4), arterial and venous stasis ulcers, postsurgical incisions, donor sites, trauma wounds, diabetic ulcers, and dermal lesions

Contraindications

- Contraindicated for dry to lightly exuding wounds
- Contraindicated in patients with known sensitivity to calcium alginate or with other known allergic conditions

Application

- Prepare the wound according to facility policy, or as directed. Make sure the skin is clean and dry.
- Measure the wound with a wound-measuring guide.
- Apply the dressing to the wound surface. Loosely pack deep wounds with rope dressing.
- Cover the dressing with a secondary dressing, and secure it.

Removal

- Remove the secondary dressing according to facility policy.
- Remove the Restore CalciCare dressing.
- If necessary, gently rinse away the remaining gel or dressing fibers, using Restore Wound Cleanser or normal saline solution.

ALGINATES

SeaSorb Soft Alginate
Coloplast Corporation

How supplied
Dressing: 2" × 2"; A6196
              4" × 4"; A6196
              6" × 6"; A6197
Rope: 1" × 17¹/₂"; A6199

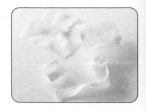

Action
SeaSorb is a sterile, fiber-free, highly absorbent dressing composed of a unique combination of calcium alginate and carboxymethylcellulose. On contact with wound exudate, the dressing forms a moist gel through ion exchange. SeaSorb Soft dressing is easy to apply and remains intact after absorbing exudate, allowing one-piece removal.

Indications
To manage wounds with heavy exudate, such as leg ulcers and pressure ulcers; may also be used in clinically infected wounds, for which concurrent systemic antibiotic therapy may be given if indicated

Contraindications
- Contraindicated for dry wounds and third-degree burns
- Contraindicated for deep, undermined ulcers in which wound edges are at risk for collapsing
- Contraindicated in patients allergic to one or more of the components
- Physician consultation needed before use of this product on wounds with a high risk of infection or on lesions caused by syphilis, tuberculosis, leprosy, or cancer
- Must be removed before the start of long-term radiation treatment (with X-rays, ultrasound, diathermy, or microwaves)

Application
- Choose a dressing large enough to allow an overlap of ³/₄" (2 cm) onto the surrounding skin. SeaSorb Soft dressing may be cut to size if necessary.
- Use a secondary dressing, such as Comfeel Plus Clear Dressing or Biatain Foam Dressing.

Removal
- Change the dressing when it's saturated with exudate and has reached maximum absorption capacity.
- Change the dressing every 7 days or more often if necessary (may be required for the first few days). As granulation occurs, however, exudation decreases, and fewer changes are needed.

ALGINATES

SilverCel Antimicrobial Alginate Dressing

Johnson & Johnson
Wound Management
A division of ETHICON, Inc.

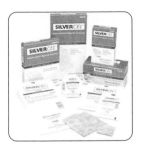

How supplied

Dressing: 2" × 2"; A6196
4¼" × 4¼", 4" × 8"; A6197
1" × 12"; A6199

Action

SilverCel Dressing is a primary dressing that is an effective barrier to bacterial penetration, which may help reduce infection in moderate to heavily exuding partial and full-thickness wounds. Combining the potent broad-spectrum antimicrobial action of silver with the enhanced exudate management properties of alginate technology, SilverCel Dressing not only protects the healing environment, but also provides superior tensile strength for easy removal.

Indications

SilverCel Antimicrobial Alginate Dressing is a primary dressing that is an effective barrier to bacterial penetration; the barrier functions of the dressing may help reduce infection in moderate to heavily exuding partial- and full-thickness wounds including pressure ulcers, venous ulcers, diabetic ulcers, donor sites, and traumatic and surgical wounds

Contraindications

- Not indicated for third-degree burns
- Not indicated for patients with known sensitivity to alginates or silver
- Not indicated to control heavy bleeding

Application

- Apply SilverCel Antimicrobial Alginate Dressing directly to wound, covering the entire wound bed. The dressing forms a gel on contact with exudate or through saline hydration.
- Cover with a nonocclusive secondary dressing to maintain a moist healing environment.
- Dressing may be reapplied daily or as directed by the physician. Frequency of reapplication depends on amount of exudate.

Removal

- The dressing may adhere if used on lightly exuding wounds. If the dressing isn't easily removed, moisten it with sterile saline before removing it. The dressing performance may be impaired by excess use of ointments with a petroleum jelly base.

ALGINATES

Sorbsan Topical Wound Dressing

Mylan Bertek Pharmaceuticals Inc.

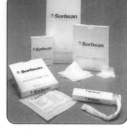

How supplied

Pad: 2″ × 2″, 3″ × 3″, 4″ × 4″; A6196
          4″ × 8″; A6197
Rope: ¹/₂″ × 12″; A6199

Action

When in immediate contact with wound exu-
date, the surface of Sorbsan Topical Wound Dressing forms a soft, hydrocolloid gel. This gel maintains a physiologically moist microenvironment
at the wound surface that is conducive to granulation tissue formation,
rapid epithelialization, and healing. The gel provides a nonadherent interface with the wound bed, allows for exchange of gases to and from the
wound surface, is strongly hydrophilic and wicks exudate into the wound
dressing, and provides a physical barrier against inadvertent contamination of the wound. For wounds prone to bleeding, such as donor sites and
wounds that have been mechanically or surgically debrided, calcium alginate is absorptive and has been shown to aid in the control of minor bleeding.

Indications

For the local management of exuding wounds, including infected and noninfected pressure ulcers, venous ulcers, arterial ulcers, diabetic ulcers, donor
sites and other bleeding surface wounds, dermal lesions, trauma injuries
or incisions

Contraindications

- Not intended for third-degree burns

Application

- If present, eschar or necrotic tissue should be surgically or mechanically removed or debrided with an appropriate agent before Sorbsan is applied to the wound site.
- Irrigate wound site with normal saline solution, and dry surrounding
  area.
- Remove the dressing from the package, and apply it to the moist wound
  surface.
- When using Sorbsan Wound Packing, gently place it into the wound,
  layering it by folding it back and forth onto itself, taking care not to pack
  the wound tightly.
- Cover the dressing with an appropriate secondary dressing.

Dressing change

- The frequency with which Sorbsan should be changed will depend on
  the volume of exudate.

- Reapply when saturation of Sorbsan is indicated by wetting of secondary dressing or leakage from under the semipermeable film. A heavily exuding wound may require one or two dressing changes daily. Clinically infected wounds should be dressed at least daily.
- As the wound begins to heal and exudation lessens, change the dressing every 2 to 4 days or as directed by a health care professional.

Removal

- Gently lift the secondary dressing, remove and discard the nongelled Sorbsan.
- For wounds with minimal exudate, it may be necessary to dampen the dressing with normal saline prior to dressing removal.
- Irrigate the wound thoroughly with normal saline solution to wash away the remaining gel without disrupting granulation tissue.
- Redress the moist wound site as directed previously.
- Care should be taken to prevent the gel from drying.

ALGINATES

3M Tegaderm High Integrity Alginate Dressing

3M Tegaderm High Gelling Alginate Dressing
3M Health Care

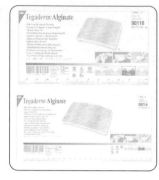

How supplied
High Integrity
Pad: 2″ × 2″, 4″ × 4″; A6196
          4″ × 8″; A6197
Rope: 12″; A6199
High Gelling
Pad: 2″ × 2″, 4″ × 4″; A6196
          4″ × 8″; A6197
Rope: 12″; A6199

Action
3M Tegaderm is a gel-forming, absorbent, versatile alginate, which provides for optimum wound healing. 3M Tegaderm High Integrity offers high integrity for quick dressing changes. 3M Tegaderm High Gelling offers high-gelling properties, which may be preferable for gentle removal of the dressing from fragile tissue.

Indications
To manage wounds with moderate to heavy exudate, pressure ulcers, arterial ulcers, venous ulcers, diabetic ulcers, trauma wounds, and other dermal lesions

Contraindications
- Contraindicated for surgical implantation
- Contraindicated for third-degree burns

Application
Pad
- Moisten the wound site with normal saline solution or other sterile irrigation solution, according to facility policy. Dry the periwound skin.
- If the patient's skin is fragile or wound drainage may contact the periwound skin, apply 3M No-Sting Barrier Film around the wound.
- Select the appropriate dressing size for the wound. Tegaderm HG and HI alginate dressings may be trimmed to fit the wound site.
- Apply the dressing to the wound bed with minimal overlap to the periwound skin.
- Loosely pack deep wounds.
- Cover the dressing with an appropriate secondary dressing.

Rope
- Fluff the rope dressing as needed for light packing.
- Make sure the dressing lightly contacts all wound surfaces, including areas of undermining.
- Loosely pack deep wounds by fluffing and layering the dressing back and forth into the wound.
- Cover the rope dressing with an appropriate secondary dressing.
- Extend the cover dressing at least 1" (2.5 cm) beyond the edge of the wound.

Removal
- Remove secondary dressing and nongelled alginate dressing. Rinse away remaining gel with gentle irrigation.
- If the dressing appears dry, saturate it with sterile saline solution to help remove it.
- Dressing may be removed using sterile forceps or gentle irrigation.

ALGINATES

Antimicrobials

Action
Antimicrobial dressings are topical wound care products derived from agents such as silver, iodine, and polyhexethylene biguanide. These products combine active ingredients with a dressing to deliver an antimicrobial or antibacterial action to the wound. Silver dressings come in various delivery systems as well as shapes and sizes. The silver is activated from the dressing to the wound's surface based on the amount of exudate and bacteria in the wound. Silver dressings are available in foams, hydrocolloids, alginates, barriers layers, charcoal cloth dressings, or a combination of different forms. Silver dressings may be used with select topical and adjunctive therapies to, among other things, decrease the bacterial load and manage exudate, and as a result, optimize the appearance of the wound's granulation tissue.

Gauze products containing antibacterial properties have been designed to provide a barrier to specific organisms but also inhibit the growth of bacteria within the dressing, thus protecting the wound and potential spread of bacteria from the dressed site.

Indications
Antimicrobial dressings are intended for use in draining, exuding, and non-healing wounds where protection from bacterial contamination is desired. These dressings may be used as primary or secondary dressings to manage various amounts of exudate (minimal, moderate, or heavy) for both acute and chronic wounds, including burns, surgical wounds, diabetic foot ulcers, pressure ulcers, and leg ulcers. Select dressings may also be used under compression.

Advantages
- Provides a broad range of antimicrobial or antibacterial activity
- Reduces infection
- Prevents infection
- May alter metalloproteinases within wounds with select dressings

Disadvantages
- May cause staining on wound and intact skin with silver dressings
- May cause stinging or sensitization
- Development of resistant organisms not yet known

HCPCS code overview
Each product under this category description has been assigned a different code based on its physical size and characteristics; or the manufacturer hasn't yet received or applied for a code. Please refer to individual product listings for further information about each product.

Acticoat 3

Smith & Nephew, Inc.
Wound Management

How supplied

Pad: $2'' \times 2''$, $5'' \times 5''$; A9270

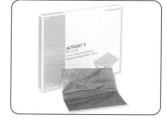

Action

Acticoat 3 (with SILCRYST Nanocrystals) consists of a rayon/polyester core that helps manage moisture level. The sustained release of broad-spectrum ionic silver actively protects the dressing from bacterial contamination, whereas the inner core maintains the moist environment needed for wound healing. Acticoat 3 delivers 3 days of uninterrupted antimicrobial activity.

Indications

An effective barrier to bacterial penetration; may help reduce infection in partial- and full-thickness wounds, including decubitus ulcers, venous stasis ulcers, diabetic ulcers, first- and second-degree burns, and donor sites; may be used over debrided and grafted partial-thickness wounds

Contraindications

- Not for use on patients with sensitivity to silver
- Not for use on patients during magnetic resonance imaging (MRI) examination
- For external use only
- Incompatible with oil-based products such as petrolatum
- Not for contact with electrodes or conductive gels during electronic measurements, for example, EEG and ECG
- Not for exposure to temperatures above $50°$ C, protect from light
- Not for use if product color isn't uniform
- Not for use if pack is opened or damaged

Application

- Follow standard protocol to cleanse wound; don't use oil-based cleansing agents. Where required, wound cleansing should be performed according to local clinical protocol using sterile water only.

For heavily exudative wounds:

- Remove the Acticoat 3 dressing from the package and cut to size.
- Apply the dry Acticoat 3 dressing to the wound, either side down, as the exudate will be sufficient to activate the dressing.
- Cover the Acticoat 3 dressing with an absorbent secondary dressing.
- Complete the dressing with appropriate gauze wrappings if necessary.

For all other wounds:

- Remove the Acticoat 3 dressing from the package and cut to shape.
- Moisten the dressing with sterile water (don't use saline).

- Allow the dressing to drain on an absorbent surface in a sterile field for at least 2 minutes.
- Apply the Acticoat 3 dressing to the wound surface, either side down.
- Cover the dressing with a moist absorbent secondary dressing that may be prepared by saturating gauze with sterile water and wringing out the excess water.
- Complete the dressing with appropriate gauze wrappings if necessary.

Removal

- Change the dressing depending on the amount of exudate present and the condition of the wound. Avoid using oil-based cleansing agents. The dressing may be worn for up to 3 days.
- Remove the secondary dressing, and then remove Acticoat 3 from the wound bed. Make sure the dressing is moist before removing it.
- Avoid forceful removal of the dressing and disruption of the healing wound.
- Keep in mind that the dressing may cause transient discoloration.

ANTIMICROBIALS

Acticoat 7
Smith & Nephew, Inc.
Wound Management

How supplied
Pad: 4″ × 5″, 6″ × 6″, 2″ × 2″; A9270

Action
Acticoat 7 (with SILCRYST Nanocrystals)
consists of two layers of an absorbent, rayon/polyester inner core sandwiched between three layers of silver-coated, polyethylene netting. The sustained release of broad-spectrum ionic silver actively protects the dressing from bacterial contamination, whereas the inner core maintains the moist environment needed for wound healing. Acticoat 7 delivers 7 days of uninterrupted antimicrobial activity.

Indications
An effective barrier to bacterial penetration; may help reduce infection in partial- and full-thickness wounds, including decubitus ulcers, venous stasis ulcers, diabetic ulcers, first- and second-degree burns, and donor sites; may be used over debrided and grafted partial thickness wounds

Contraindications
- Not for use on patients with a sensitivity to silver
- Not for use on patients during magnetic resonance imaging (MRI) examination
- For external use only
- Incompatible with oil-based products such as petrolatum
- Avoid contact with electrodes or conductive gels during electronic measurements, for example, electroencephalography and electrocardiography
- Avoid exposure to temperatures above 50° C; protect from light
- Not for use if product color isn't uniform
- Not for use if pack is opened or damaged

Application
- Follow standard protocol to cleanse wound; don't use oil-based cleansing agents. Where required, wound cleansing should be performed according to local clinical protocol using sterile water only.

For heavily exudative wounds:
- Remove the Acticoat 7 dressing from the package and cut to size.
- Apply the dry Acticoat 7 dressing to the wound, either side down, as the exudate will be sufficient to activate the dressing.
- Cover the Acticoat 7 dressing with an absorbent secondary dressing.
- Complete the dressing with appropriate gauze wrappings if necessary.

For all other wounds:
- Remove the Acticoat 7 dressing from the package and cut to shape.
- Moisten the dressing with sterile water (don't use saline).

ANTIMICROBIALS

- Allow the dressing to drain on an absorbent surface in a sterile field for at least 2 minutes.
- Apply the Acticoat 7 dressing to the wound surface, either side down.
- Cover the dressing with a moist absorbent secondary dressing that may be prepared by saturating gauze with sterile water and wringing out the excess water.
- Complete the dressing with appropriate gauze wrappings if necessary.

Removal

- If the dressing dries and adheres to the wound, moisten or soak the dressing prior to removal.
- Change the dressing depending on the amount of exudate present and the condition of the wound. Avoid using oil-based cleansing agents. The dressing may be worn for up to 7 days.
- Remove the secondary dressing, and then remove Acticoat 7 from the wound bed. Make sure the dressing is moist before removing it.
- Avoid forceful removal of the dressing and disruption of the healing wound.
- Keep in mind that the dressing may cause transient discoloration.

ANTIMICROBIALS

Acticoat Absorbent Antimicrobial Alginate Dressing

Smith & Nephew, Inc.
Wound Management

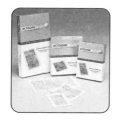

How supplied
Pad: 4″ × 5″; A6197
Rope: ³⁄₄″ × 12″; A6199

Action
Acticoat Absorbent absorbs excess wound fluid to form a gel that maintains a moist environment for optimal wound healing. The sustained release of broad-spectrum ionic silver actively protects the dressing from bacterial contamination. Acticoat Absorbent delivers 3 days of uninterrupted antimicrobial activity.

Indications
To protect wounds from bacterial penetration; the barrier function of the dressing may help reduce infection in partial- and full-thickness wounds with moderate to heavy exudate, including decubitus, venous, and diabetic ulcers, and surgical and traumatic wounds

Contraindications
- Contraindicated in patients with sensitivity to silver
- Not for use on third-degree burns
- Incompatible with oil-based products such as petroleum jelly

Application
- Cleanse the wound using conventional, non-oil-based techniques, and leave the wound moist.
- Apply the dressing to the wound, either side down, and secure with an appropriate secondary dressing that will maintain a moist environment.
- Keep the dressing moist but not so wet that tissue maceration occurs.

Removal
- Change the dressing depending on the amount of exudate present and the condition of the wound. Avoid using oil-based cleansing agents. The dressing may be worn for up to 3 days.
- Remove the secondary dressing, then remove Acticoat Absorbent from the wound bed. Make sure the dressing is moist before removing it.
- If the dressing dries and adheres to the wound, moisten or soak the dressing before removing it.
- Avoid forceful removal of the dressing and disruption of the healing wound.
- Remember that the dressing may cause transient discoloration.

ANTIMICROBIALS

Acticoat Burn Antimicrobial Dressing
Smith & Nephew, Inc.
Wound Management

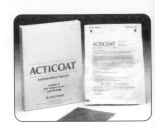

How supplied
Pad: 4″ × 4 , 4″ × 8″, 8″ × 16″,
         16″ × 16″; A9270
Roll: 4″ × 48″; A9270

Action:
Acticoat Burn consists of a rayon/polyester core that helps manage moisture level and control silver release. The silver-coated high-density polyethylene mesh facilitates the passage of silver through the dressing. The nanocrystalline coating of pure silver delivers antimicrobial barrier activity within 30 minutes—faster than other forms of silver.

Indications
An effective barrier to bacterial penetration; may help reduce infection in partial, and full-thickness wounds, including decubitus ulcers, venous stasis ulcers, diabetic ulcers, first- and second-degree burns, and donor sites; may be used over debrided and grafted partial-thickness wounds

Contraindications
- Contraindicated in patients with sensitivity to silver
- Not for use on third-degree burns
- Incompatible with oil-based products, such as petroleum jelly

Application
- Cleanse the wound using conventional, non-oil-based techniques, and leave the wound moist.
- Remove Acticoat Burn from the package.
- Apply the dressing to the wound, either side down, and secure with an appropriate secondary dressing that will maintain a moist environment.
- Keep the dressing moist but not so wet that tissue maceration occurs.

Removal
- Change the dressing depending on the amount of exudate present and the condition of the wound. Avoid using oil-based cleansing agents. The dressing may be worn for up to 3 days.
- Remove the secondary dressing, then remove Acticoat Absorbent from the wound bed. Make sure the dressing is moist before removing it.
- If the dressing dries and adheres to the wound, moisten or soak the dressing before removing it. Avoid forceful removal of the dressing and disruption of the healing wound.
- Remember that the dressing may cause transient discoloration.

New Product

Acticoat Moisture Control Dressing
Smith & Nephew, Inc.
Wound Management

How supplied
Pad: 2″ × 2″; 4″ × 4″ A6209
         4″ × 8″; A6210

Action
Acticoat Moisture Control (with SILCRYST Nanocrystals) is an absorbent three-layer dressing providing an effective barrier to bacterial penetration. Consisting of a nanocrystalline silver-coated wound contact layer, a white polyurethane foam layer, and a blue waterproof top film layer, the dressing will help maintain a moist wound environment in the presence of exudate. The dressing may be left in place over a wound for up to 7 days.

Indications
For use in light to moderately exuding partial- and full-thickness wounds, including pressure ulcers, diabetic ulcers, partial-thickness burns, and donor sites; may be used over debrided and partial-thickness wounds

Contraindications
- Not for use on patients with a sensitivity to silver
- Not for use on patients during magnetic resonance imaging
- For external use only
- Incompatible with oil-based products, such as petroleum jelly
- May not be compatible with topical antimicrobials
- Incompatible with oxidizing agents (for example, Eusol) because these can break down the absorbent polyurethane component of the dressing
- Not for contact with electrodes or conductive gels during electronic measurements, for example, electroencephalography and electrocardiography
- Not for use if reddening or sensitization occurs
- Not intended to provide treatment for infected wounds; may be used on infected wounds that are being managed in accordance with institutional clinical protocols for infection abatement as an adjunct to the standard treatment regimen to provide a barrier to bacterial penetration

Application
- Where required, wound cleansing should be performed according to local clinical protocol using sterile water only.
- Choose a dressing that is larger than the wound.
- Remove the Acticoat Moisture Control Dressing from the pack using aseptic technique.
- Cut to shape as necessary for awkward areas.

ANTIMICROBIALS

- The dressing shouldn't be moistened before use because it's indicated for use on exuding wounds.
- Place the silver layer in intimate contact with the wound bed, ensuring the entire surface is covered.
- Secure with an appropriate secondary retention dressing.
- Acticoat Moisture Control may be used under compression bandages. Cut dressing to the size of the wound, check regularly and change as needed.

Removal

- The dressing may be left in place up to 7 days, but will require earlier changing if a strikethrough of exudate occurs.
- The dressing may adhere if used on lightly exuding wounds. If the dressing isn't easily removed, moisten or soak to assist removal and avoid disruption of the wound.

Actisorb Silver 220 Antimicrobial Binding Dressing

Johnson & Johnson
Wound Management
A division of ETHICON, Inc.

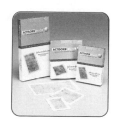

How supplied
Dressing: 2¹/₂" × 3³/₄"; A6206
4¹/₈" × 4¹/₈", 4¹/₈" × 7¹/₂"; A6207

Action
A combination of silver and activated charcoal for the care of chronic wounds. Silver particles embedded in the charcoal kill bacteria and fungi; porous activated charcoal layer binds toxins and odor-causing molecules.

Indications
To provide an effective barrier to bacterial penetration, to absorb offending odor resulting from wounds, and to trap bacteria, bacterial toxins, and odor; to help reduce infection in partial- and full-thickness wounds, including pressure ulcers, venous and diabetic ulcers, first- and second-degree burns, donor sites, and surgical wounds; suitable for use under compression bandages, such as DYNA-FLEX Multi-Layer Compression System

Contraindications
- Contraindicated for third-degree burns
- Contraindicated in patients with sensitivity to silver

Application
- Prepare the wound bed according to protocol, removing all necrotic tissue. The dressing may be used wet or dry, but excess use of ointments with a petroleum jelly base can impair dressing performance.
- Place either side of the dressing against the wound, ensuring direct contact. If the wound is deep, pack the dressing loosely.
- Use a nonadherent wound contact layer along with the dressing, if necessary. Keep in mind, however, that the outer nylon sleeve facilitates dressing removal with minimal adherence to the wound bed.
- Secure the dressing as appropriate for the indication. Depending on the amount of exudate, use an absorbent secondary dressing on top.

Removal
- The dressing may be left in place for up to 7 days, depending on the wound and the amount of exudate. Initially, it may be necessary to change the dressing every 24 hours to ensure optimum performance. Change the secondary absorbent dressing as required.
- Avoid cutting the dressing, otherwise particles of activated charcoal may get into the wound and cause discoloration.

ANTIMICROBIALS

New Product

Algidex Ag
DeRoyal

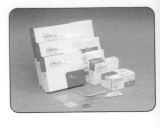

How supplied
Foam Back: 2″ × 2″, 4″ × 4″; A6209
4″ × 5″, 6″ × 6″; A6210
8″ × 8″; A6211

Thin Sheet: 2″ × 2″, 4″ × 4″; A6196
4″ × 8″, 6″ × 6″; A6197
8″ × 8″, 8″ × 16″, 16″ × 16″; A6198

Paste: 10 cc; A6261

Action
Algidex Ag provides slow, extended release of active ionic silver for broad antimicrobial effectiveness. The unique matrix formulation of silver, alginate, and maltodextrin allows Algidex Ag to absorb wound exudates, decrease surface wound contaminates, decrease wound odor, and create a moist environment conducive to healing. The maltodextrin creates an environment that helps the body's own cells to carry out the task of granulation tissue formation while eliminating wound odor. Algidex Ag isn't absorbed systemically.

Indications
For use in infected and noninfected wounds of all types; dermal ulcers (leg ulcers, pressure ulcers); diabetic ulcers; abdominal wounds; superficial wounds; lacerations, cuts, and abrasions; donor sites; second-degree burns; and dry, moist, or wet wounds

Contraindications
- Not for use on third-degree burns
- Not for use on ulcers resulting from infections
- Contraindicated for lesions associated with active vasculitis
- Contraindicated for patients with sensitivity to alginates

Application
For Algidex Ag Foam
- Thoroughly cleanse wound with normal saline.
- Apply Algidex Ag with silver matrix touching the wound.
- Secure dressing in place with retention dressing such as gauze, transparent film, or tape.
- Algidex Ag is antimicrobial for up to 7 days and may be worn until dressing has reached saturation.

For Algidex Ag Thin Sheet
- Thoroughly cleanse wound with normal saline.
- Remove backing from Algidex Ag Thin Sheet.

- Place Algidex Ag Thin Sheet over shallow wounds, or pack into deep wounds.
- Cover with appropriate secondary dressing based on wound drainage.
- Algidex Ag Thin Sheet is antimicrobial for up to 7 days and may be worn until secondary dressing requires changing.

For Algidex Ag Paste
- Thoroughly cleanse wound with normal saline.
- Apply $1/4''$ thickness of paste to shallow wounds, or completely fill deep wounds.
- Cover with appropriate secondary dressing based on wound drainage.
- Algidex Ag Paste is antimicrobial for up to 7 days and may be worn until secondary dressing requires changing.

Removal

For Algidex Ag Foam
- Remove retention dressing, if applicable.
- Gently lift Algidex Ag from the wound. If dressing adheres to wound, gently irrigate with saline to help loosen dressing.
- Discard according to institutional policy.
- Once dressing is removed, thoroughly cleanse wound with normal saline to remove any residue or debris from the wound.

For Algidex Ag Thin Sheet or Paste
- Remove secondary dressing.
- Gently irrigate wound with saline to help loosen Algidex Ag.
- Continue to thoroughly cleanse wound to remove wound drainage or any residue left from Algidex Ag.

ANTIMICROBIALS

Arglaes Antimicrobial Barrier

Medline Industries, Inc.

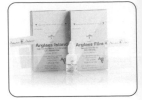

How supplied

Film dressing: $2^{3}/8''$ × $3^{1}/8''$
              $4''$ × $4^{3}/4''$
              $4^{3}/4''$ × $10''$
              $3''$ × $14''$ (postop)
Film with Alginate pad: $2^{3}/8''$ × $3^{1}/8''$ ($1''$ × $2''$ pad)
                        $4''$ × $4^{3}/4''$ ($2''$ × $2''$ pad)
                        $4^{3}/4''$ × $10''$ ($2^{3}/4''$ × $8''$ pad)

Action

Arglaes Antimicrobial Barrier applies the principle of moist wound healing and also serves as a potent antimicrobial barrier that remains effective for 7 days. Arglaes technology uses sustained release of ionic silver that's antibacterial and antifungal but remains completely noncytotoxic. Arglaes Antimicrobial Barrier has a high moisture vapor transfer rate and is available as a transparent film dressing, with or without an alginate pad.

Indications

To manage superficial wounds, lacerations, cuts, and abrasions, leg ulcers, pressure ulcers (stages 2, 3, and 4), donor sites, partial- and full-thickness wounds, infected and noninfected wounds, wounds with light to heavy drainage, and wounds with serosanguineous or purulent drainage

Contraindications

- Contraindicated for third-degree burns
- Contraindicated in patients with hypersensitivity to silver or heavy metals

Application

- Clean the application site with normal saline solution or another appropriate cleanser, such as Skintegrity Wound Cleanser. Dry the surrounding skin to ensure it's free from any greasy substance. Allow any skin preparation to dry completely.
- Select an appropriate-sized dressing that allows $1^{1}/4''$ to $1^{1}/2''$ (3 to 4 cm) of attachment to healthy periwound skin.
- With one hand, hold the dressing's white tab with the printed side facing up. With the other hand, take hold of the loose film flap, and gently peel off the release sheet.
- Hold the dressing on both ends, then turn it over so the adhesive surface is facing the wound. Ensure that both edges of the white tab are held together.
- Apply the dressing, pressing firmly and smoothing down. Make sure the edges of the dressing are firmly fixed in place.
- Take hold of the second release sheet at the end of the dressing opposite the white tab, and gently peel away and discard.

- For moderately to heavily draining wounds, use the O-Technique. It involves cutting small openings into the dressing before removing the carrier sheet. Excess drainage is allowed to pass through the dressing onto an absorbent secondary dressing. The technique is also helpful when using Arglaes under a compression dressing.

Removal

- Gently lift up one corner of the dressing, and begin stretching it horizontally along the skin surface to break the adhesive bond.
- When two sides of the dressing are partially removed, grasp both sides and stretch the dressing horizontally, parallel to the skin.

ANTIMICROBIALS

Arglaes Antimicrobial Barrier Powder Dressing
Medline Industries, Inc.

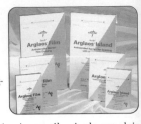

How supplied
Bottle: 5 g, 10 g, 10 g in sterile O.R. packaging; A6262

Action
Arglaes Antimicrobial Barrier Powder Dressing is a sterile, single-use alginate powder containing ionic silver, making it ideal for difficult to dress, highly exuding wounds. Using controlled-release polymers that are activated by moisture, Arglaes Powder delivers a constant stream of antimicrobial silver ions into the wound. Continuous delivery, at a constant rate, means that only minute quantities of silver ions are required to maintain a continuous antimicrobial barrier without cytotoxicity. The sustained-release effect remains constant until Arglaes Powder is removed from the wound site (up to 5 days). In addition, Arglaes Powder contains alginate to aid in fluid handling. As the powder mixes with wound exudate, it turns into a gel that adheres to the wound bed and is easily removed during wound irrigation. Arglaes Powder has been shown to be effective against a broad range of fungi, gram-positive, and gram-negative bacteria, including *Staphylococcus aureus, Pseudomonas aeruginosa, Escherichia coli, Candida albicans, Aspergillus niger*, methicillin-resistant *Staphylococcus aureus*, and vancomycin-resistant *enterococcus*.

Indications
To manage infected or noninfected wounds, such as pressure ulcers, arterial ulcers, venous ulcers, diabetic ulcers, donor sites and other bleeding surface wounds, dermal lesions, trauma injuries or incisions, and minor burns

Contraindications
- Not intended for use on dry wounds or wounds that are completely covered with black necrotic tissue
- Not intended for surgical implantation
- Not intended for use on third-degree burns
- Not intended for use on patients with sensitivity to silver
- Not for use if the packaging has been damaged
- Not for use on infected wounds except at the health care provider's discretion
- Not for use with topical antibiotics or antiseptics
- Not for use before eschar is debrided

Application
- Clean the wound site with sterile saline or appropriate wound cleanse such as Skintegrity Wound Cleanser.

- One 10-g bottle of Arglaes Powder is sufficient to dress a wound area of up to 4″ × 4″ (10 cm × 10 cm).
- Gently dry the surrounding area.
- Shake bottle thoroughly, then open Arglaes Powder by removing the tamper-evident collar and screw cap.
- Apply the dressing by squeezing the bottle (gently tap bottle if flow is blocked) and "puffing" the powder into the wound bed. Apply until wound surfaces are completely covered to a depth of not less than 1 mm.
- Cover site with an appropriate secondary dressing. Heavily exuding wounds may require a more absorbent secondary dressing, such as Maxorb Alginate covered with a Stratasorb Composite Island Dressing.
- Arglaes Powder should be changed when the secondary dressing is wet or if there is any sign of leakage. Heavily draining wounds may require more than one change per day. Dressing may remain in place up to 5 days.

Removal

- To remove Arglaes Powder, gently lift and discard the secondary dressing. Irrigate the wound thoroughly with normal saline or appropriate wound cleanser, such as Skintegrity Wound Cleanser. Continue irrigating until all gelled or ungelled powder is removed.
- Redress the wound as appropriate.

ANTIMICROBIALS

Contreet Foam Adhesive Antimicrobial Barrier Dressing with Silver

Coloplast Corporation

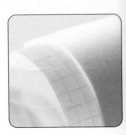

How supplied

Dressing: 5″ × 5″ with 3″ × 3″ pad; A6212
7″ × 7″ with 5″ × 5″ pad; A6213

Action

Contreet Foam combines an effective, sustained silver-release technology with moist wound healing to effectively prepare problem wounds for healing. Contreet Foam Adhesive Dressings are antibacterial wound dressings with ionic silver as the active component homogeneously dispersed throughout the foam. Silver is released from the dressing into the wound bed when in contact with wound exudate. Depending on the amount of exudate, the release continues for up to 7 days.

Indications

To manage wounds with moderate to high amounts of exudate or with a risk for infection; to progress wounds that exhibit delayed healing due to bacteria

Contraindications

- Contraindicated in patients with sensitivity to silver
- Must be removed before radiation treatment or examinations that include X-rays, ultrasonic treatment, diathermy, or microwaves

Application

- Rinse the wound with physiologic saline or Sea-Clens Wound Cleanser. Gently dry the skin surrounding the wound.
- Select a dressing that overlaps the wound edge by a minimum of 1″ (2.5 cm).
- Remove the paper carrier from the dressing, center the dressing over the site, and apply to skin using a "rolling" motion.
- Smooth the dressing into place, especially around edges, and hold in place for 5 seconds to maximize adhesive qualities. If necessary, use tape around the edges to avoid rollup.

Removal

- Dressing should be changed when clinically indicated or when visible signs of transparency approach ¾″ (2 cm) from the edge of the dressing.
- Dressing may be left in place for up to 7 days, depending on the condition of the wound.

Contreet Foam Cavity Dressing with Silver
Coloplast Corporation

How supplied
Dressing: 2″ × 3″; A6209

Action
Contreet Foam Cavity Dressings combine an effective, sustained silver-release technology with moist wound healing to effectively prepare problem wounds for healing. Contreet Foam Cavity Dressings are antibacterial wound dressings with ionic silver as the active component homogeneously dispersed throughout the foam. Silver is released from the dressing when in contact with wound exudate. Depending on the amount of exudate, the release will continue for up to 7 days.

Indications
To manage wounds with moderate to high amounts of exudate or with a risk for infection; to progress wounds that exhibit delayed healing due to bacteria

Contraindications
- Contraindicated in patients with known sensitivity to silver
- Must be removed before radiation treatment or examinations that include x-rays, ultrasonic treatment, diathermy, microwaves, or magnetic resonance imaging

Application
- Rinse the wound with physiologic saline or Sea Clens Wound Cleanser. Gently dry the skin surrounding the wound.
- Remove the product from the packaging and the paper backing.
- Mold Contreet Cavity Dressing to the wound shape by loosely folding the product along the perforations or by rolling the dressing. The dressing can be cut to fit the wound. Fill half the volume of the wound. On absorption of exudate, the foam expands to fill the cavity over a short period of time.
- For fixation and covering, use a separate dressing such as Biatain Foam Adhesive Dressing or Comfeel Plus Clear Hydrocolloid Dressing.

Removal
- Dressing should be changed when clinically indicated or when visible signs of transparency approach ¾″ (2 cm) from the edge of the dressing.
- Dressing may be left in place for up to 7 days, depending on the condition of the wound.

ANTIMICROBIALS

Contreet Foam Non-Adhesive Antimicrobial Barrier Dressing with Silver

Coloplast Corporation

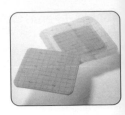

How supplied

Dressing: 4″ × 4″; A6209
6″ × 6″; A6210

Action

Contreet Foam combines an effective, sustained silver-release technology with moist wound healing to effectively prepare problem wounds for healing. Contreet Foam Non-Adhesive Dressings are antibacterial wound dressings with ionic silver as the active component homogeneously dispersed throughout the foam. Silver is released from the dressing into the wound bed when in contact with wound exudate. Depending on the amount of exudate, the release will continue for up to 7 days.

Indications

To manage wounds with moderate to high amounts of exudate or with a risk for infection; to progress wounds that exhibit delayed healing due to bacteria

Contraindications

- Contraindicated in patients with sensitivity to silver
- Must be removed before radiation treatment or examinations that include X-rays, ultrasonic treatment, diathermy, or microwaves

Application

- Rinse the wound with physiologic saline or Sea-Clens Wound Cleanser. Gently dry the skin surrounding the wound.
- Select a dressing that overlaps the wound edge by a minimum of 1″ (2.5 cm).
- Remove the paper carrier from the dressing, center the dressing over the site, and apply to skin.
- Use tape or appropriate secondary dressing to hold in place.

Removal

- Dressing should be changed when clinically indicated or when visible signs of transparency approach ³/₄″ (2 cm) from the edge of the dressing.
- Dressing may be left in place for up to 7 days, depending on the condition of the wound.

Contreet Hydrocolloid Antimicrobial Barrier Dressing with Silver
Coloplast Corporation

How supplied
Dressing: 4" × 4"; A6234
6" × 6"; A6235
8" × 8"; A6236

Action
Contreet Hydrocolloid Dressings combine an effective silver-release technology with moist wound healing to effectively prepare the problem wounds for healing. Contreet Hydrocolloid Dressings are antibacterial wound dressings with ionic silver as the active component homogeneously dispersed throughout the hydrocolloid. Silver is released from the dressing when in contact with wound exudate. Depending on the amount of exudate, the release will continue for up to 7 days.

Indications
To manage wounds with moderate to high amounts of exudate or with a risk for infection; to progress wounds that exhibit delayed healing due to bacteria

Contraindications
- Contraindicated in patients with known sensitivity to silver
- Must be removed before radiation treatment or examinations that include x-rays, ultrasonic treatment, diathermy, microwaves, or magnetic resonance imaging

Application
- Rinse the wound with physiologic saline or Sea-Clens Wound Cleanser. Gently dry the skin surrounding the wound.
- Select a dressing that overlaps the wound edge by a minimum of 1" (2.5 cm).
- Remove the paper carrier from the dressing, center the dressing over the site, and apply to skin using a "rolling" motion.
- Smooth the dressing into place, especially around edges, and hold in place for 5 seconds to maximize adhesive qualities. If necessary, use tape around the edges to avoid rollup.

Removal
- Dressing should be changed when clinically indicated or when visible signs of transparency approach ³⁄₄" (2 cm) from the edge of the dressing.
- Dressing may be left in place for up to 7 days, depending on the condition of the wound.

ANTIMICROBIALS

Excilon AMD
Tyco Healthcare/Kendall

How supplied
Drain sponge: 4″ × 4″; A6222
I.V. sponge: 2″ × 2″; A6222

Action
Excilon AMD helps prevent deadly and expensive infections. It resists bacterial colonization within the dressing and reduces bacterial penetration through the dressing. Broad-spectrum effectiveness protects against gram-positive and -negative microorganisms, including methicillin-resistant Staphylococcus aureus (MRSA) and vancomycin-resistant *enterococcus* (VRE). Superior absorbency and fast wicking action lead to fewer dressing changes. Unique precut T-Slit conforms snugly.

Indications
To protect against bacteria and manage drains, catheters, chest tubes, I.V. sites, and tracheotomies

Contraindications
None provided by the manufacturer

Application
■ Apply Excilon AMD as a primary dressing.

Removal
■ Gently remove dressing.

ANTIMICROBIALS

Kerlix AMD Antimicrobial Bandage Roll

Kerlix Antimicrobial Super Sponge

Tyco Healthcare/Kendall

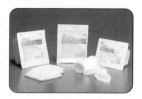

How supplied
Bandage roll: 4.50 × 4.1 yards (1 per tray)
Super sponge: Medium (2, 5, or 10 per tray)

Action
Help protect against methicillin-resistant *Staphylococcus aureus* (MRSA) and vancomycin-resistant *enterococcus* infections (VRE), and other wound infections with no change to protocol. Kerlix bandage rolls and super sponges resist bacterial colonization within the dressing and reduce bacterial penetration through the dressing as well. Broad-spectrum effectiveness provides protection against gram-positive and -negative microorganisms, including, and fungi and yeasts. Kerlix also limits cross-contamination from patient to patient, patient to clinician, and patient to the environment.

Indications
To manage pressure ulcers (stages 1, 2, 3, and 4), partial- and full-thickness wounds, tunneling wounds, infected and noninfected wounds, draining wounds, and red, yellow, or black wounds

Contraindications
- Contraindicated for third- and fourth-degree burns

Application
- Apply Kerlix as a primary or secondary dressing.

Removal
- Gently remove the dressing.

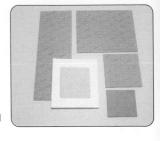

PolyMem Silver QuadraFoam Non-Adhesive Wound Dressings*

PolyMem Silver QuadraFoam Adhesive Cloth Wound Dressings*

Ferris Manufacturing Corporation

How supplied

Non-Adhesive Silver Dressing pad: 4.25″ × 4.25″; A6209
　　　　6.5″ × 7.5″, 4.25″ × 12.5″; A6210
Cloth-Backed Adhesive Silver Dressing: 6″ × 6″ island dressing with
　　　　3.5″ × 3.5″ pad; A6212

Action

PolyMem Silver dressings belong to an innovative class of adaptable wound dressings called QuadraFoam. QuadraFoam dressings effectively cleanse, fill, absorb, and moisten wounds throughout the healing continuum.

　　PolyMem Silver Wound Dressing is composed of a patented hydrophilic polyurethane membrane matrix. The membrane pad is covered with a semipermeable continuous thin film backing, which is optimized for oxygen and moisture vapor permeability and is a barrier to liquids. The PolyMem silver formulation is the only dressing formulation that contains a safe, nontoxic cleanser (F68 surfactant), a moisturizer (glycerol, also known as glycerin), an absorbing agent (superabsorbent starch copolymer), and silver (124 µg/cm^2 minimum), all in the pad matrix. The silver protects the dressing from microbial contamination. Both F68 and glycerol are soluble in wound fluid and skin moisture. The superabsorbent starch copolymer contained in the PolyMem formulation draws wound fluid, which is known to contain natural growth factors and nutrients, to the wound site.

Indications

For the management of pressure ulcers (stages 1 through 4), venous stasis ulcers, acute wounds, leg ulcers, donor and graft sites, skin tears, diabetic ulcers, dermatologic disorders, first- and second-degree burns, and surgical wounds; PolyMem formulation dressings are suitable for use when visible signs of infection are present if proper medical treatment that addresses the cause of the infection has been implemented

Contraindications

- Incompatible with hypochlorite solutions (bleach) such as Dakin's solution
- Not for use on patients with sensitivity to any ingredient

ANTIMICROBIALS

Application

- Prepare the wound according to facility policy or as directed by a physician or other ordering clinician. With subsequent dressing changes, cleaning the wound isn't recommended unless infection or gross contamination is present.
- Select a PolyMem Silver dressing of appropriate size. The silver membrane should be ¼" to 2" (0.6 to 5 cm) larger than the wound area.
- Apply the dressing film side and printed side out.
- Topical treatments aren't recommended for use with PolyMem Silver dressings.

Removal

- A dramatic increase in wound fluid may be observed during the first few days.
- Keep the dressing dry when bathing the patient. Change the dressing if it gets wet.
- Change the dressing before exudate, visible through the dressing, reaches the periwound area (wound edges). If the wound fluid reaches the the edge of the dressing membrane pad, change immediately. For a mildly exuding wound in an otherwise healthy patient, the dressing may remain in place for up to 7 days. As with other dressings, more frequent changes may be indicated if the patient has a compromised immune system, diabetes, or infection at the wound site.
- Gently remove the dressing. Don't disturb the wound bed. Don't clean the wound or flush with saline or water unless the wound is infected or contaminated. PolyMem Silver dressings contain a mild, nontoxic wound cleanser and leave no residue. Additional cleaning of the wound may injure regenerating tissues and delay the wound-healing process.
- Apply a new PolyMem Silver dressing.

*See package insert for complete information.

ANTIMICROBIALS

New Product

PolyMem Wic Silver QuadraFoam Cavity Wound Filler Dressing*

Ferris Manufacturing Corporation

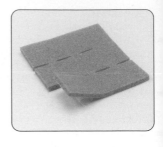

How supplied

Cavity filler pad: 3" × 3"; A6215

Action

PolyMem formulation dressings belong to an innovative class of adaptable wound dressings called QuadraFoam. QuadraFoam dressings effectively cleanse, fill, absorb, and moisten wounds throughout the healing continuum.

PolyMem Wic Silver cavity filler is composed of a hydrophilic polyurethane membrane, which may be placed into open wounds to eliminate dead space, absorb exudate, and maintain a moist wound surface. PolyMem Wic Silver Filler minimizes the need to disturb the wound bed. PolyMem Wic Silver Filler is the only dressing that contains a safe, nontoxic wound cleanser (F68 surfactant), a moisturizer (glycerin), an absorbing agent (superabsorbent starch copolymer), and silver (186 $\mu g/cm^2$ minimum), all in the polyurethane matrix. Both F68 and glycerin are soluble in wound fluid and skin moisture. Silver protects the dressing from microbial contamination. PolyMem Wic Silver is placed in the wound bed; it provides fast wicking and absorbent capacity to accommodate large amounts of exudate. PolyMem Wic Silver Filler expands to fill dead space and allows extended times between dressing changes. PolyMem Wic Silver Filler is perforated so that 1"-wide strips can be detached or easily folded, or it can be placed as is into a cavity. PolyMem Wic Silver Cavity Filler is to be covered with a secondary PolyMem formulation dressing or another suitable secondary dressing.

Indications

To manage moderately to heavily exuding wounds associated with pressure ulcers (stages 3 and 4), vascular ulcers, acute wounds, diabetic ulcers; suitable for use when visible signs of infection are present if proper medical treatment that addresses the cause of the infection has been implemented

Contraindications

■ Incompatible with hypochlorite solutions (bleach) such as Dakin's solution
■ Not for use on patients with sensitivity to any ingredient

Application

■ Prepare the wound according to facility policy or as directed by a physician or other ordering clinician. With subsequent dressing changes, cleaning the wound isn't recommended unless infection or gross contamination is present.

- Ensure that PolyMem Wic Silver is 30% smaller than the wound diameter. PolyMem Wic Silver will expand as it wicks and absorbs fluid. Avoid overfilling the wound, because overfilling may increase pressure on the tissue in the wound bed, potentially causing additional damage.
- Lightly place the wound filler in the middle of the wound, either side up. PolyMem Wic Silver is perforated so that 1"-wide strips can be detached, cut, folded, or placed as is into the cavity.
- Cover the wound and the PolyMem Wic Silver with a PolyMem formulation dressing or another suitable secondary dressing.

Removal

- Change PolyMem Wic Silver and secondary dressing when exudate reaches the periwound area. Change daily if the patient has a compromised immune system, diabetes, or an infection at the wound site.
- Gently remove the wound filler in one piece. (It won't adhere to the wound.) Don't disturb the wound bed. Don't clean the wound or flush with saline or water unless the wound is infected or contaminated. Additional cleaning of the wound may injure regenerating tissues and may delay the wound-healing process.
- Apply a new PolyMem Wic Silver dressing with a suitable secondary dressing.

*See package insert for complete information.

ANTIMICROBIALS

SeaSorb-Ag Alginate Dressing with Silver
Coloplast Corporation

How supplied
Dressing: 2″ × 2″, 4″ × 4″; A6196
6″ × 6″; A6197
1″ × 17½″; A6199

Action
SeaSorb-Ag Alginate Dressing with Silver is a unique mix of calcium alginate and highly absorbent carboxymethylcellulose with the addition of an
ionic silver complex, which releases silver ions in the presence of wound
exudate. As exudate is absorbed, the dressing forms a soft, cohesive gel that
intimately conforms to the wound surface. Silver ions protect the dressing
from a broad spectrum of microorganisms over a period of up to 4 days.

Indications
To manage moderate to heavily exuding wounds such as pressure ulcers,
leg ulcers, diabetic ulcers, second-degree burns, grafts, donor sites, trauma
wounds, as well as cavity wounds; may be used on infected wounds under
the discretion of a health care professional

Contraindications
- Contraindicated for use on third-degree burns
- Contraindicated for use on dry or lightly exuding wounds
- Contraindicated for use on individuals with a known sensitivity to al-
  ginates or silver
- Contraindicated for control of heavy bleeding
- Contraindicated for surgical implantation

Application
- Debride when necessary, and irrigate the wound site in accordance with
  standard protocols.
- Remove excess solution from surrounding skin.
- Select a size of SeaSorb-Ag alginate dressing with silver that is slightly
  larger than the wound.
- Cut or fold the dressing to fit the wound.
- Apply to wound bed directly.
- Cover and secure with a nonocclusive secondary dressing, such as Com-
  feel Plus Clear Dressing or Biatain Foam Dressing.

Removal
- Dressing change frequency will depend on wound condition and the
  level of exudate. Initially, it may be necessary to change the dressing
  every 24 hours.

ANTIMICROBIALS

- Reapply SeaSorb-Ag Alginate Dressing with Silver when the secondary dressing has reached its absorbent capacity or whenever good wound care practice dictates that the dressing should be changed.
- Gently remove the secondary dressing. If the wound appears dry, saturate the dressing with sterile saline solution before removal.
- Gently remove the dressing from the wound bed and discard. Irrigate the wound site in accordance with standard protocols before application of a new dressing.

Shapes by PolyMem Silver QuadraFoam Dressings*

Ferris Manufacturing Corporation

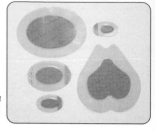

How supplied

Sacral Silver Dressing Adhesive Island Film Dressing: 7.2″ × 7.8″ with 4.5″ × 4.7″ membrane pad; A6212

#8 Oval Silver Adhesive Island Film Dressing: 6.5″ × 8.2″ oval with 4″ × 5.7″ oval membrane pad; A6213

#5 Oval Silver Adhesive Island Film Dressing: 3.5″ × 5″ oval with 2″ × 3″ oval membrane pad; A6212

#3 Oval Silver Adhesive Island Film Dressing: 2″ × 3″ oval with 1″ × 2″ oval membrane pad; A6212

#1 Oval Silver Adhesive Island Film Dressing: 2″ × 3″ oval with 1″ × 1.5″ oval membrane pad; A6212

Action

Shapes by PolyMem dressings belong to an innovative class of adaptable wound dressings called QuadraFoam. QuadraFoam dressings effectively cleanse, fill, absorb, and moisten wounds throughout the healing continuum. Shapes by PolyMem Silver dressings are easy-to use, precut dressings, contoured to fit most wounds.

Shapes by PolyMem Silver Wound Dressing is composed of a patented hydrophilic polyurethane membrane matrix with a thin film adhesive border. The membrane pad is covered with a semipermeable continuous thin film backing, which is optimized for oxygen and moisture vapor permeability and as a barrier to liquids. The PolyMem silver formulation is the only dressing formulation that contains a safe, nontoxic cleanser (F68 surfactant), a moisturizer (glycerol, also known as glycerin), an absorbing agent (superabsorbent starch copolymer), and silver (124 μg/cm^2 minimum), all in the pad matrix. The silver protects the dressing from microbial contamination. Both F68 and glycerol are soluble in wound fluid and skin moisture. The superabsorbent starch copolymer contained in the PolyMem formulation draws wound fluid, which is known to contain natural growth factors and nutrients, to the wound site.

Indications

For the management of pressure ulcers (stages 1 through 4), venous stasis ulcers, acute wounds, leg ulcers, donor and graft sites, skin tears, diabetic ulcers, dermatologic disorders, first- and second-degree burns, and surgical wounds; suitable for use when visible signs of infection are present if proper medical treatment that addresses the cause of the infection has been implemented

Contraindications

- Incompatible with hypochlorite solutions (bleach) such as Dakin's solution
- Not for use on patients with sensitivity to any ingredient

Application

- Prepare the wound according to facility policy or as directed by a physician or other ordering clinician. With subsequent dressing changes, cleaning the wound isn't recommended unless infection or gross contamination is present.
- Select a Shapes by PolyMem Silver Dressing of appropriate size. The silver membrane should be ¼" to 2" (0.6 to 5 cm) larger than the wound area.
- Apply the dressing film side and printed side out.
- Topical treatments aren't recommended for use with Shapes by PolyMem family of dressings.

Removal

- A dramatic increase in wound fluid may be observed during the first few days.
- Keep the dressing dry when bathing the patient. Change the dressing if it gets wet.
- Change the dressing before exudate, visible through the dressing, reaches the periwound area (wound edges). If the wound fluid reaches the the edge of the dressing membrane pad, change immediately. For a mildly exuding wound in an otherwise healthy patient, the dressing may remain in place for up to 7 days. As with other dressings, more frequent changes may be indicated if the patient has a compromised immune system, diabetes, or infection at the wound site.
- Gently remove the dressing. Don't disturb the wound bed. Don't clean the wound or flush with saline or water unless the wound is infected or contaminated. Shapes by PolyMem Silver Dressings contain a mild, nontoxic wound cleanser and leave no residue. Additional cleaning of the wound may injure regenerating tissues and delay the wound-healing process.
- Apply a new Shapes by PolyMem Silver Dressing.

*See package insert for complete information.

ANTIMICROBIALS

SilvaSorb
Medline Industries, Inc.

How supplied
Amorphous gel: 0.25 oz, 1.5 oz, 3 oz,
8 oz, 16 oz; A6248
Cavity: 6-g strands
Sheet: 2″ × 2″; A6242
4.25″ × 4.25″, 4.25″ × 4.25″ perforated, 4″ × 8″, 4″ × 10″ perforated; A6243
Site: 1″ disk with radial slit, 1.75″ disk with radial slit; A6242

Action
SilvaSorb is a sterile, single-use wound dressing for use in moist wound management, combining patented MicroLattice technology with sustained-release silver. SilvaSorb's increased fluid management and antimicrobial performance make it ideal for chronic wounds. SilvaSorb is an effective barrier to bacterial penetration. The antimicrobial barrier function of the dressing may help reduce infection by inhibiting the growth of *Staphylococcus aureus,* methicillin-resistant *S. aureus, Pseudomonas aeruginosa, Escherichia coli, Candida albicans,* vancomycin-resistant *enterococcus,* and other clinically significant microorganisms. SilvaSorb is biocompatible and won't stain or discolor tissue. It also doesn't require preconditioning or periodic irrigation.

SilvaSorb Amorphous Gel donates moisture to dry wound beds while providing antimicrobial silver. Thick, viscous formulation stays in contact with the wound bed to provide an optimally moist environment for up to 3 days.

The polyacrylate material in SilvaSorb Cavity and Sheet Dressings helps maintain a moist wound environment by either donating moisture or absorbing at least five times its weight in excess wound exudate. These dressings maintain their antimicrobial effectiveness for up to 7 days.

SilvaSorb Site offers ionic silver percutaneous site protection to help fight infection at pin, port, and catheter sites. The translucent, flexible material offers a snug fit around the indwelling device, with little or no gap where beacria could easily enter.

Indications
To manage partial- and full-thickness wounds, such as pressure ulcers, diabetic foot ulcers, leg ulcers, skin tears, first- and second-degree burns, grafted wounds and donor sites, surgical wounds, and lacerations and abrasions

Contraindications
- Not intended for use on infected wounds, except at discretion of physician
- Not for use over eschar; eschar should be debrided before use

Application

SilvaSorb Amorphous Gel

- Clean the wound using sterile saline or appropriate wound cleanser, such as Skintegrity Wound Cleanser.
- Dispense SilvaSorb to an appropriate clean applicator, such as a tongue blade or gauze, in sufficient quantities to liberally cover the wound.
- Cover the gel with an appropriate secondary dressing, such as a gauze pad, a film dressing, or nonwoven adhesive secondary dressing, such as Stratasorb.

SilvaSorb Cavity and Sheet Dressings

- Clean the wound using sterile saline or appropriate wound cleanser, such as Skintegrity Wound Cleanser.
- Remove the dressing from the package and blue liners. For the perforated version, prestretch the sheet to open the perforations and allow the dressing to relax.
- For the cavity dressing, adequate spacing is obtained by loosely filling one-half to two-thirds of the wound deficiency. For the sheet dressing, place either side of the dressing in contact with the wound base, making sure that greater than $1/2''$ (1.3 cm) is covering the periwound skin.
- If the cavity or sheet style is too large for the wound, tear or cut the dressing to the appropriate size.
- Cover the dressing with an appropriate secondary cover like a transparent film such as SureSite, Medline Bordered Gauze, or a composite island dressing such as Stratasorb. Your secondary dressing selection and wear time will depend on the amount of exudate and the condition of the periwound skin.
- The dressing may remain in place for up to 7 days, depending on the amount of exudate. Change the dressing if the wound exudate begins to pool within the wound or significant strikethrough occurs on the secondary dressing. Generally, dressings should be changed more frequently for heavily exuding wounds.

SilvaSorb Site

- Prepare the site per facility protocol.
- Wrap dressing around insertion site.
- Cover and secure with transparent film (such as Sureview IV dressings).
- Remove every 7 days (or more often if heavy exudate is present).

Removal

- Carefully remove the secondary dressing and SilvaSorb from the wound.
- SilvaSorb Sheets and Cavity Dressings are normally nonadherent to the wound, but they can be remoistened with saline or wound cleanser to ease removal.
- Gently clean the wound with sterile saline or an appropriate wound cleanser, such as Skintegrity Wound Cleanser.
- Follow the directions for reapplying a new SilvaSorb dressing, if appropriate.

ANTIMICROBIALS

New Product

SilverDerm7
DermaRite Industries, LLC

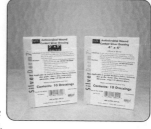

How supplied
Dressing: 2″ × 2″, 4″ × 4″

Action
SilverDerm7 antimicrobial dressings are
nonadherent, absorbent wound dressings.
They provide a sustained release of ionic silver from a silver-plated rayon
fabric. Only ionic silver is released without the deposition of metallic silver in the wound. Silver ions are released within 30 minutes and aid in
pain reduction.

Indications
To help reduce infection and to encourage draining by wicking fluid from
body cavity, infected areas or abscess; may also be used for control of local wound bleeding and nasal hemorrhage

Contraindications
- Contraindicated on patients with sensitivity to silver
- Use on third-degree burns not yet evaluated

Application
- Clean the wound with sterile water. Moisten the dressing with water.
  Don't use saline solution.
- Apply in direct contact with wound, overlapping wound margins by ³/₈″
  to ³/₄″ (1 to 2 cm).
- Cover dressing with conventional techniques.

Removal
- Change dressing based on exudate buildup and wound condition.
- Rinse the dressing with sterile water and reapply if clear of exudates and
  debris.
- If the dressing dries and adheres to the wound, moisten with sterile wa-
  ter before removing.

Silverlon Breast Pads
Argentum Medical, LLC

How supplied
Breast Pad: 5″ diameter with moisture-
control pouch

Action
Silverlon Breast Pads are designed to re-
lieve mastitis, laceration irritation, postmastectomy pain, as well as other
breast and nipple inflammation or infection.

Indications
For over-the-counter or professional use; to manage partial-thickness burns,
incisions, skin grafts, donor sites, lacerations, abrasions, and stages 1 through
4 dermal ulcers

Contraindications
■ Not for use on patients with sensitivity to silver or nylon or those with
third-degree burns

Application
■ Moisten the dressing (sterile or drinking water preferred;, avoid saline),
place in intimate contact with all affected wound surfaces, and secure
with conventional techniques.
■ Rear moisture control pouch utilizes standard disposable absorbent lactation pads and should be changed when saturated.

Removal
■ Saturate with water and gently lift

ANTIMICROBIALS

New Product

Silverlon CA
Argentum Medical, LLC

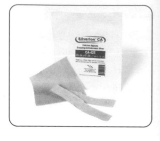

How supplied
Pads: 2″ × 2″; A6196
         4.25″ × 4.25″, 4″ × 8″; A6197
         8″ × 12″; A6198
         ³/₄″ × 12″; A6199

Action
Silverlon CA Advanced Antimicrobial Alginate Dressings are durable non-woven pads composed of High M (manuronic acid) alginate and a Silverlon mesh core. In the presence of moisture, the silver ions provide an antimicrobial barrier that protects the dressing from bacterial contamination. The dressings absorb exudates, maintain a moist wound environment, and feature easy one-piece removal.

Indications
Effective barrier to microbial penetration for moderate to heavily exuding partial- and full-thickness wounds, including pressure ulcers, venous ulcers, diabetic ulcers, donor and graft sites, traumatic and surgical wounds, and first- and second-degree burns; for external use only

Contraindications
■ Not for use on patients with sensitivity to silver or nylon

Application
■ Select a size of Silverlon CA that is slightly larger than the wound. Cut using clean scissors, or fold the dressing to fit the wound.
■ Loosely pack deep wounds, ensuring the dressing doesn't overlap the wound margins.
■ For heavily exuding wounds, apply to the wound bed directly.
■ For wounds with minimal exudates, apply to wound bed moistened with sterile water or saline.
■ Cover and secure Silverlon CA dressing with a nonocclusive secondary dressing.

Removal
■ Based on professional discretion, removal will depend on patient condition and the level of exudates.
■ First, gently remove the secondary dressing. If the wound appears dry, saturate the Silverlon CA dressing with sterile water or normal saline solution before removal.
■ Gently grasp the Silverlon mesh core, remove the dressing from the wound bed, and discard.

New Product

Silverlon Lifesaver Dressing

Argentum Medical, LLC

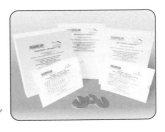

How supplied

Catheter dressing: 1″ diameter, 1.5 mm, 4 mm × 7 mm; A6251

Action

Silverlon technology uses the sustained release of ionic silver, offering effective antimicrobial and antifungal spectrum of activity for up to 7 days of use.

Indications

For over-the-counter as well as professional use; primary antimicrobial dressing to prevent local infection; placed around I.V. insertion sites, catheters, dialysis catheters, drain tubes, and external fixator pins

Contraindications

■ Not for use on patients with sensitivity to silver or nylon

Application

■ Moisten and place tubing through the center hole.
■ Secure directly to entry site, silver side down.

Removal

■ Saturate with clean water, then gently lift.

New Product

Silverlon Negative Pressure Dressing

Argentum Medical, LLC

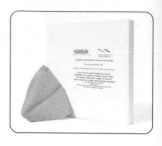

How supplied
Dressing: 2″ × 2″, 4″ × 5″; A6206
5″ × 8″; A6207
5″ × 12″, 12″ × 12″; A6208

Action

Silverlon Negative Pressure Dressing (NPD) is designed for use with negative-pressure wound therapy systems. The unique design with built-in dual flow ports allows for easy flow of fluid and particles through the dressing, while providing sustained release of ionic silver from a stable silver-plated fabric. Silverlon NPD offers an effective antibacterial and antifungal spectrum of activity for up to 7 days of use. Only ionic silver is released, without the deposition of metallic silver into the wound. In a moist environment, the fabric's high conductivity provides analgesia.

Indications

For use in partial-thickness burns, incisions, skin grafts and flaps, donor sites, lacerations, abrasions, stages 1 through 4 dermal ulcers (vascular, venous, pressure, and diabetic), and acute, traumatic, or dehisced wounds

Contraindications
- Contraindicated on patients with sensitivity to silver or nylon

Application
- Wet dressing with sterile or clean water.
- Apply either side of dressing in direct contact with the wound, overlapping wound margins by ³/₈″ to ³/₄″(1 to 2 cm).
- Cover Silverlon with foam or fill media of choice, then cover with drape or film according to manufacturer's instructions.
- Based on professional discretion, Silverlon NPD can be used for up to 7 days.

Removal
- Gently remove secondary dressings. If the wound appears dry, saturate the Silverlon dressing with sterile water or normal saline solution before removal.
- Gently remove the dressing from the wound bed and discard.

ANTIMICROBIALS

Silverlon Surgical Wound Pad and Island Dressing

Argentum Medical, LLC

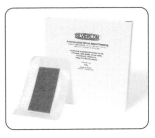

How supplied

Pad dressing: 2″ × 2″, 2″ × 3″, 2″ × 6″,
2″ × 8″; A6251
2″ × 10″, 2″ × 12″, 3″ × 8″,
3″ × 10″, 3″ × 16″,
4″ × 4.5″; A6252

Island dressing: 2″ × 3″ (1″ × 2″ pad), 4″ × 4″ (2″ × 2″ pad); A6254
4″ × 6″ (2″ × 4″ pad), 4″ × 10″ (2″ × 8″ pad), 4″ × 12″
(2″ × 10″ pad), 6″ × 6″ (4″ × 4.5″ pad); A6255
4″ × 14″ (2″ × 12″ pad); A6256

Adhesive strip: 1″ × 3″ (1″ × 1″ pad); A6254

Action

The Silverlon Pad Dressing is a multilayer sterile dressing combining a Silverlon wound contact layer, an absorbent rayon pad layer, and a clear semipermeable film top layer. The island dressings include an additional top layer of adhesive tape. The Silverlon Island and Adhesive Strip Dressings are multilayer dressings with a semipermeable polyurethane tape backing layer overlapping the pad circumferentially and providing adhesion to the surrounding skin.

Indications

For over-the-counter as well as professional use; to manage partial-thickness burns, incisions, skin grafts, donor sites, lacerations, abrasions, and stages 1 to 4 dermal ulcers (vascular, venous, pressure, and diabetic)

Contraindications

- Contraindicated on patients with sensitivity to silver or nylon

Application

- Clean the wound with the fluid of choice.
- Wet dressing with clean water, and place the silver side in direct contact with wound surface, overlapping periwound skin by 1″ (2.5 cm).
- For the pad dressing, secure with conventional techniques.

Removal

- Change the dressing depending on the amount of exudate present and the condition of the wound.
- Based on professional discretion, and if clear of exudate and debris, the dressing may be used for up to 7 days.
- If the dressing dries and adheres to the wound, saturate with clean water before removing.

ANTIMICROBIALS

Silverlon Wound and Burn Contact Dressings and Gloves

Argentum Medical, LLC

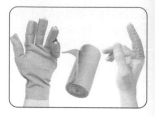

How supplied

Wound contact dressing: 2" × 2"; A6206
4" × 4.5", 4" × 12"; A6207
10" × 12", 4" × 66"; A6208

Burn contact dressing: 4" × 4", 4" × 8", 8" × 16", 16" × 16", 24" × 24"; A9270

Compressive burn wrap: 4" × 66", 6" × 108"; A9270

Acute burn glove: Pediatric, Small, Medium, Large, X-Large; A9270

Action

Silverlon technology uses the sustained release of ionic silver from a stable, highly comformable and comfortable silver nylon substrate and offers effective antibacterial and antifungal spectrum of activity for up to 7 days. Since only ionic silver is released, without the deposition of metallic silver in the wound, Silverlon won't stain wound tissue. In a moist environment, it has been reported that the fabric's high conductivity provides analgesic activity.

Indications

For over-the-counter as well as professional use; to manage partial-thickness burns, incisions, skin grafts, donor sites, lacerations, abrasions, and stages 1 through 4 dermal ulcers (vascular, venous, pressure, and diabetic)

Contraindications

- Contraindicated on patients with sensitivity to silver or nylon

Application

- Clean the wound with fluid of choice.
- Cut dressing to fit the wound base, overlapping periwound skin by 1" (2.5 cm).
- Wet the dressing with clean water, and place either side in direct contact with the wound surface, overlapping periwound skin by 1".
- Cover Silverlon with gauze, hydrocolloid, hydrogel, foam, hydrogel, or the vacuum-assisted closure, to maintain a moist environment.

Removal

- Change the dressing depending on the amount of exudate present and the condition of the wound.
- The dressing may be moistened with a wound cleanser, or rinsed with clean water, and reapplied to the wound surface if the dressing is clear of exudate and debris.
- Based on professional discretion, and if clear of exudate and debris, the dressing may be used for up to 7 days.
- If the dressing dries and adheres to the wound, saturate with clean water or normal saline before removing.

ANTIMICROBIALS

Silverlon Wound Packing Strips

Argentum Medical, LLC

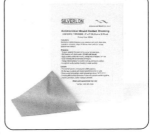

How supplied
Strips: 1″ × 12″, 1″ × 24″; A4649

Action
The Silverlon Wound Packing Strips are sterile, nonadherent, wound dressings. They provide a sustained release of ionic silver from a stable silver nylon substrate and offer effective antibacterial and antifungal spectrum of activity for up to 7 days. Because only ionic silver is released, without the deposition of metallic silver in the wound, Silverlon won't stain wound tissue. The durable ribbonlike format encourages the drainage and wicking of fluids from a body cavity, infected area, or abscess, and features easy one-piece removal.

Indications
For professional use only, to help control local wound bleeding and nasal hemorrhage and to encourage draining by wicking fluids from a body cavity, infected area, or abscess

Contraindications
- Contraindicated on patients with sensitivity to silver or nylon

Application
- Clean the wound with the fluid of choice.
- Wet the dressing with clean water.
- Loosely pack from the origin of the sinus or tunnel to the surface.
- Cover with dressing of choice.

Removal
- Change the dressing depending on the amount of exudate present and the condition of the wound.
- The dressing may be sprayed with a wound cleanser, rinsed with sterile water, and reapplied if clear of exudate and debris.
- The secondary dressing is changed depending the amount of exudate or debris on the surface of the dressing.
- If the dressing dries and adheres to the wound, saturate with clean water or wound cleanser before removing.

ANTIMCROBEALS

Silverlon Tubular Stretch Knit Digit Dressing
Argentum Medical, LLC

How supplied
Pediatric digit dressing: $1/2'' \times 1\,1/2''$; A4649
Pediatric multiple-digit dressing: $1/2'' \times 10''$; A4649
Adult digit dressing: $1'' \times 3\,1/2''$; A4649
Adult multiple-digit dressing: $1'' \times 15''$; A4649
Ear/hand dressing: $3'' \times 4''$; A4649

Action
The Silverlon Tubular Stretch Knit provides a sustained release of ionic silver from a stable silver-plated fabric substrate, offering effective antibacterial and antifungal spectrum of activity for up to 7 days. Only ionic silver is released, without the deposition of metallic silver in the wound. The fabric is very elastomeric and flexible, conforming to the surfaces of digits and toes, allowing range of motion.

Indications
For over-the-counter as well as professional use; to manage partial-thickness burns, incisions, skin grafts, donor sites, lacerations, abrasions, and stages 1 to 4 dermal ulcers (vascular, venous, pressure, and diabetic)

Contraindications
- Contraindicated on patients with sensitivity to silver or nylon

Application
- Clean the wound with the fluid of choice.
- Wet the dressing with sterile water, and gently stretch it around digits or toes. Allow it to conform to the surface of the digit or toe.
- Cover the Silverlon dressing and secure with conventional techniques.

Removal
- Change the dressing depending on the amount of exudate present and the condition of the wound.
- The dressing may be sprayed with a wound cleanser or rinsed with clean water and reapplied to the wound surface if the dressing is clear of exudate and debris.
- Based on professional discretion, and if clear of exudate and debris, the dressing may be used for up to 7 days.
- If the dressing dries and adheres to the wound, saturate with water or nomal saline solution before removing.

ANTIMICROBIALS

3M Tegaderm Ag Mesh
3M Health Care

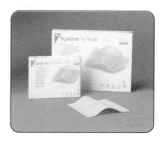

How supplied
Dressing: 2" × 2"; A6402
             4" × 5", 4" × 8"; A6403
             8" × 8", 16" × 16"; A6404

Action
3M Tegaderm Ag Mesh is a fast-acting, long-lasting antimicrobial barrier in an affordable silver dressing. 3M Tegaderm Ag Mesh is effective, patient-friendly, and ready to use. It may be used as a primary dressing, used with absorbent wound fillers, or packed into tunnels or undermined areas.

Indications
For ulcers (pressure, venous, arterial, and neuropathic), open surgical wounds, trauma wounds, superficial partial-thickness burns (second degree) and abrasions

Contraindications
None provided by the manufacturer.

Application
- Remove the dressing from the package.
- If necessary, trim or fold the dressing to fit the wound site.
- Apply the dressing to the wound bed without overlap onto the surrounding skin.
- Secure with an appropriate cover dressing to help manage the wound drainage. A moisture retentive barrier may be used as a cover dressing to help maintain a moist wound environment.

Removal
- Change the dressing as needed. Frequency of changing will depend on factors such as the type of wound and volume of drainage. The dressing remains effective for up to 7 days.
- At the time of dressing change, if the dressing is adhered to the wound surface, saturate with sterile normal saline or sterile water, allow the dressing to soften, and gently remove.
- Avoid forceful removal of the dressing to minimize disruption of the wound.

ANTIMICROBIALS

TELFA AMD
Tyco Healthcare/Kendall

How supplied
Pad: 3″ × 4″; A6222
                3″ × 8″; A6223
Island dressing: 4″ × 5″, 4″ × 8″; A6203
                4″ × 10″, 4″ × 14″; A6204

Action
TELFA AMD helps protect against methicillin-resistant *Staphylococcus aureus* (MRSA), vancomycin-resistant enterococcus (VRE), and wound infections with no change to protocol. TELFA AMD resists bacterial colonization within the dressing and reduces bacterial penetration through the dressing. Broad-spectrum effectiveness provides protection against gram-positive and gram-negative microorganisms, including MRSA and VRE. Nonadherent TELFA AMD won't disrupt healing tissue.

Indications
To protect lightly draining wounds, including surgical site wounds and central or peripheral I.V. sites

Contraindications
■ None provided by the manufacturer

Application
■ Apply TELFA AMD as a primary dressing.

Removal
■ Gently remove dressing.

ANTIMICROBIALS

Collagens

Action

Collagen, the most abundant protein in the body, is fibrous and insoluble and is produced by fibroblasts. Its fibers are found in connective tissues, including skin, bones, ligaments, and cartilage. During wound healing, collagen encourages the deposition and organization of newly formed collagen fibers and granulation tissue in the wound bed. It also stimulates new tissue development and wound debridement, creating an environment conducive to healing. Collagen dressings are manufactured as sheets, pads, particles, solutions, and gels.

Indications

Collagen dressings may be used as primary dressings for partial- and full-thickness wounds, infected and noninfected wounds, tunneling wounds, wounds with minimal to heavy exudate (depending on the form of collagen dressing), skin grafts, donor sites, and red or yellow wounds.

Advantages

- Are absorbent
- Maintain a moist, wound-healing environment
- May be used in combination with topical agents
- Conform well to a wound surface
- Are nonadherent
- Are easy to apply and remove

Disadvantages

- Aren't recommended for third-degree burns
- Aren't recommended for black wounds
- Require a secondary dressing

HCPCS code overview

The HCPCS codes normally assigned to collagen dressings are:
A6021—pad size < 16 in^2
A6022—pad size > 16 in^2 but < 48 in^2
A6023—pad size > 48 in^2.
 The HCPCS codes normally assigned to collagen wound fillers are:
A6010—wound filler, dry form, per gram of collagen
A6011—wound filler, gel/paste, per gram of collagen
A6024—wound filler, per 6" (15 cm).

BGC Matrix Wound Dressing
Brennen Medical, Inc.

How supplied
Patch: 2.5″ × 3″; A6021
Sheet: 5″ × 6″; A6022
          5″ × 12″; A6023

Action
BGC Matrix is a temporary, multifilament, mesh matrix wound dressing. It combines the highly advanced oat beta-glucan technology with collagen, which provides structural support for new cell growth. BGC Matrix provides a moist environment that supports the autolytic debridement of wounds with scattered areas of necrosis and slough.

Indications
To manage partial-thickness burns, ulcers, donor sites, chronic wounds, and other shallow or abrasive wounds

Contraindications
- Contraindicated for third-degree burns and for wounds with large amounts of eschar
- Contraindicated on patients with a sensitivity to plant extracts or collagen
- Contraindicated on patients with a history of multiple serum allergies

Application
- Prepare the wound by removing (debriding) dead or necrotic tissue, eschar, or foreign debris. Cleanse the wound with normal saline solution or other noncytotoxic wound cleanser.
- Apply the mesh side of the dressing to the wound surface, film side up. (Dressing is labeled "This Side Up.") If the wound bed is dry, or to increase dressing pliability, lightly moisten the dressing with sterile saline before application.
- Smooth the BGC Matrix into place on the wound surface. Avoid any wrinkling; the BGC Matrix should have intimate contact with the wound bed. If necessary, overlap adjoining pieces of Matrix to provide total wound coverage. Cut edges to fit wound.
- For deep wounds, cut the BGC Matrix to fit the size of the wound bed. Push it gently into the wound so dressing is in contact with wound bed. Then lightly pack the wound with dry gauze if wound is heavily exudating, or moist gauze if wound is dry.
- If the wound is exudative, apply a nonadherent absorbent secondary dressing over the BGC Matrix, and secure in place. If the wound is nonexudative, apply a secondary dressing to maintain moisture at the wound base, and secure in place.

COLLAGENS

- After 24 hours, remove the secondary dressing and inspect the wound. If the wound is still draining, leave the BGC Matrix in place and reapply a clean absorbent outer dressing. Inspect daily.
- If the BGC Matrix is adherent and the film layer is intact, see Removal.
- If any signs of infection are present, remove the BGC Matrix dressing, clean the wound site and reapply a new dressing. Treat infection per normal prescribed protocol.
- You may see an increase of exudate during the first few days of the BGC Matrix application.
- BGC Matrix may be left on the wound for up to 72 hours. Check secondary dressing every 24 hours. If "strikethrough" is evident, or outer dressing is saturated with exudate, remove outer dressing and replace. Note: The Matrix mesh will not dissolve.

Removal

- BGC Matrix will occasionally adhere to red, granulating tissue. To remove an adherent BGC Matrix dressing, apply a normal saline moistened gauze, amorphous hydrogel, or topical ointment over the BGC Matrix, then lightly cover with a nonadherent secondary dressing. Leave in place for 24 hours.
- After 24 hours, carefully lift the dressing off the wound. To prevent damage to new tissue, never force the dressing from the wound; simply reapply gauze, hydrogel, or topical ointment to remaining adherent dressing, and attempt removal in 12 to 24 hours.
- When the outer secondary dressing is removed, you may observe an accumulation of yellow exudate. You may also detect an odor. Yellow exudate and odor may be normal occurrences when using dressings containing hydrocolloid; they're not necessarily signs of infection.

Cellerate RX Gel

The Hymed Group
Wound Care Innovations

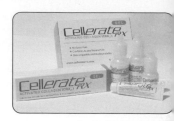

How supplied

Tube: 1 oz (28.4 g); A6011
        ¹/₄ oz (6 g); A6011

Action

Cellerate RX Gel—an all-natural product containing no preservatives, alcohol, or synthetic substances—interacts with the wound site to provide a moist environment that encourages healing. It protects the wound bed and newly formed granulation tissue by the formation of an occlusive gelatinous barrier, absorbs wound exudate, and promotes natural autolysis by rehydrating and softening necrotic tissue and eschar, which encourages autolytic debridement. It also reduces pain, soothes, and deodorizes. The product conforms to any wound site and is biocompatible and biodegradable.

Indications

To manage chronic and acute wounds and skin ulcers, such as pressure ulcers (stages 1, 2, 3, and 4), venous stasis ulcers, ulcers resulting from arterial insufficiency, surgical wounds, diabetic ulcers, traumatic wounds, superficial wounds, first- and second-degree burns, and other general dermatologic conditions

Contraindications

- None provided by the manufacturer

Application

- Clean the wound.
- Apply Cellerate RX Gel directly into the wound and onto the surrounding area.
- Cover the wound with a nonadherent dressing.

Removal

- Remove the secondary dressing, and reapply gel every 24 hours or as needed.
- To ease removal, soak the dressing in warm water.

COLLAGENS

Cellerate RX Powder

The Hymed Group
Wound Care Innovations

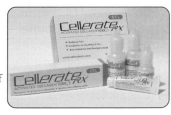

How supplied

Powder: 1 g (box of 24), 5 g (box of
          12); 20 g; 40 g; A6010

Action

A medical hydrolysate of type I collagen, Cellerate RX Powder interacts with
the wound site, forming a gel when it mixes with wound exudate and providing a moist healing environment. Naturally absorbent, Cellerate protects the wound bed and newly formed granulation tissue by forming an
occlusive gelatinous barrier, controls the evaporation of fluid, reduces pain,
and soothes and deodorizes. The product conforms to any wound site and
is biocompatible and biodegradable.

Indications

To manage chronic and acute wounds and skin ulcers, including pressure
ulcers (stages 1, 2, 3, and 4), venous stasis ulcers, diabetic ulcers, first- and
second-degree burns, ulcers resulting from arterial insufficiency, surgical
wounds, traumatic wounds, and superficial wounds

Contraindications

- None provided by the manufacturer

Application

- Clean the wound site, leaving the wound moist.
- Apply Cellerate RX Powder directly to the wound site to about ¼" (0.6
  cm) thickness.
- Cover the wound with a nonadherent dressing (gauze or polyurethane
  film).

Removal

- Change the secondary dressing, and reapply Cellerate RX Powder every
  24 hours or as needed.
- Cellerate RX Powder doesn't need to be removed with subsequent dressing changes.

COLLAGENS

FIBRACOL PLUS Collagen Wound Dressing with Alginate

Johnson & Johnson
Wound Management
A division of ETHICON, Inc.

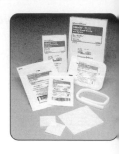

How supplied

Pad: 2″ × 2″; A6021
       4″ × 4³/₈″; A6022
       4″ × 8³/₄″; A6023
Rope: ³/₈″ × ³/₈″ × 15³/₄″; A6024

Action

FIBRACOL PLUS Collagen Wound Dressing with Alginate combines the strength and structural support of collagen and the gel-forming properties of alginate into a soft, highly absorbent, and conformable topical wound dressing. FIBRACOL PLUS Dressing is made of 90% collagen and 10% alginate. It maintains a physiologically moist microenvironment at the wound surface that is conducive to granulation tissue formation and epithelialization and enables healing to proceed at a rapid rate. FIBRACOL PLUS Dressing is versatile as a primary wound dressing. It can be cut to the exact size of the wound, multilayered to manage deep wounds, and used with either a semiocclusive or a nonocclusive secondary dressing.

Indications

To manage partial- and full-thickness wounds, including pressure ulcers, venous ulcers, ulcers with mixed vascular causes, diabetic ulcers, second-degree burns, donor sites and other bleeding surface wounds, abrasions, traumatic wounds healing by secondary intention, and dehisced surgical incisions; may be used when visible signs of infection are present in the wound area only when proper medical treatment addresses the underlying cause; may be used under compression therapy, under a physician's supervision

Contraindications

- Contraindicated for wounds with active vasculitis
- Contraindicated for third-degree burns
- Not recommended on patients with sensitivity to collagen or alginates

Application

- Debride when necessary.
- Irrigate wound site with normal saline solution.
- Cut dressing to the general size of the wound with clean scissors.
- For heavily exuding wounds, apply to the wound bed.
- Loosely pack deep wounds.
- For wounds with minimal exudate, apply to a moistened wound bed to initiate gel-forming process.

- Cover with appropriate secondary dressing based on the amount of exudate, such as TIELLE Hydropolymer Adhesive Dressing for low to moderately exuding wounds and TIELLE PLUS Hydropolymer Adhesive Dressing for moderately to heavily exuding wounds.

Removal

- Remove secondary dressing.
- Clean the wound with normal saline solution.
- May be reapplied daily or per physician's recommendation. Frequency of reapplication depends on level of exudate.

PROMOGRAN Matrix
Johnson & Johnson
Wound Management
A division of ETHICON, Inc.

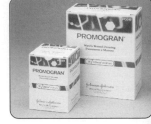

How supplied
Dressing: 4.34" × 4.34"; A6021
            19.1" × 19.1"; A6022

Action
PROMOGRAN Matrix uses a unique combination of 45% oxidized regenerated cellulose (ORC) and 55% collagen. This combination binds and inactivates matrix metalloproteases, creating an environment that results in rapid wound healing.

Indications
To manage exuding wounds, including diabetic foot ulcers, venous ulcers, pressure ulcers, ulcers of mixed vascular causes, full- and partial-thickness wounds, donor sites and other bleeding surface wounds, abrasions, traumatic wounds healing by secondary intention, and dehisced surgical wounds; may be used under compression therapy, under a physician's supervision; may be used when visible signs of infection are present in the wound area only when proper medical treatment addresses the underlying cause

Contraindications
- Not indicated for wounds with active vasculitis
- Not indicated for third-degree burns
- Not indicated for patients with sensitivity to ORC or collagen

Application
- Before applying the dressing, debride necrotic tissue and treat infection per facility protocol, if necessary.
- For wounds with low or no exudate, hydrate the dressing with saline.
- Apply the dressing directly to wound, covering the entire wound bed. (The dressing forms a gel on contact with exudate or through saline hydration.)
- Cover the dressing with a secondary dressing to maintain a moist healing environment. Choose an appropriate secondary dressing depending on amount of exudate.
- Dressing may be reapplied daily or as directed by the physician. Frequency of reapplication depends on amount of exudate.

Removal
- It's unnecessary to remove residual PROMOGRAN Matrix during dressing changes. (It's biodegradable in a moist healing environment.)

COLLAGENS

PROMOGRAN PRISMA Matrix

Johnson & Johnson
Wound Management
A division of ETHICON, Inc.

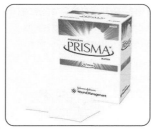

How supplied

Dressing: 28 cm² (4.34″ × 4.34″); A6021
123 cm² (19.1″ × 19.1″); A6022

Action

PRISMA Matrix is designed to provide protection and growth by addressing the continuous changes in the wound microenvironment. The unique formulation of 55% collagen, 44% oxidized regenerated cellulose (ORC), and 1% silver–ORC absorbs destructive components of chronic wound fluid and creates the optimal environment for cellular growth. Additionally, PRISMA Matrix kills clinically relevant bacteria in the dressing that helps lessen bacterial bioburden and thus may result in reduced risk of infection.

Indication

To manage exuding wounds; under the supervision of a health care professional, may be used for the management of diabetic foot ulcers, venous ulcers, pressure ulcers, and ulcers caused by mixed vascular etiologies; full-and partial-thickness wounds; donor sites and other bleeding surface wounds; abrasions, traumatic wounds healing by secondary intention, and dehisced surgical wounds; may be used under compression therapy with health care professional supervision

Contraindication

- Contraindicated for patients with third-degree burns
- Contraindicated for patients with sensitivity to silver, ORC, or collagen

Application

- Cut or tear dressing to size of wound; apply directly to whole wound bed.
- After hydration, through exposure to wound exudate or saline, the PRISMA Matrix will turn gelatinous and become intimately in contact with the wound surface.
- The biodegradable PRISMA Matrix is gradually absorbed into the body.
- In order to maintain a moist wound environment, PRISMA Matrix must be covered with a semiocclusive dressing.
- Apply daily or per physician's recommendation.
- Frequency of reapplication depends of the level of exudate.

Removal

- It isn't necessary to remove any residual PRISMA Matrix during dressing changes.

COLLAGENS

Puracol and Puracol Plus Collagen Dressings

Medline Industries, Inc.

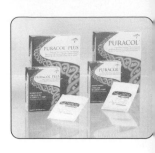

How supplied

Pad:

Puracol

    1 mm thick 2″ × 2″; A6021

    1 mm thick 4″ × 4.25″; A6022

Puracol Plus

    2 mm thick 2″ × 2.25″; A6021

    2 mm thick 4.25″ × 4.50″; A6022

Action

Puracol and Puracol Plus MicroScaffold Wound Dressing is an advanced wound care product composed of pure collagen. This unique, sterile biomaterial forms a soft, conformable moist gel sheet at the wound surface, promoting natural healing. The collagen-based, moist microenvironment provides an ideal scaffold for the infiltration, proliferation, and growth of cells involved in natural wound healing, allowing optimal levels of granular tissue formation and rapid epithelialization. The porous microstructure of the product promotes capillary action, which in turn adds to the intrinsic absorbency of native collagen. The absorbent nature of the dressing further allows for the removal of necrotic tissue fragments, exudate, and miscellaneous debris from the wound site.

The dressing can be used as a primary dressing or in combination with other traditional or advanced wound dressings of occlusive or semiocclusive nature. The dressing can be cut to any size to fit any wound. The Puracol Plus offers twice the available collagen as standard Puracol.

Indications

To manage chronic and acute, partial- and full-thickness wounds, including superficial wounds, minor abrasions, skin tears, second-degree burns, pressure ulcers, lower-extremity ulcers (venous, arterial, and mixed), diabetic ulcers, dehisced surgical wounds, and donor sites

Contraindications

- Contraindicated on patients who are allergic to collagen or who have active vasculitis; should be discontinued if signs of sensitization occur
- Not suitable for third-degree burns

Application

- Clean the wound using Skintegrity Wound Cleanser or an appropriate solution. Dry the surrounding skin to allow secure adhesion of the dressing.
- The product should be directly applied to the wound and may be moistened with saline to preform the gel if the wound bed is very dry.
- The dressing may be cut to size or shape to better match the wound area

COLLAGENS

- The product should be covered with a suitable secondary dressing (such as SureSite Film Dressings, Optifoam, or Optifoam Ag foam dressings, StrataSorb, or a bordered gauze) in order to maintain the moist wound environment.
- Change the dressing as best wound care practice suggests. A heavily exuding wound may require more frequent dressing replacement.
- The dressing may be left in the wound for up to 7 days or replaced at the discretion of the health care professional. The product is 100% pure collagen and is completely biodegradable.

Removal

- The dressing may be replaced at the discretion of the health care professional or left in place for up to 7 days or until exudate is visible and nears the edge of the dressing.
- Gently remove the outer dressing, irrigate, and reapply a new collagen dressing if appropriate.

Stimulen
Southwest Technologies, Inc.

How supplied

Powder:	1 g (10 packs/box, 10 boxes/case); A6010
	20 g (12 bottles/case); A6010
	40 g (4 bottles/case); A6010
Amorphous gel:	1 oz (12 tubes/case); A6010
	3 oz (6 tubes/case) ; A6010
Sheets:	2" × 3" (5 boxes, 40 boxes/case = 200) ; A6010
	4" × 4" (5 boxes, 20 boxes/case = 100) ; A6010
Lotion:	2 oz (12 bottles/case) ; A6010
	4 oz (6 bottles/case) ; A6010

Action
Stimulen is a new collagen line that comes in four forms: powder (which is 100% collagen), amorphous gel, sheets, and lotion are combined with glycerin to add the bacteriostatic properties. These collagen products are combined with long and short polypeptides. The long strands offer a "bridge" to connect wound edge to wound edge, providing a lattice, and the short are broken down into the amino acid form so that the body can readily use and create a healing environment especially suited for the rapid regeneration of tissue skin.

Indications
Lotion used for topical therapies such as cracked heels, herpes, facial lesions, rashes, psoriasis; sheets are soluble and will melt when in contact with wound exudate, leaving collagen and glycerin in the wound bed; amorphous gel used for deep craters or tunneling wounds; all forms used for stalled wounds or wounds in compromised patients—with diabetes, for full- and partial-thickness wounds, pressure ulcers, venous and diabetic ulcers, partial-thickness burns, acute and chronic wounds, and traumatic wounds healing by secondary intention

Contraindications
- None provided by the manufacturer

Application
Powder
- Prepare the wound site using the standard protocol. If the wound is highly contaminated, a preliminary treatment to reduce bioburden may be appropriate.
- Open the package, and apply Stimulen to the wound site. Apply a generous covering of powder over the entire wound surface, $1/32$" to $1/8$" deep.

COLLAGENS

The nature of the wound will be a factor to consider when applying the product.

■ Cover the dressing with a nonadherent secondary dressing, and secure with tape or appropriate covering.

■ Maintain a moist, not wet, wound healing environment.

■ Change the secondary dressing, and reapply the Stimulen powder daily or as needed.

Amorphous gel

■ Before use, remove cap and peel off the safety seal.

■ Cleanse the wound using standard protocol.

■ Apply a generous coating of the amorphous gel onto wound site, or fill wound cavity

■ Cover the dressing with a nonadherent secondary dressing, and secure with tape or appropriate covering.

■ Change the secondary dressing, and reapply the Stimulen powder daily or as needed.

Gel sheet

■ Prepare the wound site using the standard protocol. If the wound is highly contaminated, a preliminary treatment to reduce bioburden may be appropriate.

■ Open the package, and apply Stimulen the wound site. The nature of the wound will be a factor to consider when applying the product. Apply a gel sheet that is approximately the same size as the wound; cut to size. *Note:* The Stimulen gel sheet is soluble and will form a gel in the wound cavity.

■ Cover the dressing with a nonadherent secondary dressing, and secure with tape or appropriate covering.

■ Change the secondary dressing, and reapply the Stimulen gel daily or as needed.

Lotion

■ Before use, remove cap and peel off the safety seal.

■ Cleanse the wound using standard protocol.

■ Apply 2 to 4 drops of the lotion, and spread evenly over the affected area.

Removal

■ Remove the dressing, gel, sheet, or lotion according to your facility's policy.

COMPOSITES

Composites

Action

Composite dressings combine two or more physically distinct products and are manufactured as a single dressing with several functions. Features must include a physical (not chemical) bacterial barrier that is present over the entire dressing pad and extends out into the adhesive border; an absorptive layer other than an alginate or other fiber-gelling dressing, foam, hydrocolloid, or hydrogel; and either a semiadherent or nonadherent property over the wound site.

Indications

Composite dressings may be used as primary or secondary dressings for partial- and full-thickness wounds with minimal to heavy exudate, healthy granulation tissue, or necrotic tissue (slough or moist eschar), or mixed wounds (granulation and necrotic tissue).

Advantages

- May facilitate autolytic debridement
- Allow for exchange of moisture vapor
- Mold well
- May be used on infected wounds
- Are easy to apply and remove
- Include an adhesive border

Disadvantages

- Require a border of intact skin for anchoring the dressing

HCPCS code overview

The HCPCS codes normally assigned to composite dressings with an adhesive border are:

A6203—pad size ≤ 16 in^2

A6204—pad size > 16 in^2 but ≤ 48 in^2

A6205—pad size > 48 in^2.

Alldress
Mölnlycke Health Care

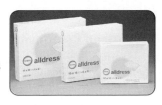

How supplied
Cover dressing: 4" × 4", 6" × 6"; A6203
6" × 8"; A6204

Action
Alldress is a multilayered, waterproof, all-in-one sterile wound dressing; each layer serves a purpose. The porous contact layer is low-adherent and protects the wound surface. An absorbent layer wicks away excess exudate and debris, minimizing exposure of intact skin to moisture and maceration. A gentle adhesive holds the dressing securely in place, and the nonwoven layer provides stability to the dressing structure for ease of application. A semipermeable film layer maintains a moist wound environment and at the same time protects the wound from external environmental contamination and doesn't let wound fluid pass through the dressing. The smooth surface reduces the friction from bed linen and clothing and potential disturbance of the dressing.

Indications
For use as a primary or secondary cover dressing through all phases of healing for pressure ulcers (stages 1, 2, 3, and 4); partial- and full-thickness wounds; tunneling wounds; infected and noninfected wounds; wounds with minimal, moderate, or heavy drainage; wounds with serosanguineous or purulent drainage; and red, yellow, or black wounds

Contraindications
- None provided by the manufacturer

Application
- If necessary, gently irrigate or flush the wound with normal saline solution or another nonirritating solution.
- Gently blot excess saline solution in the wound with sterile gauze.
- Remove one side of the dressing's backing, and place the other side on the skin. Be careful not to stretch the dressing over the wound.
- Smooth the edges to ensure secure adhesion.

Removal
- Change the dressing when it's nearly saturated (soaking is visible through the outer surface of the dressing) or as required by the product.

New Product

Borderless Composite Dressing

Medline Industries, Inc.

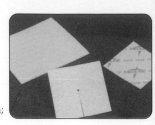

How supplied

Pad: 3″ × 3″, 3″ × 3″ with fenestration; A6200

5″ × 5″; A6201

Action

Borderless Composite Dressing is a four-layer composite dressing that absorbs exudate, protects the wound, and keeps it moist. It consists of a nonadherent wound contact layer, an absorbent soaker, and a waterproof, bacteria-resistant outer layer.

Indications

To manage pressure ulcers (stages 1, 2, 3, and 4), partial- and full-thickness wounds, tunneling wounds, infected and noninfected wounds, wounds with minimal to heavy drainage, wounds with serosanguineous or purulent drainage, and red, yellow, or black wounds

Contraindications

■ None provided by the manufacturer

Application

■ Clean the application site with normal saline solution or an appropriate cleanser, such as Skintegrity Wound Cleanser. Dry the surrounding area.
■ Select the appropriate dressing size for the wound. Make sure the dressing extends 1¼″ to 1½″ (3 to 4 cm) beyond the wound so the dressing can be attached to healthy tissue.
■ Secure with tape, elastic net, or roll gauze as appropriate.

Removal

■ Change the dressing as indicated by the wound's condition and the amount of exudate or as the primary dressing indicates.
■ Gently remove the dressing.

Comfortell
GENTELL, Inc.

How supplied
Composite dressing: 6″ × 6″; A6203

Action
Comfortell is a multilayered wound dressing designed
with four distinctive layers. Dressing combines an excellent absorbent layer with a permeable barrier that allows the wound to breathe while keeping the contaminants out.

Indications
For use as a primary or secondary dressing on a wide variety of wounds

Contraindications
- None provided by the manufacturer

Application
- Peel backing from the center to expose pad.
- Apply the pad over the wound, making sure that tape doesn't touch the wound.
- Remove the backing and smooth the dressing.

Removal
- Carefully lift edges of dressing.
- Ease dressing from the wound.

CompDress Island Dressing

Derma Sciences, Inc.

How supplied
Pad: 2″ × 2″, 4″ × 4″, 4″ × 6″, 6″ × 6″, 4″ × 8″, 4″ × 10″, 6″ × 8″, 4″ × 14″

Action
CompDress is a sterile multilayer dressing combining a nonadherent gauze pad contact layer with a dressing retention tape.

Indications
For use as a primary or secondary dressing to manage acute and chronic lightly to moderately draining wounds

Contraindications
■ None provided by the manufacturer

Application
■ Clean the wound with PrimaDerm Dermal Cleanser or solution.
■ Pat dry the skin adjacent to the wound.
■ Peel back the dressing's backing, and position dressing over the wound.
■ Smooth the dressing edges to ensure secure adhesion.

Removal
■ Gently lift the edge of the dressing.
■ Continue around the perimeter of the dressing until it lifts off easily.

Covaderm Plus
DeRoyal

How supplied
Multilayered pad with fabric tape border: 1″ pad
with 2″ tape, 1½″pad with 2½″tape,
2½″pad with 4″ tape, 2″ × 7½″ pad
with 4″ × 10″ tape; A6203
4″ pad with 6″ tape, 2½″ diameter pad
with 4″ diameter tape with 2″ radial slit;
A6203
2″ × 11″ pad with 4″ × 14″ tape, 4″ × 6″ pad with 6″ × 8″ tape;
A6204

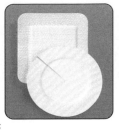

COMPOSITES

Action
Covaderm Plus is an adhesive barrier composite wound dressing that consists of a protective, nonadherent wound contact layer; a soft drainage absorption pad; a semiocclusive polyurethane film (to maintain moisture, prevent contamination, and allow vapor transmission); and a conformable adhesive tape border.

Indications
For use as a primary or secondary dressing to manage pressure ulcers (stages 1, 2, 3, and 4), leg ulcers, I.V. sites, chronic wounds, and surgical wounds; may also be used on partial- and full-thickness wounds, burns, tunneling wounds, infected and noninfected wounds, wounds with moderate drainage, wounds with serosanguineous or purulent drainage, and red, yellow, or black wounds; may also be used to cover orthopedic incisions and joint pins under casts

Contraindications
- None provided by the manufacturer

Application
- Peel the dressing's backing from the center to expose the pad.
- Apply the pad over the cleansed wound, making sure that adhesive tape doesn't touch the wound site.
- Remove the product's backing one side at a time, and smooth the dressing into place.

Removal
- Carefully lift the edges of the tape, and peel off the dressing.

COMPOSITES

Covaderm Plus VAD
DeRoyal

How supplied
Multilayered dressing: 4″ × 4″, 6″ × 6″;
                          A6203

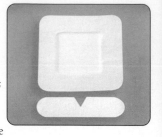

Action
The Covaderm Plus Vascular Access Device
(VAD) dressing is a multilayered dressing that provides protection, bacterial barrier, absorption, cushioning, and conformability and also has an extra tape that is uniquely shaped to seal around the vascular access catheter extension.

Indication
For use with central venous catheter sites (subclavian, jugular, femoral, and antecubital); peripheral I.V. sites; implanted parts; and midline catheters

Contraindication
- None provided by the manufacturer

Application
- Peel the dressing's backing from the center to expose the pad.
- Apply the pad over the cleansed wound, making sure that adhesive tape doesn't touch the wound site.
- Remove the product's backing one side at a time, and smooth the dressing into place.

Removal
- Carefully lift the edges of the tape, and peel off the dressing.

DermaDress
DermaRite Industries, LLC

How supplied
Dressing: 4″ × 4″, 6″ × 6″; A6203

Action
DermaDress is a multilayered waterproof
sterile dressing. A low-adherent layer protects the wound, a semiocclusive layer keeps external contamination from striking through, and a nonwoven adhesive tape holds the dressing in place.

Indications
For use as a primary or secondary dressing to manage pressure ulcers (stages 1, 2, 3, and 4); full-thickness wounds; wounds with minimal, moderate, or heavy drainage; and red, yellow, or black wounds

Contraindications
- None provided by the manufacturer

Application
- Clean the wound with DermaKlenz wound cleanser.
- Remove one side of the backing, and place the dressing over the wound.
- Remove the remaining backing to cover the wound entirely.
- Secure the edges of the dressing with gentle pressure.

Removal
- Carefully loosen the perimeter of the dressing.
- Holding down one edge of the dressing, gently lift dressing.

DuDress Film Top Island Dressing
Derma Sciences, Inc.

How supplied
Pad: 4″ × 4″, 6″ × 6″, 6″ × 8″

Action
DuDress is a sterile multilayer dressing composed of a nonadherent, gauze pad contact layer and a transparent film top layer.

Indications
For use as a primary or secondary dressing to manage acute and chronic lightly to moderately draining wounds; waterproof to allow bathing, reducing unnecessary dressing changes

Contraindications
- None provided by the manufacturer

Application
- Clean the wound with PrimaDerm Dermal Cleanser or saline solution.
- Pat dry the skin adjacent to the wound.
- Peel back the dressing's backing, and position the dressing over the wound.
- Smooth the dressing edges to ensure secure adhesion.

Removal
- Lift the edge of the dressing.
- Gently stretch the dressing to facilitate removal.
- Continue around the perimeter of the dressing until it lifts off easily.

MPM Multi-Layered Dressing (Bordered)

MPM Medical, Inc.

How supplied

Pad: 4″ × 4″, 6″ × 6″; A6203
6″ × 8″; A6204

Action

MPM Multi-Layered Dressing (Bordered) is a nonadherent, absorbent dressing with a protective adhesive backing that allows for moisture vapor transfer. The dressing provides a moist environment that facilitates wound healing

Indications

To manage pressure ulcers (stages 1, 2, 3, and 4); partial- and full-thickness wounds, surgical incisions, dehisced incisions, tunneling wounds, infected and noninfected wounds, wounds with moderate to heavy serosanguineous and purulent drainage, and red, yellow, or black wounds

Contraindications

- None provided by the manufacturer

Application

- Clean the wound with MPM Wound Cleanser or normal saline solutions.
- Peel back and release the dressing's backing to expose the pad.
- Apply the pad over the wound, and finish removing the backing.
- Smooth the dressing into place.

Removal

- Carefully lift the edge of the tape, and peel off the dressing

COMPOSITES

MPM Multi-Layered Dressing (Non-Bordered)
MPM Medical, Inc.

How supplied
Pad: 2″ × 2″, 4″ × 4″; A6200
         6″ × 6″, 8″ × 10″; A6201

Action
MPM Multi-Layered Dressing (Non-Bordered) is a nonadherent, absorbent dressing with a protective adhesive backing that allows for moisture vapor transfer. The dressing provides a moist environment that facilitates wound healing.

Indications
To manage pressure ulcers (stages 1, 2, 3, and 4); partial- and full-thickness wounds, surgical incisions, dehisced incisions, tunneling wounds, infected and noninfected wounds, wounds with moderate to heavy serosanguineous and purulent drainage, and red, yellow, or black wounds

Contraindications
- None provided by the manufacturer

Application
- Clean the wound with MPM Wound Cleanser.
- Remove pad from pouch, and, if necessary, cut to fit the wound. Adhere to patient using hypoallergenic tape.

Removal
- Remove pad from wound according to protocol or when saturated.

OpSite Post-Op Composite Dressing

Smith & Nephew, Inc.
Wound Management

How supplied

Dressing: $2^1/2'' \times 2''$ with $1^1/2'' \times {}^1/2''$ pad, $3^1/4'' \times 3^3/8''$ with
$3'' \times 1^1/5''$ pad, $4^3/4'' \times 4''$ with $3'' \times 2''$ pad, $6^1/8'' \times 3^1/8''$ with
$5'' \times 1^1/2''$ pad, $8'' \times 4''$ with $6'' \times 2''$ pad, $10'' \times 4''$ with $8'' \times$
$2''$ pad; A6203
$11^3/4'' \times 4''$ with $10'' \times 2''$ pad, $13^1/4'' \times 4''$ with
$11^3/4'' \times 2''$ pad; A6204

Action

OpSite Post-Op Composite Dressings combine OpSite transparent film with an absorbent, nonadherent pad. Drainage can be monitored without disturbing the dressing. Moisture vapor permeability combined with non-sensitizing adhesive allows the wound and the skin under the dressing to breathe. The dressing stays in place, reducing the risk of maceration. The OpSite film is impermeable to water and body fluids. The pad is highly absorbent, minimizing the number of dressing changes. Its nonadherent surface leaves the wound site undisturbed, reducing pain and wound trauma during dressing changes.

Indications

For use as primary dressings for skin tears, pressure ulcers (stages 1, 2, and 3), postoperative and arthroscopic wounds, minor cuts, and lacerations; may also be used as secondary dressings over gels and alginates

Contraindications

■ None provided by the manufacturer

Application

■ Remove one backing tab, and place the dressing over the wound.
■ Peel off the remaining backing while smoothing the dressing onto the skin.
■ Remove the film carrier.

Removal

■ Grasp a corner of the dressing's clear film, and pull it parallel to the skin. This stretching action releases the adhesive for gentle removal.
■ Continue stretching around the circumference of the dressing, and then lift it off.

COMPOSITES

Repel Wound Dressing

MPM Medical, Inc.

How supplied

Pad: 4″ × 4″ ; A6203
          6″ × 6″, 6″ × 8″; A6204

Action

Repel Wound Dressing is a nonadherent island dressing with a waterproof protective backing and an adhesive border that allows for moisture vapor transfer. Repel Wound Dressing maintains a moist wound environment that facilitates wound healing.

Indications

To manage pressure ulcers (stages 2, 3, and 4), venous stasis ulcers, partial- and full-thickness wounds, surgical incisions, tunneling wounds, infected and noninfected wounds, and moderately to heavily draining wounds

Contraindications

- None provided by the manufacturer

Application

- Clean the wound with MPM Wound Cleanser or normal saline solution.
- Peel back the dressing's backing to expose the pad.
- Apply the pad over the wound, and finish removing the backing.
- Smooth the dressing into place.

Removal

- Carefully lift the edge of the tape, and peel off the pad.

Stratasorb
Medline Industries, Inc.

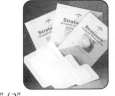

How supplied
Island dressing: 4″ × 4″ (2.5″ × 2″ pad)
6″ × 6″ (4″ × 4″ pad)
4″ × 10″ (2″ × 8″ pad); A6203
6″ × 7.5″ (4″ × 6″ pad), 4″ × 14″ (2″ × 12″ pad); A6204

Action
Stratasorb is a four-layer composite island dressing that absorbs exudate, protects the wound, and keeps it moist. It consists of a nonadherent wound contact layer, an absorbent soaker, a nonwoven adhesive border, and a waterproof, bacteria-resistant outer layer.

Indications
To manage pressure ulcers (stages 1, 2, 3, and 4), partial- and full-thickness wounds, tunneling wounds, infected and noninfected wounds, wounds with minimal to heavy drainage, wounds with serosanguineous or purulent drainage, and red, yellow, or black wounds

Contraindications
■ None provided by the manufacturer

Application
■ Clean the application site with normal saline solution or an appropriate cleanser, such as Skintegrity Wound Cleanser. Dry the surrounding area to ensure that it's free from any greasy substance.
■ Select the appropriate dressing size for the wound. Make sure the dressing extends 1¼″ to 1½″ (3 to 4 cm) beyond the wound so the dressing can attach to healthy tissue.
■ Remove one side of the dressing's paper backing, and apply the exposed adhesive to the skin.
■ Remove the second side of the paper backing, and apply the remaining adhesive, being careful not to stretch the dressing.

Removal
■ Change the dressing as indicated by the wound's condition and the amount of exudate or as the primary dressing indicates.
■ Lift the dressing by one edge, and peel it back while holding the skin edge.
■ Repeat cleansing procedure before applying a new dressing.

COMPOSITES

Suresite 123 + Pad Composite Island Film Dressing
Medline Industries, Inc.

How supplied
Island dressing: 2.4″ × 2.8″ (1.3″ × 1.6″ pad), 4″ × 4.8″ (2.4″ × 3.2″ pad)

Action
Suresite 123 + Pad is a composite island dressing constructed with a nonadherent, absorbent center pad and transparent film, waterproof adhesive border. This dressing absorbs exudate, protects the wound, and keeps it moist.

Indications
To manage pressure ulcers (stages 1, 2, 3, and 4), partial- and full-thickness wounds, tunneling wounds, infected and noninfected wounds, wounds with minimal to heavy drainage, wounds with serosanguineous or purulent drainage, and red, yellow, or black wounds

Contraindications
- None provided by the manufacturer

Application
- Clean the application site with normal saline solution or an appropriate cleanser, such as Skintegrity Wound Cleanser. Dry the surrounding area to ensure that it's free from any greasy substance.
- Select the appropriate dressing size for the wound. Make sure the dressing extends 1¼″ to 1½″ (3 to 4 cm) beyond the wound so the dressing can attach to healthy tissue.
- Remove one side of the dressing's paper backing, and apply the exposed adhesive to the skin.
- Remove the second side of the paper backing, and apply the remaining adhesive, being careful not to stretch the dressing.
- Remove the top, paper liner from the center S-curve split.

Removal
- Change the dressing as indicated by the wound's condition and the amount of exudate or as the primary dressing indicates.
- Lift the dressing by one edge, stretch laterally to the skin surface to release the adhesive from the skin.

TELFA Adhesive Dressing
Tyco Healthcare/Kendall

How supplied
Pad: 2″ × 3″, 3″ × 4″

Action
TELFA Adhesive Dressing is made of highly absorbent, nonwoven cotton fabric on both sides. Adhesive strips keep the dressing intact. The nonadherent surface permits nontraumatic removal.

Indications
For use as a primary dressing on lightly draining wounds; may also be used on pressure ulcers (stages 1 and 2), partial-thickness wounds, infected and noninfected wounds, wounds with minimal drainage, and red wounds

Contraindications
- Contraindicated for heavily draining wounds

Application
- Clean the wound with normal saline solution or a cleansing agent.
- Apply the dressing over the wound, and smooth the adhesive onto the periwound skin.

Removal
- Gently remove the soiled dressing, taking care not to disturb the wound bed.

COMPOSITES

TELFA Island Dressing

Tyco Healthcare/Kendall

How supplied

Pad: 2" × 3³/₄" 4" × 4", 4" × 5"; A6219
         4" × 8", 4" × 10", 6" × 6"; A6220
         4" × 14"; A6221

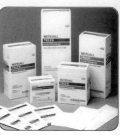

Action

TELFA Island Dressing has a soft, nonwoven backing that conforms to the wound and seals all four sides. The dressing protects the wound from the external environment, and the nonadherent surface allows nontraumatic removal.

Indications

To manage lightly draining wounds and to act as a securing dressing for central and peripheral I.V. sites; may also be used on pressure ulcers (stages 1 and 2), infected and noninfected wounds, partial-thickness wounds, wounds with minimal drainage, and red wounds

Contraindications

■ Contraindicated for heavily draining wounds

Application

■ Clean the wound with normal saline solution or a cleansing agent.
■ Apply the dressing over the wound.
■ Secure the dressing with an appropriate material, such as tape.

Removal

■ Gently remove the soiled dressing, taking care not to disturb the wound bed.

Pressure ulcers

Stage 1

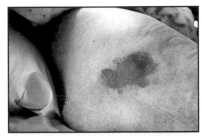

Stage 2

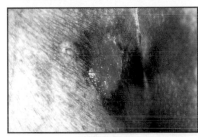

Stage 3

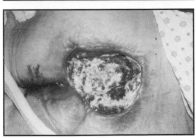

Stage 4

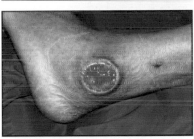

Pressure ulcers *(continued)*

Stage 4, hip prosthesis exposed

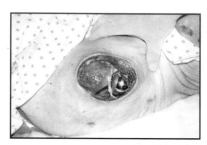

Unstageable, with slough and surrounding erythema

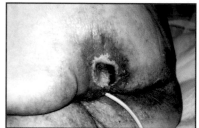

Unstageable, with eschar

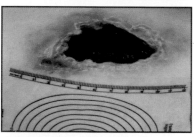

Deep tissue injury

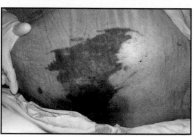

Wound healing by primary, secondary, or tertiary intention

Surgical wound healing by primary intention

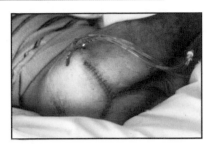

Full-thickness surgical wound healing by secondary intention

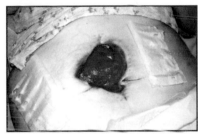

Pressure ulcer healing by secondary intention

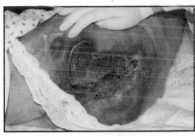

Surgical wound healing by tertiary intention

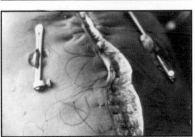

Lower leg and foot wounds

Arterial wound

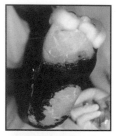

Venous ulcer

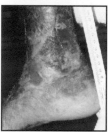

Vascular disease of the arteries and veins

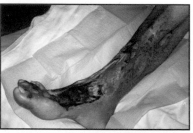

Diabetic foot ulcer

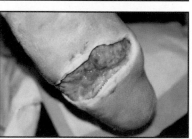

Wound types

Partial-thickness wound with skin tear

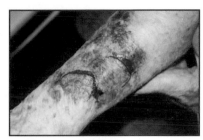

Full-thickness surgical wound (failed skin graft secondary to osteomyelitis)

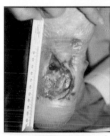

Full-thickness abdominal wound

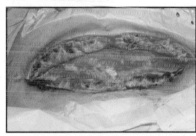

Full-thickness surgical wound

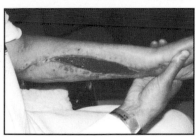

Wound tissue types

Granulation tissue

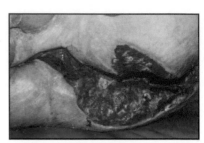

Slough with peri-wound erythema

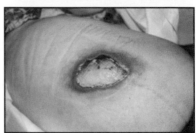

Eschar

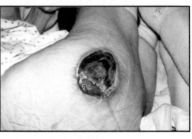

Hypergranulation tissue

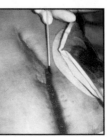

Skin conditions

Bruising

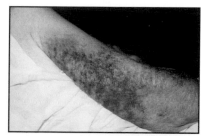

Candidiasis (yeast infection)

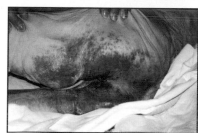

Xerotic skin around a partial-thickness wound

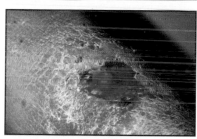

Hemosiderin staining

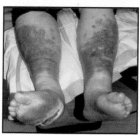

Measuring wounds

Measuring length

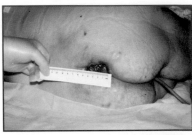

Measuring width

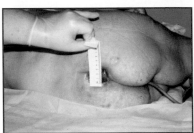

Measuring depth

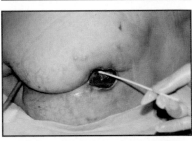

Measuring tunneling

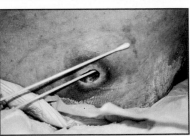

TELFA PLUS Island Dressing
Tyco Healthcare/Kendall

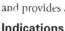

How supplied
Pad: 4″ × 6″; A6203
6″ × 7″, 6″ × 10″, 8″ × 8″; A6204

Action
TELFA PLUS Island Dressing absorbs moderate amounts of fluid, doesn't adhere to wounds, and provides a barrier to fluid and bacteria.

Indications
For use as a primary or secondary dressing and securing layer to manage surgical incisions, lacerations, central and peripheral I.V. sites, pressure ulcers (stages 1, 2, and 3), partial-thickness wounds, stasis ulcers, arterial ulcers, and diabetic ulcers. May also be used for wounds with light to moderate drainage, noninfected wounds, and red wounds

Contraindications
- Contraindicated for stage 4 pressure ulcers
- Contraindicated for full-thickness wounds, tunneling wounds, infected wounds, and heavily draining wounds

Application
- Clean the wound with a nontoxic cleansing solution, such as Constant Clens Wound Cleanser or normal saline solution.
- To remove excess cleanser or saline solution, gently pat the wound and surrounding skin with a sterile 4″ × 4″ gauze sponge. Be sure the surrounding skin is thoroughly dry to ensure a good seal between the skin and the dressing adhesive.
- Remove the dressing's release liners from the center out, position and apply the dressing over the wound, and then smooth the adhesive borders to ensure contact.

Removal
- Carefully peel back the island border and pad, taking care not to tear fragile skin or disturb the wound bed.

THINSite Hydrogel Dressing TRANSORBENT
Swiss-American Products, Inc.

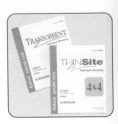

How supplied
THINSite Hydrogel Dressing
Sterile sheet: 4" × 4", 1 1/4" circular; A6203
6" × 6"; A6204
8" × 8"; A6205

TRANSORBENT
Sterile pad: 4" × 4"; A6203
6" × 6"; A6204
8" × 8"; A6205

Action
THINSite Hydrogel Dressing is a sterile, semiocclusive dressing made of a combination of super-thin layers. An adhesive layer bonds the dressing to intact skin around the wound to keep it in position until removal. The middle layer is an absorbent hydrogel that transfers exudate away from the wound and captures it to maintain a moist environment. The outermost layer is a semipermeable polyurethane film that allows moisture vapor to escape, reduces friction, and provides a smooth, easy-to-clean surface.

TRANSORBENT is a sterile, semiocclusive, multilayered dressing. Its adhesive layer bonds to intact skin to keep the dressing in position until removal. An absorbent hydrogel layer transfers exudate away from the wound and captures it to maintain a moist environment. A foam layer provides a pathway for the escape of moisture vapor and also makes the dressing soft and pliable, cushioning the wound. The outermost layer is a semipermeable polyurethane film that reduces friction and provides a smooth, easy-to-clean surface.

Indications
To manage partial- and full-thickness wounds, pressure ulcers (stages 1, 2, 3, and 4), and arterial and venous stasis leg ulcers; to aid in the prevention of skin breakdown; also indicated for use on postsurgical wounds, laparoscopic and biopsy sites, suture and drainage tube sites, minor abrasions, lacerations, and partial- and full-thickness dermatologic sites

Contraindications
- Contraindicated for ulcers resulting from infection, such as tuberculosis or syphilis, or deep fungal infections
- Not for use on third-degree burns

Application
- Clean the wound area thoroughly with normal saline solution or a similar wound-cleansing solution to ensure that the wound is free from foreign debris.

- Ensure that the surrounding skin is clean and dry and free from greasy material.
- Allow at least $1\frac{1}{4}''$ (3.2 cm) perimeter around the wound site for attachment.
- Grasping the dressing tab, position the dressing over wound site with tab sides downward.
- Peel away the tab from one side of dressing, and roll the dressing over the wound site.
- Remove the other tab.
- Secure the dressing by gently applying pressure to ensure that the wound surface comes in contact with the dressing.
- Framing the sides of the dressing with $1''$ (2.5 cm) hypoallergenic tape may improve wear time. Don't overlap dressings.
- Check the dressing daily for leakage or other problems.

Removal

- The dressing may be left in place for up to 1 week.
- To remove, gently press down on the skin, and carefully free the dressing edges one at a time.

COMPOSITES

3M Tegaderm + Pad Transparent Dressing with Absorbent Pad

3M Health Care

How supplied

Island: 2" × 2³/₄" (1" × 1¹/₂" pad);
2³/₈" × 4" (1" × 2³/₈" pad),
3¹/₂" × 4" (1³/₄" × 2³/₈" pad), 6" × 6" (4" × 4" pad),
3¹/₂" × 6" (1³/₄" × 4" pad), 3¹/₂" × 8" (1³/₄" × 4" pad),
3¹/₂" × 10" (1³/₄" × 8"); A6203
3¹/₂" × 13³/₄" (1³/₄" × 11³/₄" pad); A6204

Oval: 3¹/₂" × 4¹/₈" (1³/₄" × 11³/₄" pad); A6203

Action

The 3M Tegaderm + Pad Transparent Dressing with Absorbent Pad is a waterproof, bacterial barrier dressing that consists of a nonadherent, absorbent pad bonded to a larger thin film backing with a border of hypoallergenic, water-resistant adhesive.

Indications

To manage acute wounds, cuts, burns, abrasions, I.V. catheter sites, and surgical incisions; may also be used for superficial and partial-thickness chronic wounds

Contraindications

■ Not for replacing sutures or other primary wound closures

Application

■ Prepare the site for wound dressing or catheter insertion according to facility policy. To ensure dressing adhesion, clip excess hair at the site, but don't shave. Allow all preparation liquids to dry completely before applying the dressing.
■ Peel the paper liner from the paper-framed dressing, exposing the adhesive surface. Position the framed window over the wound site or catheter insertion site; apply the dressing.
■ Remove the paper frame from the dressing while smoothing down the dressing edges and sealing them securely around the wound or catheter.

Removal

■ Grasp the edge gently, and slowly peel the dressing from the skin in the direction of hair growth.

3M Tegaderm Absorbent Clear Acrylic Dressing
3M Health Care

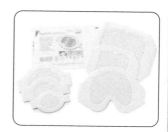

How supplied

Oval: $1^1/_2'' \times 2^1/_4''$, $2^3/_8'' \times 3''$,
           $3^3/_8'' \times 4^1/_4''$; A6203

Sacral: $4^1/_2'' \times 5''$; A6204

Square: $3^7/_8'' \times 4''$; A6203
           $5^7/_8'' \times 6''$; A6204

Action

3M Tegaderm Absorbent Clear Acrylic Dressing is a transparent, absorbent dressing for optimal clinical performance and wear time by allowing wound monitoring without changing the dressing. 3M Tegaderm Absorbent Clear Acrylic Dressing provides a moist wound environment, which promotes autolytic debridement. It's conformable, comfortable for patients, and easy to apply and remove.

Indications

For use on pressure ulcers, skin tears, abrasions, donor sites, and superficial burns

Contraindications

None known

Application

- Hold the dressing by a tab, and peel the liner from the dressing, exposing the adhesive surface.
- Hold the dressing by the tabs, and center the dressing over the wound, adhesive side down. Avoid stretching the dressing.
- Gently position the dressing in place, smoothing from the center outward.
- Slowly remove the paper frame while pressing down and smoothing the film border to ensure good adhesion.

Removal

- Carefully lift the film edges from the skin. If there is difficulty lifting the dressing, apply tape to the edge and use tape to lift.
- Continue lifting the film until all edges are free from the skin surface. Remove the dressing slowly, folding it over itself. Pull carefully in the direction of hair growth.

Contact layers

Action
Contact layers are manufactured as single layers of a woven (polyamide) net that acts as a low-adherence material when placed in contact with the base of the wound. These materials allow wound exudate to pass to a secondary dressing. May be used with topical medications. Contact layers aren't intended to be changed with each dressing change.

Indications
Contact layers may be used as primary dressings for partial- and full-thickness wounds; wounds with minimal, moderate, and heavy exudate; donor sites; and split-thickness skin grafts.

Advantages
- Can protect wound bases from trauma during dressing changes
- May be applied with topical medications, wound fillers, or gauze dressings

Disadvantages
- Aren't recommended for stage 1 pressure ulcers; wounds that are shallow, dehydrated, or covered with eschar; or wounds that are draining a viscous exudate
- Require secondary dressings

HCPCS code overview
The HCPCS codes normally assigned to contact layer dressings are:
A6206—pad size $\leq$ 16 in^2
A6207—pad size > 16 in^2 but $\leq$ 48 in^2
A6208—pad size > 48 in^2.

Conformant 2 Wound Veil

Smith & Nephew, Inc.
Wound Management

How supplied

Sterile sheet: 4″ × 4″; A6206
4″ × 12″; A6207
12″ × 12″, 12″ × 24″, 24″ × 36″; A6208

Sterile roll: 3″ × 5 yards, 4″ × 3 yards, 6″ × 2 yards, 6″ × 4 yards; A6206

Action

Conformant 2 is a single, transparent, nonadherent wound veil made of perforated high-density polyethylene. It's used to line wounds or to place under packing materials. It's easy to remove and assists in the removal of other products placed over the veil. Because it's transparent, Conformant 2 allows visualization of the wound bed.

Indications

To prevent skin breakdown and to manage pressure ulcers (stages 1, 2, 3, and 4), partial- and full-thickness wounds, infected and uninfected wounds, draining wounds, and red, yellow, or black wounds; may also be applied directly to the wound as a liner or used with any topical preparation or ointment

Contraindications

■ Contraindicated for tunneling wounds

Application

■ Place the sheet over the wound and surrounding tissue, and affix it with tape or roll gauze.

Removal

■ Remove the tape or roll gauze.
■ Gently lift one corner of the sheet, and peel it back from the wound.

CONTACT LAYERS

DERMANET Wound Contact Layer

DeRoyal

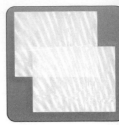

How supplied

Sheet: 3″ × 3″; A6206
       5″ × 4″; A6207
       8″ × 10″, 20″ × 15″, 24″ × 36″; A6208
Roll: 6″ × 72″; A6208

Action

DERMANET Wound Contact Layer is a lightweight net made from high-density polyethylene that forms a porous fine-mesh structure. It's non-linting, inert (totally nonreactive), soft, air- and fluid-permeable, and non-adherent. It conforms to the shapes of wounds and may be used as a primary dressing, coated with ointment for burns, or used as a liner for deep wounds that need to be packed (thus allowing easy removal of packing material).

Indications

For use as a primary dressing to protect burns, graft sites, donor sites, and granulating dermal ulcers and to line deep wounds before packing

Contraindications

- None provided by the manufacturer

Application

- After cleaning the wound and applying topical medications, as prescribed, carefully apply DERMANET Wound Contact Layer.
- Cover the contact layer with a secondary dressing.
- Alternatively, apply medications directly to DERMANET Wound Contact Layer, and place it over the wound before applying a cover dressing.
- For deep, open wounds, line the wound with DERMANET Wound Contact Layer, pack the wound with appropriate packing material, and then apply a cover dressing.

Removal

- Gently lift the dressing off or out of the wound.

Glucan II Wound Dressing

Brennen Medical, Inc.

How supplied

Dressing: 5″ × 6″; A6207
5″ × 12″, 10″ × 15″; A6208

Action

The Glucan II Wound Dressing is a film-backed, mesh-reinforced wound dressing consisting of b-D Glucan. This temporary wound dressing provides an optimum gas-permeable, semiocclusive covering for the wound site, decreases pain by providing a cover for sensory nerve terminals; reduces the need for painful dressing changes; decreases fluid loss; reduces heat loss; forms a barrier against bacterial contamination; may permit early physical therapy; and provides cover for donor sites. It may provide a soothing interface at the wound surface.

Indications

To manage partial-thickness burns, ulcers, donor sites, and other shallow or abrasive wounds. May be used as a wound covering immediately after initial cleansing and removal of broken blisters (unbroken blisters may be left intact)

Contraindications

- Contraindicated for third-degree burns and for wounds with large amounts of eschar
- Contraindicated on patients with sensitivity to plant extracts and patients with a history of multiple serum allergies

Application

- Using aseptic technique, prepare the wound site. If necessary, debride or excise the wound, removing broken blisters, eschar, necrotic tissue, and foreign debris.
- Apply the dressing to the wound surface. (Dressing is labeled "THIS SIDE UP.") Smooth the Glucan II Wound Dressing into place on the wound surface to ensure intimate contact of the dressing with the wound. If necessary, moisten the dressing with sterile saline for easier manageability. Remove any wrinkles or creasing of the dressing.
- Staples may be used when applying the dressing to donor sites.
- Apply an absorbent dressing over the Glucan II Wound Dressing, and secure in place with a flexible net, gauze, or similar dressing.
- Protect the wound from movement for 30 to 60 minutes after the dressing has been applied to ensure adherence to the wound. Dressing perforations allow normal wound drainage.
- Inspect covered areas daily to detect the formation of purulent accumulations, suggesting infection. Take appropriate measures, possibly including removal of the dressing.

CONTACT LAYERS

- Abrupt temperature elevation may occasionally be observed immediately following the application of the Glucan II Wound Dressing. If the elevated temperature persists, an infection may be present and appropriate measures should be taken. Removal of the dressing may be indicated.

Removal

- Inspect the wound after 24 hours to assess status.
- Remove the absorbent outer dressing. Leave the Glucan II Wound Dressing open, or wrap lightly with a flexible net, gauze, or similar dressing. If any signs of infection are present, remove the Glucan II Wound Dressing, clean the wound site, and apply a new dressing. If the Glucan II Wound Dressing adheres to the wound and/or the wound is re-epithelializing, the dressing may remain on the wound as a simple barrier or protective dressing until healing is complete.
- When dressing becomes very dry and healing appears complete, apply a topical cream (such as GlucanPro Cream) over the Glucan II Wound Dressing and leave in place overnight. Easily lift the Glucan II Wound Dressing off the healed wound at next dressing change.

Mepitel Soft Silicone Wound Contact Layer

Mölnlycke Health Care

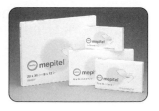

How supplied

Sheet: 2″ × 3″, 3″ × 4″; A6206
4″ × 7.2″; A6207
8″ × 12″; A6208

Action

Mepitel is a soft silicone wound contact layer featuring Safetac technology, which is nonadherent to moist wound beds, yet adheres gently to dry skin. Mepitel prevents the outer dressing from sticking to the wound and therefore minimizes trauma and pain associated with dressing changes. This results in less trauma to the wound and less pain to the patient, which ensures undisturbed wound healing.

Indications

To manage a wide range of painful wounds and wounds with compromised or fragile surrounding skin, such as skin tears, chronic wounds, traumatic wounds, contact layer for protection of fragile granulation tissue, fixation of grafts, partial-thickness burns, and painful skin conditions with blisters such as epidermolysis bullosa

Contraindications

- None provided by the manufacturer

Application

- Clean the wound area.
- If necessary, cut the dressing to the appropriate shape.
- Remove the release film. (*Note:* To avoid sticking when handling Mepitel once the backing has been removed, moisten gloves with saline or water.)
- Apply Mepitel to the wound, overlapping dry skin by at least ³/₈″ (1 cm).
- Apply outer absorbent dressing. Mepitel can be left in place through several outer-dressing changes.

Removal

- Gently lift one corner of the sheet, and peel back from the wound.

CONTACT LAYERS

N-TERFACE Interpositional Surfacing Material
Winfield Laboratories, Inc.

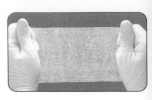

How supplied
Roll: 4" × 10"; A6208
Sheet: 4" × 4"; A6206
         4" × 12"; A6207
         12" × 12", 12" × 24"; A6208

Action
N-TERFACE Interpositional Surfacing Material is a patented, lightweight, extruded, high-density polyurethane sheeting material that can be used as the primary wound contact layer to prevent adherence of secondary dressings or to line deep wounds for easy removal of packing material. It's nonreactive, translucent, nonlinting, air- and fluid-permeable, and nonadherent. It allows visual examination of the wound as well as cleaning and medicating through the material. It may be changed daily or after several days. It's useful under an Unna boot to prevent its sticking to wounds or grafts.

Indications
As a wet or dry dressing and postoperatively, to manage pressure ulcers (stages 1, 2, 3, and 4), partial- and full-thickness wounds; skin graft sites; donor sites, skin conditions; fungating neoplasms; burns; tunneling wounds; infected and noninfected wounds; wounds with heavy, serosanguineous, or purulent drainage; minor lacerations; and red, yellow, or black wounds

Contraindications
- Contraindicated for preventing skin breakdown
- Contraindicated for third-degree burns

Application
- Select a dressing size that covers the wound and periwound area.
- Apply the desired topical agent to the wound or to the dressing before placing the dressing on the wound.
- Apply the dressing dry, or dip it in normal saline solution for better conformability.
- Apply a secondary dressing.
- Secure with stretch netting, roll gauze, or tape.

Removal
- Change the dressing as required.
- Gently lift the dressing off the wound.
- If the wound has dried or is very bloody, or if the contact layer sticks to the wound, rinse the wound with normal saline solution, leaving the contact layer in place. Then remove the contact layer, or leave this layer in place to protect fragile epithelium.
- If the contact layer is left in place for longer than 24 hours, clean the wound through the N-TERFACE contact layer when the secondary absorptive dressing is changed.

CONTACT LAYERS

Profore WCL

Smith & Nephew, Inc.
Wound Management

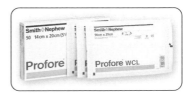

How supplied
Sheet: 5¹/₂″ × 8″; A6207

Action
Profore WCL (wound contact layer) is a dressing made of knitted viscose rayon. It provides physical separation between the wound and external environments to assist in preventing bacterial contamination of the wound. It also aids in the creation and maintenance of a moist wound environment. Moist wound environments have been established as optimal environments for the management of the wound.

Indications
To act as a nonadherent interface between the granulating wound surface and conventional absorbent dressings; also for use in conjunction with Profore, Profore LF and Profore Lite, the Multi-Layer Compression Bandage Systems

Contraindications
■ Not for use if reddening or sensitization occurs; discontinue use and consult a health care professional

Application
■ CAUTION: Don't use contents if pouch is opened or damaged.
■ Use a clean technique to remove the wound contact layer from the pack and apply directly to the wound.
■ Either side of the WCL can be placed in contact with the wound.
■ Make sure that the ulcerated area is covered.
■ Use extra WCL as required.

Removal
■ Gently lift the layer out of the wound.

ProGuide WCL
Smith & Nephew, Inc.
Wound Management

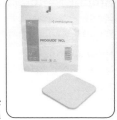

How supplied
Sheet: 4″ × 4″; A6207

Action
ProGuide WCL (wound contact layer) is a unique
dressing based on Trilaminate Hydrocellular Foam
Technology. The dressing is a centrally located absorbent hydrocellular pad
sandwiched between two perforated wound contact layers.

Indications
To absorb exudate and manage partial- to full-thickness wounds; to help
create and maintain a moist wound environment; and to provide physical
separation between the wound and external environments to assist in preventing bacterial contamination of the wound

Contraindications
- Not for use with oxidizing agents such as hypochlorite solutions (such
  as Eusol, Dakins) or hydrogen peroxide, as these can break down the
  absorbent hydrocellular component of the dressing
- Not for use if reddening or sensitization occurs; discontinue use and
  consult a health care professional

Application
- Use a clean technique to remove the wound contact layer from the pack
  and apply directly to the wound.
- Either side of the WCL can be placed in contact with the wound.
- Make sure that the ulcerated area is covered.
- Use extra WCL as required.
- Don't use contents if pouch is opened or damaged.

Removal
- Gently lift the layer out of the wound.

CONTACT LAYERS

Silon-TSR Temporary Skin Replacement
Bio Med Sciences, Inc.

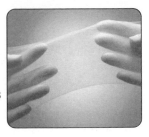

How supplied
Dressing:	5″ × 5″; A6207
	5″ × 10″, 11″ × 12″; A6208
Face mask:	Irregular
Face mask kit:	Irregular
Roll:	5″ × 48″

Action
Silon-TSR (temporary skin replacement) is a semiocclusive silicone membrane that provides a moist environment for rapid healing. Unique surface properties include a self-cling effect without adhesives and a nonadherent surface that won't integrate into the wound. Silon is very thin and transparent, permitting continuous monitoring of the wound without removal of the dressing, thus reducing patient discomfort.

Indications
To manage partial-thickness wounds (laser resurfacing wounds, dermabrasion wounds, donor sites, second-degree burns, skin tears), and autograft sites (meshed autografts, sheet autografts)

Contraindications
- Contraindicated for infected wounds
- Contraindicated in patients with allergies or sensitivities to silicone

Application
- Remove eschar, necrotic tissue, and foreign debris from the wound, and carefully irrigate the site with cleansing solution.
- While gripping the product by the "butterfly" folds of the release liners, peel the liners away while applying the dressing to the wound site. Overlap beyond the edges of the wound by at least 1″ (2.5 cm).
- Apply a gauze pad as a secondary dressing. Wound exudate will pass through the Silon-TSR and collect in the gauze. Secondary dressings may be changed periodically to prevent strikethrough of blood and exudate.
- Mastisol may be applied around the perimeter of the wound to enhance fixation. Adhesive tape may be used at points around the perimeter to prevent rollup or shifting position. Silon-TSR may remain in place for up to 10 days.

Removal
- Inspect the wound periodically.
- Remove the dressing after the first 1 to 2 days, cleaning the area, and reapplying a new dressing for the remainder of the healing process. Superficial wounds, such as laser resurfacing wounds, may not require dressing replacement.

CONTACT LAYERS

Telfa Clear
Tyco Healthcare/Kendall

How supplied
Sheet: 3″ × 3″, 4″ × 5″, 4″ × 12″,
       12″ × 12″, 12″ × 24″

Action
Telfa Clear makes re-epithelialization possible without interrupting the healing
process, and it can be removed without causing pain.

Indications
For use as a primary dressing on lightly, moderately, or heavily draining
wounds; allows the freedom to choose the most appropriate absorbent secondary dressing

Contraindications
- None provided by the manufacturer

Application
- Clean the wound and surrounding skin according to facility policy.
- Carefully apply the dressing to the wound.
- Apply any prescribed medications directly over the dressing.
- Cover the contact layer with an appropriate wound dressing.

Removal
- Dressing may be left in place for several days.
- Gently lift the contact layer off the wound.

CONTACT LAYERS

3M Tegaderm Wound Contact Material

3M Health Care

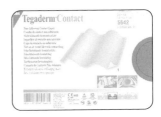

How supplied

Sheet: 3" × 4"; A6206
3" × 8"; A6207
8" × 10"; A6208

Action

3M Tegaderm Wound Contact Material minimizes disruption of granulating tissue and recepithelialized surfaces. It lessens patient pain during dressing changes, maintains a moist wound environment for healing, and can be left on a wound for up to 7 days. It's woven nylon fabric with sealed edges. It's lint-free, nonadherent, nontoxic, nonirritating, and hypoallergenic, and it's to be used on wounds along with an appropriate outer dressing. Intimate contact of the dressing's wound contact material with the wound allows the flow of exudate away from the wound, preventing pooling of fluids that can cause maceration.

Indications

For use directly over wounds, including partial- and full-thickness wounds, clean closed surgical incisions, second-degree burns, donor sites, graft fixation sites, skin tears, traumatic and chronic wounds, and dermatologic lesions

Contraindications

- Not designed, sold, or intended for use except as indicated

Application

- Debride, clean, or irrigate the wound and surrounding skin as necessary according to facility policy.
- Topical treatment with ointments or medicaments, if indicated, can be applied to the wound surface before applying the wound contact material, or they can be applied on top of the material after it has been placed on the wound.
- If the dressing material must be cut to fit, remove all frayed or loose fibers.
- When wound drainage is minimal, moisten the dressing's wound contact material with sterile saline solution to facilitate positioning and to ensure complete contact with the wound surface.
- Gently position the material over the entire wound, including a margin of healthy skin. The material should extend at least ½" (1.3 cm) beyond the edge of the wound, and the cut edges of the material should not be placed directly over the wound bed.
- Dress the wound with an outer dressing of gauze, a transparent dressing, a hydrocolloid, or another suitable wound dressing.

CONTACT LAYERS

Removal

- Dressing may remain undisturbed on the wound for up to 7 days. If the wound is infected, change the dressing according to facility policy for infected wounds.
- Change gauze dressings as needed, or at least every 24 hours. During gauze dressing changes, moisten 3M Tegaderm Wound Contact Material, if necessary, to maintain a moist healing environment.
- When a transparent or hydrocolloid dressing is used as the outermost dressing, follow facility policy for dressing changes.
- Gently lift 3M Tegaderm Wound Contact Material off the wound. When this material is maintained in a moist environment, it's nonadherent and its removal is virtually pain-free.
- If the wound surface is dry, soak the dressing with normal saline solution, and then gently remove it.

Foams

Action
Foam dressings are nonlinting and absorbent. They vary in thickness and have a nonadherent layer, allowing nontraumatic removal. Some have an adhesive border and may have a film coating as an additional bacteria barrier. Foam dressings provide a moist environment and thermal insulation. They're manufactured as pads, sheets, and pillow (cavity) dressings.

Indications
Foam dressings may be used as primary and secondary dressings for partial- and full-thickness wounds with minimal, moderate, or heavy drainage, as primary dressings for absorption and insulation, or as secondary dressings for wounds with packing. They may also be used to provide additional absorption and to absorb drainage around tubes.

Advantages
- Are nonadherent
- May repel contaminants
- Are easy to apply and remove
- Absorb light to heavy amounts of exudate
- May be used under compression

Disadvantages
- Aren't effective for wounds with dry eschar
- May macerate periwound skin if they become saturated
- May require secondary dressing, tape, wrap, or net

HCPCS code overview
The HCPCS codes normally assigned to foam wound covers without an adhesive border are:

A6209—pad size ≤ 16 in^2

A6210—pad size > 16 in^2 but < 48 in^2

A6211—pad size > 48 in^2.

The HCPCS codes normally assigned to foam wound covers with an adhesive border are:

A6212—pad size ≤16 in^2

A6213—pad size > 16 in^2 but < 48 in^2

A6214—pad size > 48 in^2.

The HCPCS code normally assigned to foam wound fillers is:

A6215—per gram.

Allevyn Adhesive Hydrocellular Foam Dressing

Smith & Nephew, Inc.
Wound Management

How supplied

Allevyn Plus Adhesive Dressing: 5″ × 5″; A6212
7″ × 7″, 5″ × 9″;
A6213

Allevyn Adhesive Dressing: 3″ × 3″, 5″ × 5″; A6212
7″ × 7″; A6213
9″ × 9″; A6214

Allevyn Adhesive Sacrum Dressing: 6³/₄″ × 6³/₄″, 9″ × 9″; A6213

Action

Allevyn Adhesive Hydrocellular Foam Dressing is a sterile, absorbent foam dressing with a nonadherent wound contact layer and a semipermeable polyurethane film top layer. It maintains a moist environment and helps prevent bacterial contamination. The dressing absorbs well under compression, conforms well in areas that are awkward to dress, and absorbs up to four times more than a hydrocolloid dressing of similar size. The adhesive dressings now incorporate a dynamic breathable top film that maintains a moist wound environment for low to highly exuding wounds. In low to moderate exudate, moisture is locked into the dressing so that the wound doesn't dry out. In moderate to high exudate, there is an increased rate of moisture vapor transmission rate as fluid reaches the top film.

Indications

To manage exudate in pressure ulcers (stages 2, 3, and 4), leg ulcers, donor sites, partial- and full-thickness wounds, wounds with moderate drainage, wounds with serosanguineous drainage, and red or yellow wounds

Contraindications

■ Not intended for use on nonexuding wounds

Application

■ Apply the foam dressing directly to the wound surface.

Removal

■ Pull corner of the dressing up and then remove.
■ Soak the wound site, and then remove the fixative tape.
■ The dressing will come off without leaving residue in the wound.

Allevyn Cavity Wound Dressing

Allevyn Plus Cavity Wound Dressing

Smith & Nephew, Inc.
Wound Management

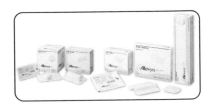

How supplied

Allevyn Cavity Wound Dressing
Circular pad: 2", 4"; A6215
Tubular pad: 3½" × 1", 4¾" × 1½"; A6215
Allevyn Plus Cavity Wound Dressing
Sheet: 2" × 2⅜", 4" × 4", 6" × 8"; A6215

Action

Allevyn Cavity Wound and Plus Cavity Dressings absorb exudate when used to pack heavily exuding cavity wounds.

Indications

To manage exudate in deep chronic wounds or separated surgical wounds; may be used on pressure ulcers (stages 2, 3, and 4), full-thickness wounds, tunneling wounds, infected (when appropriate antibiotic therapy is prescribed) and noninfected wounds, wounds with heavy drainage, wounds with purulent drainage, and red or yellow wounds

Contraindications

■ Contraindicated for nonexuding wounds

Application

■ Choose the appropriate dressing size. (Allevyn Plus Cavity can be cut or shaped into place.)
■ Press the dressing into the wound, filling about 80% of the cavity (Allevyn Cavity).
■ For Allevyn Plus Cavity, only fill up to 50%, because this dressing expands as it absorbs exudate.
■ Secure the dressing with a transparent film dressing or nonwoven retention tape.

Removal

■ Lift the dressing out of the wound.

FOAMS

Allevyn Non-Adhesive Hydrocellular Foam Dressing

Smith & Nephew, Inc. Wound Management

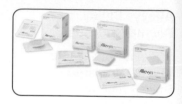

How supplied

Pad:	2″ × 2″, 4″ × 4″; A6209
	6″ × 6″; A6210
	8″ × 8″; A6211
Heel:	A6210
Tracheostomy:	3½″ × 3½″; A6209

Action

Allevyn Hydrocellular Foam Dressing is a sterile, absorbent foam dressing with a nonadherent wound contact layer and a semipermeable polyurethane film top layer. It maintains a moist environment and helps prevent bacterial contamination. The dressing absorbs well under compression, conforms well in areas that are awkward to dress, and absorbs up to four times more than a hydrocolloid dressing of similar size.

Indications

To manage exudate in pressure ulcers (stages 2, 3, and 4), leg ulcers, donor sites, partial- and full-thickness wounds, wounds with moderate drainage, wounds with serosanguineous drainage, and red or yellow wounds

Contraindications

- Not intended for use on nonexuding wounds

Application

- Apply the foam dressing directly to the wound surface.
- Secure the foam dressing with dressing retention tape, regular surgical tape, or waterproof tape.

Removal

- Soak the wound site, and then remove the fixative tape.
- The dressing will come off without leaving residue in the wound.

Allevyn Thin Polyurethane Dressings

Allevyn Compression Polyurethane Dressings

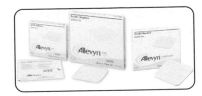

Smith & Nephew, Inc. Wound Management

How supplied
Allevyn Thin
Dressing: $2'' \times 2^3/8''$, $4'' \times 4''$; A6209
              $6'' \times 8''$; A6210
Allevyn Compression
Dressing: $2'' \times 2^3/8''$, $4'' \times 4''$; A6209
              $6'' \times 8''$; A6210

Action
Allevyn Thin and Allevyn Compression Polyurethane Dressings are sterile, absorbent foam dressings with a mild, low-tac adhesive layer and a semipermeable polyurethane film top layer. They maintain a moist environment and help prevent bacterial contamination. The dressings absorb well under compression, conform well in areas that are awkward to dress, and absorb up to four times more than a hydrocolloid dressing of similar size.

Indications
For use on fragile skin or skin tears, or to manage exudate in pressure ulcers (stages 2 and 3), leg ulcers, donor sites, partial and full-thickness wounds, wounds with moderate drainage, wounds with serosanguineous drainage, and red or yellow wounds

Contraindications
■ Not intended for use on nonexuding wounds

Application
■ Apply the foam dressing directly to the wound surface.
■ For extra security, apply with dressing retention tape, regular surgical tape, or waterproof tape.

Removal
■ Soak the wound site, and then remove the fixative tape.
■ The dressing will come off without leaving residue in the wound.

FOAMS

Biatain Adhesive Foam Dressing
Biatain Non-Adhesive Foam Dressing
Coloplast Corporation

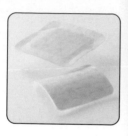

How supplied

Adhesive foam dressing:	5″ × 5″; A6212
	7″ × 7″; A6213
Sacral dressing:	9″ × 9″; A6213
Heel dressing:	7¹/₂″ × 8″; A6212
Nonadhesive foam dressing:	4″ × 4″, 2″ round, 3″ round; A6209
	4″ × 8″; A6210
	6″ × 6″; A6210
	8″ × 8″; A6211

Action

Biatain Adhesive Foam Dressing and Biatain Non-Adhesive Foam Dressing provide an exudate-handling system for wounds with light to heavy exudate. They're highly absorbent, three-dimensional, polymer dressings. Biatain Adhesive Foam Dressing has a hydrocolloid adhesive border and a central 3-D polymer absorbent pad with a waterproof, semipermeable film backing. Biatain Non-Adhesive Foam Dressing is especially suitable for use on fragile skin because it doesn't have an adhesive.

Indications

To manage leg ulcers, skin tears, and diabetic and pressure ulcers with light to heavy exudate; may be used on patients with systemic infections; may be used throughout the healing process to provide padding and protection for all types of wounds

Contraindications

- Contraindicated for use with hypochlorite solutions or hydrogen peroxide
- Must be removed before radiation therapy

Application

- Rinse the wound with Sea-Clens or normal saline solution. Gently pat dry the surrounding skin.
- Choose a dressing that overlaps each side of the wound by 1″ (2.5 cm).
- Biatain Adhesive Foam Dressing may be used with Purilon Gel to encourage natural debridement of necrotic tissue.

Removal

- Biatain Adhesive Foam Dressing and Biatain Non-Adhesive Foam Dressing may be left in place for up to 7 days, depending on the amount of exudate and the condition of the dressing. Change when clinically indicated or when the exudate reaches 1″ (2.5 cm) from the edge of the dressing.

CarraSmart Foam Dressing
Carrington Laboratories, Inc.

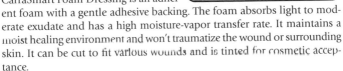

How supplied
Pad: 2″ × 3″, 4″ × 4″; A6257
        6″ × 8″; A6258

Action
CarraSmart Foam Dressing is an adherent foam with a gentle adhesive backing. The foam absorbs light to moderate exudate and has a high moisture-vapor transfer rate. It maintains a moist healing environment and won't traumatize the wound or surrounding skin. It can be cut to fit various wounds and is tinted for cosmetic acceptance.

Indications
To manage pressure ulcers (stages 1 and 2), venous stasis ulcers, first- and second-degree burns, cuts, abrasions, skin irritations, and partial- and full-thickness wounds with low to medium exudate as well as wounds with serosanguineous drainage and red or yellow wounds; may be used as a secondary dressing to cover wounds with fillers or packing or absorb drainage from around tubes; may also be cut and applied as a primary dressing around tubes, such as gastrostomy tubes

Contraindications
- Contraindicated for third-degree burns

Application
- Flush the wound with a suitable cleanser, such as CarraKlenz, UltraKlenz, or MicroKlenz.
- Apply the dressing to the wound bed by holding it and pressing it into place.

Removal
- Change the dressing as the wound condition and amount of exudate dictate or as directed by the primary care provider. Dressing may remain in place for up to 7 days.
- Gently lift the dressing to remove.

FOAMS

COPA "Ultra Soft" Foam Dressing

Tyco Healthcare/Kendall

How supplied

Sterile sheet: 2" × 2", 3" × 3", 4" × 4";
                     A6209
                     5" × 5", 6" × 6", 4" × 8",
                     8" × 8"; A6211

Drain sponge (fenestrated):   3.5" × 34"; A6209

Island dressing: 4" × 4"; A6212
                     6" × 6"; A6213
                     8" × 8"; A6214

Action

COPA Ultra Soft Foam Dressing provides an ideal healing environment for a variety of wounds. This highly absorbent dressing offers physical protection against external fluids and bacteria. The soft, gentle, nonadherent surface conforms to body contours. COPA has superior softness and absorbency. This product is available also in "Plus" with a unique backsheet.

Indications

To manage postsurgical incisions, pressure ulcers (stages 1, 2, and 3), venous stasis ulcers, diabetic foot wounds, donor sites, tubes, and drains

Contraindications

- Contraindicated for dry wounds
- Contraindicated for third-degree burns

Application

- Clean the wound.
- Apply the dressing to the wound. For best results, leave a margin of at least 1" (2.5 cm) around the wound. For improved fit around tubes and drains, the dressing may be cut.

Removal

- Change the dressing as often as necessary.

FOAMS

DermaLevin
DermaRite Industries, LLC

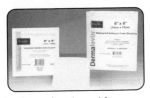

How supplied
Dressing: 4″ × 4″, 6″ × 6″

Action
DermaLevin is a sterile, waterproof, adhesive foam dressing with a non-adherent contact layer and a semipermeable polyurethane film top layer that maintains a moist healing environment and helps prevent bacterial contamination. DermaLevin absorbs four times more than hydrocolloids and conforms to awkward dress areas.

Indications
To manage chronic and acute wounds (stages 2, 3, and 4) with low to moderate exuding, partial- and full-thickness wounds, leg ulcers, and donor sites

Contraindications
■ Contraindicated for nonexuding wounds

Application
■ Clean the wound area with DermaKlenz wound cleanser.
■ Remove the release paper from the dressing, and smooth gently into place.

Removal
■ Carefully loosen the perimeter of the dressing, and lift it gently.

FOAMS

Flexzan Topical Wound Dressing

Mylan Bertek Pharmaceuticals Inc.

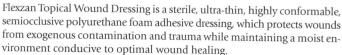

How supplied

Dressing: 2″ × 3″, 4″ × 4″; A6209
            4″ × 8″; A6210
            8″ × 8″; A6211

Action

Flexzan Topical Wound Dressing is a sterile, ultra-thin, highly conformable, semiocclusive polyurethane foam adhesive dressing, which protects wounds from exogenous contamination and trauma while maintaining a moist environment conducive to optimal wound healing.

Flexzan is constructed of an open-cell foam with a closed-cell outer surface and a patterned adhesive coating on the patient contact surface. Excess moisture from the wound passes readily through the adhesive pattern and is absorbed into the open cells of the foam. The closed-cell outer surface provides a barrier to moisture, bacteria, and contaminants, but has a high moisture vapor permeability, allowing evaporation of excess moisture from the foam to help prevent fluid accumulation under the dressing. Flexzan has moisture-management capabilities that make dry to moist wounds—even in areas difficult to dress—easy and comfortable to manage.

Indications

To manage skin tears, abrasions, lacerations, incisions, and other dermal lesions; donor sites; and superficial burns; may be used also on pressure ulcers, venous and diabetic ulcers, partial-thickness wounds, and dermatologic and plastic surgery procedures; may be used as a secondary dressing for alginates and other wound fillers

Contraindications

- Contraindicated for third-degree burns
- Contraindicated for wounds showing signs of infection

Application

- Irrigate the wound with normal saline solution or water, and dry the surrounding area.
- Remove the backing and place the dressing over the wound as desired, leaving at least a 1″ (2.5 cm) margin over intact skin. Cut or overlap the dressing to accommodate wound size and body contour.
- Secure the dressing by applying gentle hand pressure over it for about 20 seconds.

Removal

- Change the dressing at least every 5 to 7 days, or if leakage occurs.

FOAMS

- The dressing may become discolored because of wound exudate absorption, but it doesn't need to be removed unless clinical signs of infection are present.
- For laser resurfaced areas, it's recommended that a dressing change be performed by postoperative day two.

FOAMS

New Product

Gentleheal Non-Adhesive Foam Dressing
Medline Industries, Inc.

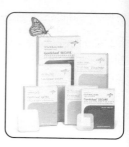

How supplied

Standard pad (3-mm thick):	4″ × 4″; A6209
	4″ × 8″; A6210
Extra pad (5-mm thick):	4″ × 4″; A6209
	4″ × 8″; A6210

Action
Gentleheal Dressings feature the Exulock technology of superabsorbent polymer channels in a polyurethane foam core that locks in exudate even under compression. The Sensil technology provides a silicone facing layer that permits atraumatic removal of dressings and protects the periwound skin from maceration and adhesive skin stripping. The waterproof, outer film expands as the dressing absorbs exudate, helping to prevent the dressing from lifting. Furthermore, the dressing's waterproof outer layer helps to maintain an optimally moist healing environment, prevent strike-through, and aid in preventing bacterial contamination of the wound.

Indications
Ideally for use under compression bandaging, to manage chronic and acute, moderately to extra heavily exuding, partial- and full-thickness wounds, including superficial wounds, minor abrasions, skin tears, second-degree burns, pressure ulcers, lower-extremity ulcers (including those of venous, arterial, and mixed etiology), diabetic ulcers, and donor sites

Contraindications
- May be used in visibly infected wounds only when proper medical treatment addresses the underlying cause

Application
- Clean the wound using Skintegrity Wound Cleanser or an appropriate solution. Dry the surrounding skin.
- Select the appropriate size dressing to allow the foam to cover all breached or compromised skin. Dressing shouldn't be cut.
- Apply the dressing, and secure it with elastic net, gauze roll, or tape.

Removal
- The dressing may be left in place for up to 7 days or until exudate is visible and nears the edge of the dressing.
- Gently remove the dressing.

FOAMS

New Product

Gentleheal Secure Foam Island Dressings
Medline Industries, Inc.

How supplied
Island dressing: 3" × 3" with 1.6" × 1.6" pad; A6212
5" × 5" with 3.3" × 3.3" pad; A6213

Action
Gentleheal Dressings feature the Exulock technology of superabsorbent polymer channels in a polyurethane foam core that locks in exudate even under compression. The Sensil technology provides a silicone facing layer that permits atraumatic removal of dressings and protects the periwound skin from maceration and adhesive skin stripping. Zoned-silicone adhesive provides a more secure adhesive border and gentler tack over the wound surface. The waterproof, outer film expands as the dressing absorbs exudate, helping to prevent the dressing from lifting. Also, the dressing's waterproof outer layer helps to maintain an optimally moist healing environment, prevent strike-through, and aid in preventing bacterial contamination of the wound.

Indications
To manage chronic and acute, moderately to extra-heavily exuding, partial- and full-thickness wounds, including superficial wounds, minor abrasions, skin tears, second-degree burns, pressure ulcers, lower-extremity ulcers (including those of venous, arterial, and mixed etiology), diabetic ulcers, and donor sites; ideally suited for use under compression bandaging; may also serve as an absorbent secondary dressing over a primary dressing, such as an alginate, to reduce frequency of dressing changes

Contraindications
■ May be used in visibly infected wounds only when proper medical treatment addresses the underlying cause

Application
■ Clean the wound using Skintegrity Wound Cleanser or an appropriate solution. Dry the surrounding skin to allow secure adhesion of the dressing.
■ Select the appropriate size dressing to allow the foam island to cover all breached or compromised skin. Dressing shouldn't be cut.
■ Remove the outermost release paper, and anchor the dressing at one side.
■ Smooth the dressing over the wound, and remove remaining release paper. Make sure the dressing is securely adhered without wrinkles in the adhesive border or stretching of the skin.

FOAMS

Removal

- The dressing may be left in place for up to 7 days or until exudate is visible and nears the edge of the dressing.
- Gently press down on the skin, and lift an edge of the dressing.
- Carefully lift all edges of the dressing to promote pain-free removal.

HydraFoam
DermaRite Industries, LLC

How Supplied
Pad: 2" × 2", 4" × 4", 6" × 6"

Action
HydraFoam is a foam dressing with a nonadherent contact layer that maintains a moist healing environment and helps prevent bacterial contamination. HydraFoam absorbs four times more than hydrocolloids and conforms to awkward-to-dress areas.

Indications
To manage chronic and acute wounds (stages 2, 3 and 4) with low to moderate exudation, partial- and full-thickness wounds, leg ulcers, and donor sites

Contraindications
■ Contraindicated for nonexudating wounds

Application
■ Clean the wound area with DermaKlenz wound cleanser. Remove the foam dressing from packaging and place on wound. Cover dressing with conventional techniques.

Removal
■ Carefully loosen any adherent dressing such as tape, bordered gauze, or transparent dressing, and remove foam dressing. If foam dressing sticks to the wound, moisten with sterile water and lift gently.

FOAMS

HydroCell Adhesive Foam Dressing
Derma Sciences, Inc.

How supplied
Adhesive foam pad: 4″ × 4″, 6″ × 6″

Action
HydroCell Adhesive Foam Dressing is a highly absorptive, nonadherent, polyurethane foam pad and an adhesive protective film covering to protect the wound from outside contaminants, without the need for a secondary dressing.

Indications
To manage moderately to highly exuding wounds

Contraindications
- Contraindicated for third-degree burns

Application
- Clean the wound with PrimaDerm Dermal Cleanser or saline solution. Pat dry the skin adjacent to the wound.
- Position the HydroCell Adhesive Foam Dressing pad directly on the wound.
- Smooth the edges of the adhesive border to ensure secure adhesion.

Removal
- Remove the dressing gently.
- Removal may be facilitated by gently stretching the adhesive film border.

FOAMS

HydroCell Foam Dressing
Derma Sciences, Inc.

How supplied
Sheet: 4″ × 4″, 6″ × 6″

Action
HydroCell Foam Dressing is a nonadherent, highly absorptive, polyurethane foam sheet with protective film covering to protect the wound from outside contaminants. A secondary dressing is required to hold this dressing in place.

Indications
To manage moderately to highly exuding wounds

Contraindications
■ Contraindicated for third-degree burns

Application
■ Clean the wound with PrimaDerm Dermal Cleanser or saline solution. Pat dry the skin adjacent to the wound.
■ Position HydroCell Foam Dressing directly on the wound.
■ Secure with an appropriate secondary dressing.

Removal
■ Remove the secondary dressing.
■ Remove the HydroCell Foam Dressing.

FOAMS

HydroCell Thin Adhesive Foam Dressing
Derma Sciences, Inc.

How supplied
Sheet: 2″ × 3″, 4″ × 4″

Action
HydroCell Thin Adhesive Foam Dressing is an absorptive polyurethane foam sheet with a nonadherent foam pad and an adhesive protective film covering to protect the wound from outside contaminants without the need for a secondary dressing.

Indications
To manage lightly exuding wounds

Contraindications
- Contraindicated for third-degree burns

Application
- Clean the wound with PrimaDerm Dermal Cleanser or saline solution. Pat dry the skin adjacent to the wound.
- Position the HydroCell Thin Adhesive Foam Dressing pad directly on the wound.
- Smooth the edges of the adhesive border to ensure secure adhesion.

Removal
- Gently remove the HydroCell Thin Adhesive Foam Dressing.
- Removal may be facilitated by gently stretching the adhesive film border.

FOAMS

Hydrofera Blue Bacteriostatic Heavy Drainage Wound Dressing
Hydrofera, LLC

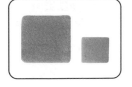

How supplied
Bacteriostatic foam dressing heavy drainage: 4″ × 4″, 6″ × 6″, 6″ × 6″ (thick)

Action
Hydrofera Blue Bacteriostatic Foam Dressing is a sterile absorptive foam dressing made of Hydrofera Polyvinyl alcohol sponge, methylene blue, and crystal violet. The product inhibits the growth of microorganisms on the foam for up to 7 days. Hydrofera Blue has a natural negative pressure and binds 100% of all endotoxins within 4 hours, providing pain relief and increased patient comfort. It's effective against many microorganisms including methicillin-resistant *Staphylococcus aureus* (MRSA) and vancomycin-resistant enterococci (VRE).

Indications
To manage pressure ulcers, venous stasis ulcers, arterial ulcers, diabetic ulcers, donor sites, abrasions, lacerations, radiation burns, postsurgical incisions, and other wounds caused by trauma

Contraindications
- Contraindicated for third-degree burns

Application
- Before the initial application of Hydrofera Blue Bacteriostatic Wound Dressing, the wound should be debrided of any necrotic tissue. The wound should be cleaned with normal saline or with an appropriate cleansing solution, or both.
- Open the Hydrofera Foam package, and moisten the dressing with either sterile saline of sterile water. Wring out the excess.
- Place the dressing on or in the wound, and secure with the appropriate secondary dressing.

Removal
- Change the dressing every 1 to 3 days. Don't let the dressing completely dry out. Rehydrate as necessary depending on amount of drainage.
- The dressing must be changed if it turns white where it's making intimate contact with the wound or upon strike-through.

FOAMS

Hydrofera Blue Bacteriostatic Wound Dressing

Hydrofera, LLC

How supplied

Bacteriostatic foam dressing: 2″ × 2″, 3″ × 3″, 4″ × 4″; A6209 4.25″ × 4.25″, 6″ × 6″; A6210

Bacteriostatic foam dressing (thick): 6″ × 6″; A6210

Bacteriostatic tunneling dressing: 9-mm diameter × 6″ long, 12-mm diameter × 6″ long; A6215

Bacteriostatic G-tube site dressing: 4″ × 4″; A6209

Bacteriostatic packing: 10 cm long, 4.5 cm long; A6209

Bacteriostatic ostomy dressing: 26-cm diameter; A6209

Bacteriostatic nail avulsion dressing: 26-mm diameter

Action

Hydrofera Blue Bacteriostatic Foam Dressing is a sterile absorptive foam dressing made of Hydrofera Polyvinyl alcohol sponge, methylene blue, and crystal violet. The product inhibits the growth of microorganisms on the foam for up to 7 days. Hydrofera Blue has a natural negative pressure and binds 100% of all endotoxins within 4 hours, providing pain relief and increased patient comfort. It's effective against many microorganisms including MRSA and VRE.

Indications

To manage pressure ulcers, venous stasis ulcers, arterial ulcers, diabetic ulcers, donor sites, abrasions, lacerations, radiation burns, postsurgical incisions, and other wounds caused by trauma.

Contraindications

- Contraindicated for third-degree burns

Application

- Before the initial application of Hydrofera Blue Bacteriostatic Wound Dressing, the wound should be debrided of any necrotic tissue. The wound should be cleansed with normal saline and/or an appropriate cleansing solution.
- Open the Hydrofera Foam package, and moisten the dressing with either sterile saline or sterile water. Wring out the excess.
- Place the dressing on or in the wound, and secure with the appropriate secondary dressing.

Removal

- Change the dressing every 1 to 3 days. Don't let the dressing completely dry out. Rehydrate as necessary depending on amount of drainage.
- The dressing *must* be changed if it turns white where it's making intimate contact with the wound or upon strike-through.

FOAMS

Hydrofera Blue Bacteriostatic Wound Dressing with Film
Hydrofera, LLC

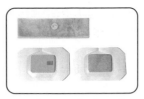

How supplied

Bacteriostatic foam dressing with film backing: 4.25″ × 4.25″, 2″ × 8″
Bacteriostatic ostomy dressing with film backing: 26 mm

Action

Hydrofera Blue Bacteriostatic Wound Dressing with Film is a sterile absorptive foam dressing made of Hydrofera Polyvinyl alcohol sponge, methylene blue, and crystal violet. The product inhibits the growth of microorganisms on the foam for up to 7 days. Hydrofera Blue has a natural negative pressure and binds 100% of all endotoxins within 4 hours, providing pain relief and increased patient comfort. It's effective against many microorganisms including MRSA and VRE.

Indications

To manage pressure ulcers, venous stasis ulcers, arterial ulcers, diabetic ulcers, donor sites, abrasions, lacerations, radiation burns, postsurgical incisions, and other wounds caused by trauma

Contraindications

■ Contraindicated for third degree burns

Application

■ Before the initial application of Hydrofera Blue Bacteriostatic Wound Dressing, the wound should be debrided of any necrotic tissue. The wound should be cleansed with normal saline and/or an appropriate cleansing solution.
■ Open the Hydrofera Foam package, and moisten the dressing with either sterile saline or sterile water. Wring out the excess.
■ Place the dressing on or in the wound, and secure with the appropriate secondary dressing.

Removal

■ Change the dressing every 1 to 3 days. Don't let the dressing completely dry out. Rehydrate as necessary depending on amount of drainage.
■ The dressing *must* be changed if it turns white where it's making intimate contact with the wound or upon strike-through.

FOAMS

LO PROFILE FOAM Plus
Wound Dressing
GENTELL, Inc.

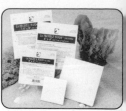

How supplied
Dressing: 4″ × 4″ with 2″ × 2″ pad; A6212
6″ × 6″ with 4.5″ × 4.5″ pad; A6213

Action
LO PROFILE FOAM is a highly absorbent foam dressing that protects and insulates the wound while promoting a moist healing environment. One side of the dressing has a waterproof polyurethane layer that's an effective barrier to outside bacteria and contaminants. This layer also prevents wound drainage from striking through. The hydrophilic foam provides gradual lateral wicking for maximum absorption, which helps minimize maceration of healthy surrounding tissue. LO PROFILE FOAM easily conforms to bony prominences, and because it's less bulky than other absorptive dressings, it doesn't bunch up.

Indications
For use as a primary dressing for minimally to moderately draining wounds and for skin tears and other superficial wounds; as a secondary absorptive dressing in conjunction with a primary dressing such as calcium alginate; may also be used around drainage tubes

Contraindications
- None provided by the manufacturer

Application
- Irrigate the wound with Gentell Wound Cleanser or a similar nontoxic cleanser.
- Gently dry the skin surrounding the wound site.
- Select the dressing size that will provide a minimum margin of 1″ (2.5 cm) around the edges of the wound.
- Place LO PROFILE FOAM Plus dressing directly over the wound surface.

Removal
- Gently roll back the adhesive border from the skin.
- Ease the dressing from the wound.

FOAMS

LYOFOAM Polyurethane Foam Dressing*

LYOFOAM A Adhesive Polyurethane Foam Dressing*

LYOFOAM C Polyurethane Foam Dressing with Activated Carbon*

LYOFOAM T Polyurethane Foam Dressing*

LYOFOAM Extra Polyurethane Foam Dressing*

ConvaTec

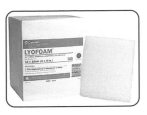

How supplied

LYOFOAM Polyurethane Foam Dressing
Sterile dressing: 3" × 3", 4" × 4"; A6209
                       7" × 4", 10" × 4", 8" × 6"; A6210
                       12" × 10", 27⅝" × 15¾"; A6211

LYOFOAM A Adhesive Polyurethane Foam Dressing
Sterile dressing: 2" × 2", 4" × 4"; A6212

LYOFOAM C Polyurethane Foam Dressing with Activated Carbon
Sterile dressing: 4" × 4"; A6209
                       8" × 6"; A6210

LYOFOAM T Polyurethane Foam Dressing
Sterile dressing: 3½" × 2½"; A6209

LYOFOAM Extra Polyurethane Foam Dressing
Dressing: 4" × 4"; A6209
                       7" × 4", 8" × 6"; A6210
                       12" × 10"; A6211

FOAMS

Action

LYOFOAM dressing is used on cutaneous wounds with exudate. It's applied directly onto clean wounds and wounds with minimal necrosis during the granulating or epithelializing phases of healing. LYOFOAM A dressing is used for lightly exuding wounds, such as sacral ulcers and cutaneous wounds. LYOFOAM C dressing is used for lightly or moderately exuding wounds to absorb and neutralize offensive odors. LYOFOAM T dressing is used for tracheostomy and other intubation sites, cannula insertion procedures, and external bone fixators.

Indications

To manage cutaneous wounds with exudate and wounds with minimal necrosis during the exuding, granulating, or epithelializing stages of healing

Contraindications

- Not recommended for dry, superficial wounds, and shouldn't be left in position on shallow, drying wounds for extended periods because of the possibility of adherence
- Shouldn't be applied to wounds covered by a dry scab or hard black necrotic tissue until the scab or tissue has been removed using other approved methods

Application

To apply LYOFOAM and LYOFOAM EXTRA Dressings:

- Clean and prepare the wound and dry the surrounding skin, leaving the wound surface moist. When cleaning the wound and during dressing changes, be careful not to disturb any newly formed tissue at the edges and in the base of the wound.
- Select a dressing large enough to overlap the wound area by 1" (2.5 cm) all around. If necessary, cut the dressing to the shape required. Place the smooth, shiny side of the dressing directly over the wound surface.
- Where compression is required, a suitable compression bandage, such as Setopress, may be used to secure the dressing. For other applications, LYOFOAM dressing can be secured with adhesive tape or a suitable dressing retention bandage, such as Tubifast.
- Don't fully cover LYOFOAM dressing with adhesive films or tapes because they reduce water vapor transmission, which can reduce the effectiveness of the dressing.

To apply LYOFOAM A Dressing:

- Clean the wound with SAF-Clens AF dermal wound cleanser or other appropriate cleansing solution, and dry the surrounding skin, leaving the wound surface moist.
- Remove LYOFOAM A dressing from the foil pouch, and peel off the backing sheet from one side. Place the dressing over the wound, ensuring that the central pad of the dressing overlaps the wound by about 1" on all sides. Gently smooth the adhesive border into position.
- Remove the second sheet of backing paper. Smooth the adhesive border gently into position, ensuring complete contact all around wound to avoid leakage or contamination.

To apply LYOFOAM C Dressing:

- Irrigate the wound with SAF-Clens AF dermal wound cleanser or other appropriate cleansing solution to remove as much necrotic material as possible. Dry the surrounding skin, leaving the wound surface moist.

- Select the appropriate size of LYOFOAM C dressing. Remove LYOFOAM C dressing from the pouch, and position it over the wound surface, allowing an overlap of about 1″ (2.5 cm) around wound margins. Secure with a conforming retention bandage, such as Tubifast.
- Don't fully cover LYOFOAM C dressing with occlusive films or tapes because they reduce water vapor loss, which can impair the effectiveness of the dressing.

To apply LYOFOAM T Dressing:

- After tube, cannula, or pin insertion, remove LYOFOAM T dressing from the foil pouch, and locate the precut "cross."
- Position the dressing carefully around the tube, cannula, or pin; then secure.
- Don't fully cover LYOFOAM T dressing with occlusive films or tapes because they reduce water vapor loss, which can impair the effectiveness of the dressing.

Removal

- For lightly exuding wounds, change the dressing every 2 to 3 days initially. Then extend the changing period to 4 to 7 days as the amount of exudate decreases.
- For moderately exuding wounds, changes may be needed daily or on alternate days for the first few days of wound management. After the initial period, granulation should begin, and the interval between dressing changes can be extended.
- The interval between dressing changes is determined by the amount of exudate and the nature and condition of the wound. The goal is to change the dressings at weekly intervals to minimize disturbance of the wound and optimize healing.
- If the absorbent surface becomes completely saturated, exudate will be visible around the edges of the dressing. This clearly indicates that the dressing should be changed, regardless of how recently it was applied.
- Gently remove the dressing.
- Dispose of the soiled dressing according to facility guidelines.

*See package insert for complete instructions for use.

FOAMS

Mepiform Soft Silicone Gel Sheeting
Mölnlycke Health Care

How supplied
Gel sheeting: 2″ × 3″, 4″ × 7″, 1.6″ × 12″

Action
Mepiform is a self-adherent soft silicone gel sheeting for scar management, featuring Safetac technology that is is breathable, comfortable, and waterproof. Mepiform is thin, flexible, and discreet and can be worn during all daily activities.

Indications
To manage old and new hypertrophic and keloid scars; can be used on closed wounds, where it may prevent the formation of hypertrophic and keloid scars; may be used prophylactically for 2 to 6 months, depending on the condition of the scar

Contraindications
- None provided by the manufacturer

Application
- Clean the scar tissue or closed wound with mild soap and water. Rinse and pat dry. Make sure the scar and surrounding skin are dry.
- If necessary, cut the dressing to the appropriate shape. No extra fixation is needed.
- Remove the release film, and apply the dressing to the scar without stretching the dressing.
- Avoid the use of creams or ointments under Mepiform.

Removal
- Optimally, Mepiform should be worn 24 hours/day. It's recommended that Mepiform be removed once a day for showering or bathing and reapplied.
- Change the dressing when it begins to lose its adherent properties. Dressing wear time varies by person.

FOAMS

Mepilex Border Lite
Mölnlycke Health Care

How supplied
Self-adherent soft silicone thin foam dressing:
> 1.6 " × 2", 2" × 5", 3" × 3",
> 4" × 4"; A6212
> 6" × 6"; A6213

Action
Mepilex Border Lite self-adherent soft silicone thin foam dressing is a highly conformable dressing that absorbs exudate, maintains a moist wound environment, and minimizes the risk for periwound maceration. The Safetac soft silicone layer allows for atraumatic removal, which prevents trauma to the wound and surrounding skin and prevents pain to the patient upon removal.

Indications
To manage a wide range of nonexuding to low exuding wounds, painful wounds, and wounds with compromised or fragile surrounding skin including lower extremity wounds, pressure ulcers, and traumatic wounds such as abrasions, cuts, finger injuries, blisters, and skin tears; can also be used for protection of compromised and/or fragile skin

Contraindications
■ None provided by the manufacturer

Application
■ Clean the wound area. Make sure the surrounding skin is dry.
■ Remove the release film, and apply the dressing to the wound. Don't stretch the dressing.

Removal
■ Mepilex Border can be left in place for 5 to 7 days, depending on the condition of the wound and the surrounding skin, or as indicated by accepted clinical practice. Mepilex Border should be changed when exudate is present at the pad edges.

FOAMS

Mepilex Border
Self-Adherent Soft Silicone Foam
Dressing
Mölnlycke Health Care

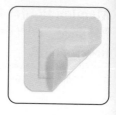

How supplied
Pad: 3" × 3" (pad 1.77" × 1.77"),
4" × 4" (pad 2.56" × 2.56"); A6212
6" × 6" (pad 4.33" × 4.33"), 6" × 8" (pad 4.33" × 6.30"); A6213

Action
Mepilex Border Self-Adherent Soft Silicone Foam Dressing absorbs exudate effectively, minimizes the risk of periwound skin maceration, and helps to maintain a moist environment for optimum wound healing. The Safetac soft silicone properties allow the dressing to be changed without causing additional trauma to the wound and surrounding skin or pain to the patient.

Indications
Designed for a wide range of exuding wounds, painful wounds, and wounds with compromised or fragile surrounding skin, including pressure ulcers, lower-extremity ulcers (such as diabetic ulcers), and traumatic wounds such as skin tears

Contraindications
- None provided by the manufacturer

Application
- Clean the wound area. Make sure the surrounding skin is dry.
- Remove the release film, and apply the dressing to the wound. Don't stretch the dressing.

Removal
- Mepilex Border can be left in place for 5 to 7 days, depending on the condition of the wound and the surrounding skin, or as indicated by accepted clinical practice. Mepilex Border should be changed when exudate is present at the pad edges.

FOAMS

Mepilex Heel
Mölnlycke Health Care

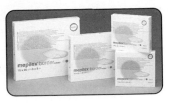

How supplied
Soft silicone absorbent foam heel dressing:
5″ × 8″

Action
Mepilex Heel is a soft silicone, absorbent, foam dressing featuring Safetac technology and specifically designed for use on the heel. It's shaped to fit any heel so there is no need for measuring or cutting. The Safetac soft silicone technology provides a good seal to reduce the risk of maceration and minimizes the trauma and pain at dressing changes.

Indications
Designed for a wide range of exuding wounds, painful wounds, and wounds with compromised or fragile periwound skin, including pressure ulcers, venous ulcers, and diabetic ulcers

Contraindications
- None provided by the manufacturer

Application
- Clean the wound area. Make sure the surrounding skin is dry.
- Remove the longer release film.
- Fix the dressing under the foot, and release the shorter release film.
- Mold the dressing around the heel, and bring edges together.
- Mepilex Heel should overlap the wound bed by at least 1″ (2.5 cm) onto the surrounding skin.

Removal
- Leave Mepilex in place for several days, depending on the condition of the wound and the surrounding skin or facility policy.

FOAMS

Mepilex Lite Absorbent Soft Silicone Thin Foam Dressing
Mölnlycke Health Care

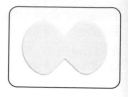

How supplied
Dressing: 2.4" × 3.4", 4" × 4"; A6209
6" × 6"; A6210
8" × 20"; A6211

Action
Mepilex Lite is a highly conformable, soft silicone foam dressing that absorbs exudates and helps maintain a moist wound environment. The Safetac layer seals around the wound edges, deterring exudate from leaking onto the surrounding skin, which minimizes the risk for maceration and ensures atraumatic dressing changes. Mepilex Lite can be cut to suit various wound shapes and locations.

Indications
Mepilex Lite may be used as a primary or secondary dressing for the management of a wide range of low to moderate exuding wounds, such as leg and foot ulcers, partial-thickness burns, radiation skin reactions, and epidermolysis bullosa (EB); Mepilex Lite can also be used for protection of compromised and/or fragile skin and may be used under compression bandaging

Contraindications
- None provided by the manufacturer

Application
- Clean the wound area. Make sure the surrounding skin is dry.
- Select an appropriate dressing size. For best results, Mepilex Lite should overlap the surrounding skin by at least ³⁄₄" (2 cm). If necessary, cut the dressing to fit.
- Remove the release film, and apply the dressing with the adherent side toward the wound. Don't stretch the dressing.
- Secure the dressing with a bandage or other fixation when necessary.

Removal
- Leave Mepilex in place for several days, depending on the condition of the wound and the surrounding skin or facility policy.

FOAMS

Mepilex Soft Silicone Absorbent Foam Dressing

Mölnlycke Health Care

How supplied
Pad: 4″ × 4″; A6209
         4″ × 8″, 6″ × 6″; A6210
         8″ × 8″; A6211

Action
Mepilex is a soft silicone absorbent foam dressing featuring Safetac technology, which effectively absorbs exudate and helps maintain a moist wound environment for optimal wound healing. The Safetac soft silicone layer minimizes the risk of periwound maceration and erosion and allows the dressing to be changed without causing additional pain to the patient or trauma to the wound and surrounding skin. Mepilex can be used under compression and may be cut for customization to the wound area.

Indications
To treat a wide range of exuding wounds, painful wounds, and wounds with compromised or fragile surrounding skin, including pressure ulcers and lower-extremity ulcers, such as venous and diabetic ulcers

Contraindications
- None provided by the manufacturer

Application
- Clean the wound area. Make sure the surrounding skin is dry.
- Select an appropriate dressing size. For best results, Mepilex should overlap the surrounding skin by at least ¾″ (2 cm). If necessary, cut the dressing to fit.
- Remove the release film, and apply the dressing with the adherent side toward the wound. Don't stretch the dressing.
- Secure the dressing with a bandage or other fixation when necessary.

Removal
- Leave Mepilex in place for several days, depending on the condition of the wound and the surrounding skin or facility policy.

Mepilex Transfer
Soft Silicone Exudate
Transfer Dressing
Mölnlycke Health Care

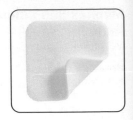

How supplied
Pad: 6″ × 8″; A6210
         8″ × 20″; A6211

Action
Mepilex Transfer is thin and conformable, enabling management of difficult-to-dress wounds. As the Safetac layer seals around the wound margins, the foam structure allows the exudate to move vertically into a secondary absorbent pad, thus protecting the surrounding skin from excess moisture and minimizing the risk of maceration. With the Safetac soft silicone layer, Mepilex Transfer ensures direct contact to the wound base and surrounding skin and helps minimize trauma and pain during dressing changes.

Indications
For a wide range of exuding wounds and difficult-to-dress wounds such as those caused by cancer, lymphedema, and Epstein-Barr virus; also used as a protective layer on minimal or low exuding wounds; cover large, awkward areas; ideal for areas with fragile skin

Contraindications
- None provided by the manufacturer

Application
- Clean the wound area. Make sure the surrounding skin is dry.
- Remove the release film, and apply the dressing to the wound, overlapping the surrounding skin by at least 2″ (5 cm).
- Dressing may be used under compression.
- Secure Mepilex Transfer with a secondary dressing. Dressing choice depends on the location and exudate amount. Options include mesh net or other nonadhesive dressing holder, Mefilm, Alldress, gauze, or Mefix.

Removal
- Mepilex Transfer can be left in place for several days, depending on the condition of the wound and the surrounding skin, or as indicated by accepted clinical practice.

FOAMS

MPM Excel Bordered Foam Barrier Dressing

MPM Medical, Inc.

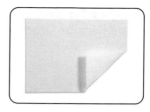

How supplied
Foam pad with border: 2″ × 2″, 4″ × 4″
Circular fenestrated pad: 2″ diameter

Action
The MPM Excel Bordered Foam Barrier Dressing is a nonadherent, highly absorptive, semiocclusive dressing with a nonwoven tape border. The dressing maintains a moist environment that's conducive to healing and resists external contaminants, such as blood and drainage.

Indications
For use as a primary or secondary dressing to manage pressure ulcers (stages 2, 3, and 4), partial- and full-thickness wounds, donor sites, tunneling wounds, infected and noninfected wounds, and draining wounds

Contraindications
- None provided by the manufacturer

Application
- Clean the wound with MPM Wound Cleanser or normal saline solution.
- Remove the release liner from the dressing.
- Place the dressing on the wound, and secure the dressing by gently pressing on the tape border.

Removal
- Carefully lift the edge of the tape, and peel off the dressing.

FOAMS

MPM Excel Non-Bordered Foam Barrier Dressing
MPM Medical, Inc

How supplied
Foam sheet: 2" × 2"

Action
MPM Excel Non-Bordered Foam Barrier Dressing is a nonadherent highly absorptive polyurethane foam sheet. A secondary dressing is required to hold this dressing in place.

Indications
To manage moderately to highly exuding wounds

Contraindications
■ Contraindicated for third-degree burns

Application
■ Clean the wound with MPM Wound Cleanser or normal saline solution.
■ Pat dry the skin adjacent to the wound.
■ Place the dressing on the wound, and secure with an appropriate secondary dressing.

Removal
■ Gently remove the tape from the patient's skin, and lift the dressing.

FOAMS

Odor-Absorbent Dressing*
Hollister Wound Care, LLC

How supplied
Pad: 4" × 4"; A6209
           6" × 10"; A6211

Action
Effectively eliminates offending odors resulting from infection or bacterial contamination in surgical, traumatic, cancerous, or gangrenous wounds, pressure ulcers, or venous stasis ulcers. The dressing is composed of a foam matrix impregnated with carbon between two layers of soft, nonwoven fabric and conforms to the contours of the patient's body.

Indications
Intended as a secondary dressing but may be used as a primary dressing over a nonexuding wound

Contraindications
- None provided by the manufacturer

Application
- Peel open the envelope; remove the Odor-Absorbent Dressing. If using the dressing as a primary dressing over a nonexuding wound, place it directly over the prepared wound surface. If it's being used as a secondary dressing, apply it over the contact layer. After placement of the dressings, complete application by taping around the perimeter.
- For particularly malodorous wounds, two or more Odor-Absorbent Dressings may be applied in layers over the same wound. For wounds that exceed dimensions of the Odor-Absorbent Dressing, two or more dressings may be overlapped and taped together.

Removal
- Remove tape securing the dressing to the skin, and lift away the dressing.

*See package insert for complete instructions for use.

FOAMS

Optifoam Adhesive Foam Island Dressing

Medline Industries, Inc.

How supplied

Island dressing: 4″ × 4″ with 2.5″ × 2.5″ pad;
A6212
6″ × 6″ with 4.5″ × 4.5″ pad;
A6213
6.1″ × 5.6″ sacral with 4″ × 4″ pad; A6212

Action

Optifoam Adhesive Foam Island Dressing is used to manage exudate in moderately to heavily draining wounds. This hydropolymer adhesive dressing is composed of a thin film backing over a hydrophilic foam island. The film backing has an adjustable moisture vapor transmission rate from 0 to 4,500 g/m2/day, depending on the fluid level in the wound. The waterproof outer layer is coated with a medical-grade adhesive that helps maintain an optimally moist environment, which supports wound healing by encouraging autolytic debridement, which enables granulation to occur. New window-frame delivery system makes application smooth and easy. New sacral shape has anatomical shape to provide better fit and longer wear.

Indications

To manage chronic and acute, moderately to heavily exudating, partial- and full-thickness wounds, including superficial wounds, minor abrasions, skin tears, second-degree burns, pressure ulcers, lower-extremity ulcers (including those of venous, arterial, and mixed causes), diabetic ulcers, and donor sites; also suitable for use under compression bandaging; may also serve as an absorbent secondary dressing over a primary dressing, such as an alginate, to reduce frequency of dressing changes

Contraindications

- Contraindicated for third-degree burns
- Contraindicated in patients with active vasculitis
- For use in visibly infected wounds only when proper medical treatment addresses the underlying cause

Application

- Clean the wound using Skintegrity Wound Cleanser or an appropriate solution. Dry the surrounding skin to allow secure adhesion of the dressing.
- Select the appropriate size dressing to allow the foam island to cover all breached or compromised skin.
- Remove the outermost release paper, and anchor the dressing at one side.

FOAMS

- Smooth the dressing over the wound, and remove remaining release paper. Make sure the dressing is securely adhered without wrinkles in the adhesive border or stretching of the skin.
- Remove the paper frame, starting at the center thumb notch, following and smoothing the dressing as you lift and remove the paper frame.

Removal

- The dressing may be left in place for up to 7 days or until exudate is visible and nears the edge of the dressing.
- Gently press down on the skin, and lift an edge of the dressing.
- Carefully stretch the dressing laterally to the skin to promote pain-free removal.
- Clean the wound again before applying a new dressing.

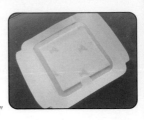

New Product

Optifoam Ag Adhesive Foam Island Dressing
Medline Industries, Inc.

How supplied
Foam island dressing: 4″ × 4″ with 2.5″ × 2.5″ pad; A6212

Action
Optifoam Ag Adhesive Foam Island Dressing provides safe, targeted release of ionic silver for an antimicrobial environment for up to 7 days. The dressing is ideal to manage exudate in moderately to heavily draining wounds. This hydropolymer adhesive dressing is composed of a thin film backing over a hydrophilic foam island. The film backing has an adjustable moisture vapor transmission rate from 0 to 4,500 $g/m^2/day$, depending on the fluid level in the wound. The waterproof outer layer is coated with a medical-grade adhesive that helps maintain an optimally moist environment, which supports wound healing by encouraging autolytic debridement, which enables granulation to occur. New window-frame delivery system makes application smooth and easy.

Indications
To manage chronic and acute, moderately to heavily exudating, partial- and full-thickness wounds, including superficial wounds, minor abrasions, skin tears, second-degree burns, pressure ulcers, lower-extremity ulcers (including those of venous, arterial, and mixed causes), diabetic ulcers, and donor sites; also for use under compression bandaging; may also serve as an absorbent secondary dressing over a primary dressing, such as an alginate, to reduce frequency of dressing changes

Contraindications
- Contraindicated for third-degree burns
- Contraindicated in patients with active vasculitis

Application
- Clean the wound using Skintegrity Wound Cleanser or an appropriate solution. Dry the surrounding skin to allow secure adhesion of the dressing.
- Select the appropriate size dressing to allow the foam island to cover all breached or compromised skin.
- Remove the outermost release paper, and anchor the dressing at one side.
- Smooth the dressing over the wound, and remove remaining release paper. Make sure the dressing is securely adhered without wrinkles in the adhesive border or stretching of the skin.

FOAMS

- Remove the paper frame, starting at the center thumb notch, following and smoothing the dressing as you lift and remove the paper frame.

Removal

- The dressing may be left in place for up to 7 days or until exudate is visible and nears the edge of the dressing.
- Gently press down on the skin, and lift an edge of the dressing.
- Carefully stretch the dressing laterally to the skin to promote pain-free removal.
- Clean the wound again before applying a new dressing.

Optifoam Ag Non-Adhesive Foam Island Dressing
Medline Industries, Inc.

How supplied
Foam pad: 4″ × 4″; A6210

Action
Optifoam Ag Non-Adhesive Foam Dressing provides safe, targeted release of ionic silver for an antimicrobial environment for up to 7 days. The dressing is ideal to manage exudate in moderately to heavily draining wounds. This hydropolymer dressing is composed of a thin film backing over a hydrophilic foam pad. The waterproof, film backing has an adjustable moisture vapor transmission rate from 0 to 4,500 g/m²/day, depending on the fluid level in the wound.

Indications
To manage chronic and acute, moderately to heavily exudating, partial- and full-thickness wounds, including superficial wounds, minor abrasions, skin tears, second-degree burns, pressure ulcers, lower-extremity ulcers (including those of venous, arterial, and mixed causes), diabetic ulcers, and donor sites; also for use under compression bandaging; may also serve as an absorbent secondary dressing over a primary dressing, such as an alginate, to reduce frequency of dressing changes

Contraindications
- Contraindicated for third-degree burns
- Contraindicated in patients with active vasculitis

Application
- Clean the wound using Skintegrity Wound Cleanser or an appropriate solution. Dry the surrounding skin to allow secure adhesion of the dressing.
- Select the appropriate size dressing to allow the foam pad to cover all breached or compromised skin.
- Place the dressing over the wound, and secure with elastic net, tape, or roll bandage.

Removal
- The dressing may be left in place for up to 7 days or until exudate is visible and nears the edge of the dressing.
- Carefully remove dressing and discard.

FOAMS

New Product

Optifoam Basic Foam Dressing
Medline Industries, Inc.

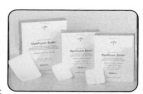

How supplied
Pad: 3″ × 3″, 3″ × 3″ with fenestration; A6209

4″ × 5″; A6210

Action
Optifoam Basic Foam Dressing is a polyurethane foam pad that provides soft, cushioning absorbency for general wound or site care.

Indications
To manage chronic and acute, light to moderately exuding, partial- and full-thickness wounds, including superficial wounds, minor abrasions, skin tears, second-degree burns, pressure ulcers, lower-extremity ulcers (including those of venous, arterial, and mixed etiology), diabetic ulcers, and donor sites; also suitable for use under compression bandaging or under tracheostomies to provide cushioning; may be cut to accommodate bony prominences or smaller wound sizes; fenestrated version accommodates a gastrostomy tube or other leaking drain tubes

Contraindications
- Contraindicated for third-degree burns
- Contraindicated in patients with active vasculitis

Application
- Clean the wound using Skintegrity Wound Cleanser or an appropriate solution. Dry the surrounding skin.
- Select the appropriate size dressing to allow the foam to cover all breached or compromised skin.
- Apply the dressing, and secure it with elastic net, gauze roll, or tape.

Removal
- The dressing may be left in place for up to 7 days or until exudate is visible and nears the edge of the dressing.
- Gently remove the dressing.
- Clean the wound again before applying a new dressing.

FOAMS

Optifoam Non-Adhesive Foam Dressing
Medline Industries, Inc.

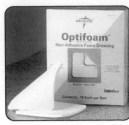

How supplied
Pad: 4″ × 4″; A6209
         6″ × 6″; A6210

Action
Optifoam Non-Adhesive Foam Island Dressing is a hydropolymer dressing consisting of a thin film backing over a hydrophilic foam pad. The dressing's waterproof outer layer helps to maintain an optimally moist healing environment, prevent strike-through, and aid in preventing bacterial contamination of the wound.

Indications
To manage chronic and acute, moderately to heavily exuding, partial- and full-thickness wounds, including superficial wounds, minor abrasions, skin tears, second-degree burns, pressure ulcers, lower-extremity ulcers (including those of venous, arterial, and mixed etiology), diabetic ulcers, and donor sites; also for use under compression bandaging or under tracheostomies to provide cushioning

Contraindications
- Contraindicated for third-degree burns
- Contraindicated in patients with active vasculitis
- For use in visibly infected wounds only when proper medical treatment addresses the underlying cause

Application
- Clean the wound using Skintegrity Wound Cleanser or an appropriate solution. Dry the surrounding skin.
- Select the appropriate size dressing to allow the foam to cover all breached or compromised skin. May be cut to accommodate bony prominences or smaller wound sizes or fenestrated to accommodate a gastrostomy tube or other leaking drain tubes.
- Apply the dressing, and secure it with elastic net, gauze roll, or tape.

Removal
- The dressing may be left in place for up to 7 days or until exudate is visible and nears the edge of the dressing.
- Gently remove the dressing.
- Clean the wound again before applying a new dressing.

FOAMS

New Product

Optifoam Site Adhesive Foam Dressing

Medline Industries, Inc.

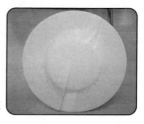

How supplied

Island dressing: 4″ round with 2″ foam pad with fenestration; A6212

Action

Optifoam Site Foam Dressing is a polyurethane foam pad that provides soft, cushioning absorbency for site care and includes a nonwoven adhesive border that is conformable even around difficult-to-dress sites. Radial slit and starburst opening easily accommodate most tube circumferences.

Indications

To manage tube sites that require cushioning, absorbency, or protection

Contraindications

- Contraindicated for third-degree burns
- Contraindicated in patients with active vasculitis

Application

- Clean the wound using Skintegrity Wound Cleanser or an appropriate solution. Dry the surrounding skin.
- Remove one side of the release paper.
- Wrap the dressing around the tube site.
- Remove the remaining release paper, and smooth the dressing border into place.

Removal

- The dressing may be left in place for up to 7 days or until exudate is visible and nears the edge of the dressing.
- Gently remove the dressing.

FOAMS

POLYDERM BORDER Hydrophilic Polyurethane Foam Dressing
DeRoyal

How supplied
Foam pad with border: $2^1/4'' \times 2^1/4''$ foam with $4'' \times 4''$ border, $3\,^3/4'' \times 3^3/4''$ foam with $6'' \times 6''$ border, $2^1/2''$ circular foam with $4''$ circular border and $2''$ radial slit; A6212

Action
POLYDERM BORDER Hydrophilic Polyurethane Foam Dressing is lint-free with a stretchable fabric border that's gentle on sensitive skin and effective for managing exuding wounds and tube sites. POLYDERM BORDER's thick foam construction provides soft, absorbent protection to painful wound sites.

Indications
For use as a primary or secondary dressing to manage pressure ulcers (stages 2, 3, and 4), partial- and full-thickness wounds, tube sites, donor sites, tunneling wounds, infected and noninfected wounds, and draining wounds; may also be used for red, yellow, and black wounds and for exuding wounds

Contraindications
None provided by the manufacturer

Application
- Clean the wound site with normal saline solution.
- Peel back the release liner from the dressing's center to expose the foam.
- Center the foam over the wound, and press it into place.

Removal
- Gently lift the edges of the border, and then peel off the dressing.

FOAMS

POLYDERM Hydrophilic Polyurethane Foam Dressing
DeRoyal

How supplied
Foam pad: $2^{1}/_{4}'' \times 2^{1}/_{4}''$; A6209
$3^{3}/_{4}'' \times 3^{3}/_{4}''$; A6212

Action
POLYDERM is a nonadherent, highly absorbent, lint-free foam dressing for the management of heavily exuding wounds.

Indications
For use as a primary or secondary dressing to manage pressure ulcers (stages 2, 3, and 4), partial- and full-thickness wounds, donor sites, second-degree burns, lacerations, cuts, abrasions, and draining wounds; may also be used for red, yellow, and black wounds and for exuding wounds

Contraindications
None provided by the manufacturer

Application
- Clean the wound site with normal saline solution.
- Center the foam over the wound.
- Secure the dressing.

Removal
- Remove any secondary dressing.
- Gently lift the foam dressing from the wound.

FOAMS

POLYDERM PLUS Barrier Foam Dressing
DeRoyal

How supplied
Foam pad with border: 2¹⁄₄″ × 2¹⁄₄″ foam with 4″ × 4″ border,
3³⁄₄″ × 3³⁄₄″ foam with 6″ × 6″ border; A6212

Action
POLYDERM PLUS is a nonadherent, highly absorbent, semiocclusive, lint-free foam dressing with a nonwoven tape border. It maintains a moist wound environment conducive to healing and resists external contaminants and blood or drainage strike-through.

Indications
For use as a primary or secondary dressing to manage pressure ulcers (stages 2, 3, and 4), partial- and full-thickness wounds, donor sites, tunneling wounds, infected and noninfected wounds, and draining wounds; may also be used for red, yellow, or black wounds and for exuding wounds

Contraindications
None provided by the manufacturer

Application
- Clean the wound with normal saline solution.
- Peel back the release liner from the dressing's center to expose the foam.
- Center the foam over the wound, and press into place.

Removal
- Gently lift the edges of the border, and then peel off the dressing.

FOAMS

PolyMem QuadraFoam Adhesive Film Dressing*

PolyMem QuadraFoam Adhesive Cloth Dressing*

PolyMem QuadraFoam Non-Adhesive Dressing*

Ferris Manufacturing Corporation

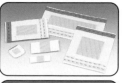
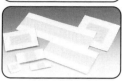
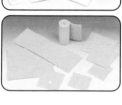

How supplied

PolyMem Adhesive Film Dressings

Sterile pad: $2'' \times 2''$ dot with $1'' \times 1''$ membrane pad, $4'' \times 5''$ island with $2'' \times 3''$ membrane pad, $6'' \times 6''$ island with $3.5'' \times 3.5''$ membrane pad, $1'' \times 3''$ strip with $1'' \times 1''$ membrane pad, $2'' \times 4''$ strip with $1.5'' \times 2''$ membrane pad; A6212

             $4'' \times 12.5''$ island with $2'' \times 10''$ membrane; A6213

PolyMem Adhesive Cloth Dressings

Sterile pad: $2'' \times 2''$ dot with $1'' \times 1''$ membrane pad, $4'' \times 5''$ island with $2'' \times 3''$ membrane pad, $6'' \times 6''$ island with $3.5'' \times 3.5''$ membrane pad, $1'' \times 3''$ strip with $1'' \times 1''$ membrane pad, $2'' \times 4''$ strip with $1.5'' \times 2''$ membrane pad; A6212

             $3'' \times 3''$ membrane pad, $4'' \times 4''$ membrane pad; A6209

             $5'' \times 5''$ membrane pad; A6210

             $6.5'' \times 7.5''$ membrane pad, $4'' \times 12.5''$ membrane pad, $4'' \times 24''$ membrane pad; A6211

Action

PolyMem dressings belong to an innovative class of adaptable wound dressings called QuadraFoam. QuadraFoam dressings effectively cleanse, fill, absorb, and moisten wounds throughout the healing continuum.

PolyMem Wound Dressing is composed of a patented hydrophilic polyurethane membrane matrix pad covered with a semipermeable continuous thin film backing that is optimized for oxygen and moisture vapor permeability and as a barrier to liquids. The PolyMem formulation is the only dressing formulation that contains a safe, nontoxic cleanser (F68 surfactant), a moisturizer (glycerol, also known as glycerin), and an absorbing agent (superabsorbent starch copolymer), all in the pad matrix. Both F68 and glycerol are soluble in wound fluid and skin moisture. The superabsorbent starch copolymer contained in the PolyMem formulation draws wound fluid, which is known to contain natural growth factors and nutrients, to the wound site.

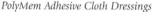

Indications

For the management of pressure ulcers (stages 1 to 4), venous stasis ulcers, acute wounds, leg ulcers, donor and graft sites, skin tears, diabetic ulcers, dermatologic disorders, first- and second-degree burns, and surgical wounds; suitable for use when signs of infection are visible if the cause of the infection has received proper medical treatment

Contraindications

- Not compatible with hypochlorite solutions (bleach) such as Dakin's solution
- Not for use on patients with sensitivity to any ingredients

Application

- Prepare the wound according to facility policy or as directed by a physician or other ordering clinician. With subsequent dressing changes, cleaning the wound isn't recommended unless infection or gross contamination is present.
- Select a PolyMem dressing of appropriate size. The pink membrane should be $1/4''$ to 2 " (0.6 to 5 cm) larger than the wound area.
- Apply the dressing film side and printed side out.
- Topical treatments aren't recommended for use with PolyMem family of dressings.

Removal

- A dramatic increase in wound fluid may be observed during the first few days.
- Keep the dressing dry when bathing the patient. Change the dressing if it gets wet.
- Change the dressing before exudate, visible through the dressing, reaches the periwound area (wound edges). If the wound fluid reaches the the edge of the dressing membrane pad, change immediately. For a mildly exudating wound in an otherwise healthy patient, the dressing may remain in place for up to 7 days. As with other dressings, more frequent changes may be indicated if the patient has a compromised immune system, diabetes, or infection at the wound site.
- Gently remove the dressing. Don't disturb the wound bed. Don't clean the wound or flush with saline or water unless the wound is infected or contaminated. PolyMem dressings contain a mild, nontoxic wound cleanser and leave no residue. Additional cleaning of the wound may injure regenerating tissues and delay the wound-healing process.
- Apply a new PolyMem dressing.

*See package insert for complete information.

FOAMS

PolyMem Max QuadraFoam Wound Dressing

Ferris Manufacturing Corporation

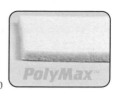

How supplied

Non-adhesive membrane pad: 4.5" × 4.5"; A6210

Action

PolyMem Max belongs to an innovative class of adaptable wound dressings called QuadraFoam. QuadraFoam dressings effectively cleanse, fill, absorb, and moisten wounds throughout the healing continuum.

PolyMem Max is the higher-profile, super-thick version of the PolyMem formulation. PolyMem Max Wound Dressing is composed of a patented hydrophilic polyurethane membrane matrix pad covered with a semipermeable continuous thin film backing that is optimized for oxygen and moisture vapor permeability and as a barrier to liquids. The PolyMem formulation is the only dressing formulation that contains a safe, nontoxic cleanser (F68 surfactant), a moisturizer (glycerol, also known as glycerin), and an absorbing agent (superabsorbent starch copolymer), all in the pad matrix. Both F68 and glycerol are soluble in wound fluid and skin moisture. The superabsorbent starch copolymer contained in the PolyMem formulation draws wound fluid, which is known to contain natural growth factors and nutrients, to the wound site.

Indications

For the management of pressure ulcers (stages 1 to 4), venous stasis ulcers, acute wounds, leg ulcers, donor and graft sites, skin tears, diabetic ulcers, dermatologic disorders, first- and second-degree burns, and surgical wounds; suitable for use when signs of infection are visible if the cause of the infection has received proper medical treatment

Contraindications

- Not compatible with hypochlorite solutions (bleach) such as Dakin's solution
- Not for use on patients with sensitivity to any ingredient

Application

- Prepare the wound according to facility policy or as directed by a physician or other ordering clinician. With subsequent dressing changes, cleaning the wound isn't recommended unless infection or gross contamination is present.
- Select a PolyMem dressing of appropriate size. The pink membrane should be ¼" to 2" (0.6 to 5 cm) larger than the wound area.
- Apply the dressing film side and printed side out.
- Topical treatments aren't recommended for use with PolyMem Max dressing.

FOAMS

Removal

- A dramatic increase in wound fluid may be observed during the first few days. Not uncommon, it indicates that the PolyMem Max dressing is working.
- Keep the dressing dry when bathing the patient. Change the dressing if it gets wet.
- Change the dressing before exudate, visible through the dressing, reaches the periwound area (wound edges). If the wound fluid reaches the the edge of the dressing membrane pad, change immediately. For a mildly exudating wound in an otherwise healthy patient, the dressing may remain in place for up to 7 days. As with other dressings, more frequent changes may be indicated if the patient has a compromised immune system, diabetes, or infection at the wound site.
- Gently remove the dressing. Don't clean the wound or flush with saline or water unless the wound is infected or contaminated. PolyMem Max dressings contain a mild, nontoxic wound cleanser and leave no residue. Additional cleaning of the wound may injure regenerating tissues and delay the wound-healing process.
- Apply a new PolyMem Max dressing.

*See package insert for complete information.

PolyMem Wic QuadraFoam Cavity Wound Filler*

Ferris Manufacturing Corporation

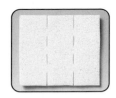

How supplied

Sterile pad: 3″ × 3″, 3″ × 12″; A6215

Action

PolyMem formulation dressings belong to an innovative class of adaptable wound dressings called QuadraFoam. QuadraFoam dressings effectively cleanse, fill, absorb, and moisten wounds throughout the healing continuum.

PolyMem Wic cavity filler is composed of a hydrophilic polyurethane membrane that may be placed into open wounds to eliminate dead space, absorb exudate, and maintain a moist wound surface. PolyMem Wic Filler minimizes the need to disturb the wound bed. PolyMem Wic Filler is the only filler that contains a safe, nontoxic wound cleanser (F68 surfactant), a moisturizer (glycerin), and an absorbing agent (superabsorbent starch copolymer), all in the polyurethane matrix. Both F68 and glycerin are soluble in wound fluid and skin moisture. PolyMem Wic is placed in the wound bed; it provides fast wicking and absorbent capacity to accommodate large amounts of exudate. PolyMem Wic Filler expands to fill dead space and allows extended times between dressing changes. PolyMem Wic Filler is perforated so that 1″ wide strips can be detached or easily folded, or it can be placed as is into a cavity. PolyMem Wic Cavity Filler is to be covered with a secondary PolyMem formulation dressing or another suitable secondary dressing.

Indications

To manage moderately to heavily exuding wounds associated with pressure ulcers (stages 3 and 4), vascular ulcers, acute wounds, and diabetic ulcers; suitable for use when signs of infection are visible if the cause of the infection has received proper medical treatment

Contraindications

- Not compatible with hypochlorite solutions (bleach) such as Dakin's solution
- Not for use on patients with sensitivity to any ingredient

Application

- Prepare the wound according to facility policy or as directed by a physician or other ordering clinician. With subsequent dressing changes, cleaning the wound isn't recommended unless infection or gross contamination is present.
- Ensure that PolyMem Wic is 30% smaller than the wound diameter. PolyMem Wic will expand as it wicks and absorbs fluid. Avoid overfill-

FOAMS

ing the wound, because overfilling may increase pressure on the tissue in the wound bed, potentially causing additional damage.

- Lightly place the wound filler in the middle of the wound, either side up. PolyMem Wic is perforated so that 1" (2.5 cm) wide strips can be detached, cut, folded, or placed as is into the cavity.
- Cover the wound and the PolyMem Wic with a PolyMem formulation dressing or another suitable secondary dressing.

Removal

- Change PolyMem Wic and secondary dressing when exudate reaches the periwound area. Change daily if the patient has a compromised immune system, diabetes, or an infection at the wound site.
- Gently remove the wound filler in one piece. (It won't adhere to the wound.) Don't disturb the wound bed. Don't clean the wound or flush with saline or water unless the wound is infected or contaminated. Additional cleaning of the wound may injure regenerating tissues and may delay the wound-healing process.
- Apply a new PolyMem Wic cavity dressing with a suitable secondary dressing.

*See package insert for complete information.

Shapes by PolyMem QuadraFoam Dressings
Ferris Manufacturing Corporation

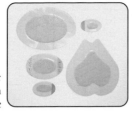

How supplied

Sacral dressing adhesive island film dressing: 7.2" × 7.8" shaped island with 4.5" × 4.7" shaped membrane pad; A6212

#8 oval adhesive island film dressing: 6.5" × 8.2" oval island with 4.0" × 5.7" oval membrane pad; A6213

#5 oval adhesive island film dressing: 3.5" × 5.0" oval island with 2" × 3" oval membrane pad; A6212

#3 oval adhesive island film dressing: 2" × 3" oval island with 1" × 2" oval membrane pad; A6212

#1 oval adhesive island film dressing: 2" × 3" oval island with 1" × 1.5"oval membrane pad; A6212

Action

Shapes by PolyMem dressings belong to an innovative class of adaptable wound dressings called QuadraFoam. QuadraFoam dressings effectively cleanse, fill, absorb, and moisten wounds throughout the healing continuum. Shapes by PolyMem dressings are easy-to use, precut dressings, contoured to fit most wounds.

Shapes by PolyMem Wound Dressing is composed of a patented hydrophilic polyurethane membrane matrix with a thin film adhesive border. The membrane pad is covered with a semipermeable continuous thin film backing that is optimized for oxygen and moisture vapor permeability and as a barrier to liquids. The PolyMem formulation is the only dressing formulation that contains a safe, nontoxic cleanser (F68 surfactant), a moisturizer (glycerol, also known as glycerin), and an absorbing agent (superabsorbent starch copolymer), all in the pad matrix. Both F68 and glycerol are soluble in wound fluid and skin moisture. The superabsorbent starch copolymer contained in the PolyMem formulation draws wound fluid, which is known to contain natural growth factors and nutrients, to the wound site.

This product is also available with silver in the membrane pad.

Indications

For the management of pressure ulcers (stages 1 to 4), venous stasis ulcers, acute wounds, leg ulcers, donor and graft sites, skin tears, diabetic ulcers, dermatologic disorders, first- and second-degree burns, and surgical wounds; suitable for use when signs of infection are visible if the cause of the infection has received proper medical treatment

FOAMS

Contraindications

- Not compatible with hypochlorite solutions (bleach) such as Dakin's solution
- Not for use on patients with sensitivity to any ingredient

Application

- Prepare the wound according to facility policy or as directed by a physician or other ordering clinician. With subsequent dressing changes, cleaning the wound isn't recommended unless infection or gross contamination is present.
- Select a Shapes by PolyMem dressing of appropriate size. The pink membrane should be $1/4''$ to $2''$ (0.6 to 5 cm) larger than the wound area.
- Apply the dressing film side and printed side out.
- Topical treatments aren't recommended for use with Shapes by PolyMem family of dressings.

Removal

- A dramatic increase in wound fluid may be observed during the first few days.
- Keep the dressing dry when bathing the patient. Change the dressing if it gets wet.
- Change the dressing before exudate, visible through the dressing, reaches the periwound area (wound edges). If the wound fluid reaches the the edge of the dressing membrane pad, change immediately. For a mildly exudating wound in an otherwise healthy patient, the dressing may remain in place for up to 7 days. As with other dressings, more frequent changes may be indicated if the patient has a compromised immune system, diabetes, or infection at the wound site.
- Gently remove the dressing. Don't disturb the wound bed. Don't clean the wound or flush with saline or water unless the wound is infected or contaminated. Shapes by PolyMem dressings contain a safe, nontoxic wound cleanser and leave no residue. Additional cleaning of the wound may injure regenerating tissues and delay the wound-healing process.
- Apply a new Shapes by PolyMem dressing.

*See package insert for complete information.

Silon Dual-Dress 20F
Bio Med Sciences, Inc.

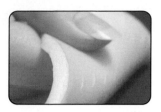

How supplied
Dressing: 5″ × 5″; A6210
5″ × 10″; A6211
11″ × 12″; A6211

Action
Silon Dual-Dress 20F is a single dressing with two different functions. One side consists of an open-celled hydrophilic foam. The other side consists of Silon-TSR semi-occlusive film. Silon is perforated to allow exudate to wick away from the wound. With the foam side of the dressing against the wound, the product provides a mildly adhesive surface for conditions where fixation is difficult. With the Silon side of the dressing against the wound, the product provides a nonadherent covering for fragile and sensitive wounds. Silon Dual-Dress 20F offers all of these features with a thicker, highly absorbent foam backing to reduce the number of dressing changes.

Indications
With the blue side of the dressing face-down for second-degree burns, skin-graft recipient sites, skin tears, and other partial-thickness wounds; with the foam side of the dressing face-down for skin-graft donor sites, abrasions, lacerations, stages 2 and 3 chronic wounds (venous stasis, pressure, and diabetic ulcers), other partial-thickness wounds and heavily exuding wounds

Contraindications
- Contraindicated for third-degree burns

Application
- Apply the appropriate side of Silon Dual-Dress 20F to the wound surface.
- Cover with a secondary gauze dressing to manage wound exudate

Removal
- Inspect periodically for signs of exudate strike-through into the gauze.
- Remove the secondary gauze dressing and Silon Dual-Dress 20F when the product becomes 80% saturated.
- Reapply new dressings as required.

FOAMS

Silon Dual-Dress 50
Bio Med Sciences, Inc.

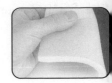

How supplied
Multifunctional dressing: 11″ × 12″, 11″ × 24″

Action
Silon Dual-Dress 50 may be used as a secondary covering over skin grafts or biosynthetic dressings or directly over clean partial-thickness wounds. The product is designed to provide and maintain a clean and moist wound healing environment and a bolster effect to maintain a slight amount of pressure on the wound surface.

Silon Dual-Dress 50 is comprised of two distinct layers: an open-cell absorbent foam and a semi-occlusive barrier film. The film is colored blue to make it easier to see. The product should be applied with the foam toward the wound and the blue film away from the wound.

Indications
For skin graft donor sites, second-degree burns, skin graft recipient sites, and other partial-thickness wounds

Contraindications
■ Contraindicated for primary coverage of third-degree burns

Application
■ Close, clean and/or dress the wound site as normal.
■ Open and remove a sheet of Silon Dual-Dress 50 using sterile technique.
■ Apply the dressing (blue side up) over the wound area and trim as required.
■ More than one sheet may be placed side by side to cover larger areas.
■ Affix the dressing(s) to the site using surgical staples around the perimeter. The dressing(s) should be stapled to the patients' skin around the perimeter but may be stapled to the next sheet if placed side by side.
■ When fixing the dressing in place, a slight amount of tension should be applied if a bolster effect is desired.

Removal
■ Inspect the wound area periodically for signs of exudate leakage.
■ The dressings may be left in place up to 5 days. Reapply as needed.

SOF-FOAM Dressing
Johnson & Johnson Wound
Management
A division of ETHICON, INC.

How supplied
Pad: 3″ × 3″; A6209
        4″ × 5″, 4″ × 8″; A6210
Fenestrated pad: 3⁵/₈″ × 3¹/₈″; A6209

Action
SOF-FOAM Dressing is a hydrophilic, polyurethane foam that's soft and nonlinting and designed to cushion and protect the wound site. When used as a primary dressing, the hydrophilic foam absorbs exudate and provides a moist healing environment. The nonadherent foam pad won't break down, making dressing changes easier. Fenestrated SOF-FOAM Dressing cushions the wound site and reduces the risk of particulate contamination.

Indications
To manage drainage around surgically induced drainage sites, such as tracheostomy and gastrostomy tubes; also for partial-thickness wounds, such as abrasions, lacerations, donor sites, and superficial burns; also for partial- and full-thickness, moderately to heavily exuding wounds, such as venous ulcers, diabetic ulcers, pressure ulcers, and surgical incisions

Contraindications
- Contraindicated for third-degree burns

Application
- Clean the wound with normal saline solution. Remove any loose necrotic tissue.
- Choose the appropriate dressing size, allowing a 1″ (2.5 cm) overlap around the wound margin.
- Apply the dressing, and secure it with adhesive tape or a bandage.

Removal
- Check the dressing for saturation and for strike-through at least once every 8 hours. Change the dressing when strike-through occurs or according to facility policy.
- Gently release the tape or wrap, and lift up the dressing.

FOAMS

SorbaCell Foam Dressing
Derma Sciences, Inc.

How supplied
Sheet: 2″ × 2″, 4″ × 4″
Strip: 1″ × 8″

Action
SorbaCell Foam Dressing is a nonadherent, highly absorptive polyurethane foam sheet that cushions and protects the wound. A secondary dressing is required to protect the wound from outside contaminants and hold the dressing in place.

Indications
To manage moderately to highly exuding wounds

Contraindications
- Contraindicated for third-degree burns

Application
- Clean the wound with PrimaDerm Dermal Cleanser or saline solution. Pat dry the skin adjacent to the wound.
- Position SorbaCell Foam Dressing directly on the wound.
- Secure with an appropriate secondary dressing.

Removal
- Remove the secondary dressing.
- Remove the SorbaCell Foam.

FOAMS

3M Tegaderm Foam Adhesive Dressing
3M Health Care

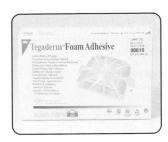

How supplied
Square: 2″ × 2″; A6212
4″ × 4″; A6212
Oval: 2½″ × 3″; A6212
4″ × 4½″; A6213
5½″ × 6¾″; A6213
Heel: 3″ × 3″; A6212

Action
3M Tegaderm Foam Adhesive Dressing is a highly absorbent, breathable wound dressing with a unique spoke delivery system that makes application easier. It's constructed from a conformable polyurethane foam pad, an additional absorbent nonwoven layer, and a top layer of transparent adhesive film. This film is moisture vapor permeable, which prevents wound exudate strike-throughs and acts as a barrier to outside contamination. The dressing maintains a moist environment, which has been shown to enhance wound healing.

Indications
For use as a primary dressing for moderately to highly exuding partial- and full-thickness dermal wounds, including pressure ulcers, venous leg ulcers, abrasions, first- and second-degree burns, donor sites, arterial ulcers, skin tears, and neuropathic ulcers

Contraindications
None provided by the manufacturer

Application
- Hold the dressing by the side tabs, and remove the printed liner, exposing the adhesive border.
- Position the dressing over the wound while holding the tabs.
- Gently press the adhesive border to the skin. Avoid stretching the dressing or skin.
- Remove the paper frame from the dressing while smoothing down the edges of the dressing.

Removal
- Carefully lift the dressing edges from the skin. If there's difficulty lifting the dressing, apply tape to the edge of the dressing and use the tape to lift. Continue lifting edges until all are free from the skin surface.

FOAMS

3M Tegaderm Foam Dressing (Nonadhesive)

3M Health Care

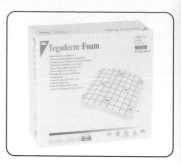

How supplied

Square:	2" × 2", 4" × 4"; A6209
	8" × 8"; A6211
Rectangle:	4" × 8"; A6210
Fenestrated:	3¹/₂" × 3¹/₂"; A6209
Roll:	4" × 24"; A6211

Action

3M Tegaderm Foam Dressing (Nonadhesive) is a highly absorbent, breathable, nonadherent wound dressing. It's constructed from conformable polyurethane foam covered with a highly breathable film backing. The film backing prevents exudate strike-through and acts as a barrier to outside contamination. The dressing maintains a moist wound environment, which has been shown to enhance wound healing. The dressing is sterile and may be cut to fit the needs of the user.

Indications

For use as a primary dressing for moderately to highly exuding partial- and full-thickness dermal wounds, including pressure ulcers, venous leg ulcers, abrasions, first- and second-degree burns, donor sites, arterial ulcers, skin tears, and neuropathic ulcers

Contraindications

None provided by the manufacturer

Application

- Remove the dressing from the package, and center it over wound, printed grid side up, with the edges overlapping onto intact skin.
- Secure the dressing with adhesive tape, elastic or cohesive wrap, or other appropriate material.

Removal

- Observe dressing frequently. As the dressing absorbs, exudates will wick to the top of the dressing, and discoloration may be noticeable. When exudates spread to the edges of dressing or dressing leaks, a dressing change is indicated.

FOAMS

TIELLE Hydropolymer Adhesive Dressing

Johnson & Johnson
Wound Management
A division of ETHICON, Inc.

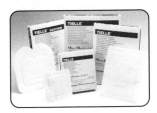

How supplied

Sterile island: $4^{1}/_{4}'' \times 4^{1}/_{4}''$; A6212
$5^{7}/_{8}'' \times 7^{3}/_{4}''$, $5^{7}/_{8}'' \times 5^{7}/_{8}''$; A6213
$5^{7}/_{8}'' \times 5^{7}/_{8}''$ (sacrum); A6254

Action

TIELLE Hydropolymer Adhesive Dressing is a fluid handling system. As exudate is absorbed by the dressing, the hydropolymer central island swells and fills any irregular contours in the wound, minimizing the buildup of exudate and the chance of maceration. Evaporation of excess moisture through the vapor-permeable polyurethane backing allows the dressing to manage additional exudate, a continuous process during wound healing.

Indications

To manage chronic and acute, low to moderately exuding, partial- and full-thickness wounds, pressure ulcers (stages 2, 3, and 4), lower-extremity ulcers (venous, arterial, and mixed etiology), diabetic ulcers, and donor sites; also for use under compression bandaging

Contraindications

- Contraindicated for third-degree burns
- Contraindicated in patients with active vasculitis
- For use in visibly infected wounds only when proper medical treatment addresses the underlying cause

Application

- Position the dressing over the wound site, making sure that the foam pad covers the wound and the smooth center portion is in place.
- One at a time, peel away the side backing papers while smoothing the film onto the intact periwound skin.

Removal

- Change the dressing when fluid is present at the edges of the hydropolymer central island. Don't allow exudate to accumulate under the backing.
- Lift one corner, and carefully peel back.
- On fragile or friable skin, water or saline solution may be used to break the adhesive seal.

FOAMS

TIELLE PLUS Hydropolymer Dressing
Johnson & Johnson Wound Management
A division of ETHICON, Inc.

How supplied
Pad: $4^1/_4'' \times 4^1/_4''$; A6212
          $5^7/_8'' \times 5^7/_8''$, $5^7/_8'' \times 7^3/_4''$; A6213

Action
TIELLE PLUS Hydropolymer Dressing is an exudate-handling system for moderately to heavily exuding wounds. This island dressing maintains a moist healing environment, encouraging autolytic debridement and enabling granulation to proceed under optimal conditions. Autolytic debridement may initially increase the wound size, which is normal and is expected before wound granulation. During use, the absorbent island gently expands as it takes up exudate.

Indications
To manage chronic and acute, moderate to heavy exuding, partial- and full-thickness wounds, including superficial wounds, such as minor abrasions, skin tears, and second-degree burns; also for use under compression bandaging; for use when signs of infection are visible in the wound area only when underlying cause is being properly treated; under a physician's supervision, to manage pressure ulcers, lower-extremity ulcers (venous, arterial, and mixed etiology), diabetic ulcers, and donor sites

Contraindications
- Contraindicated for third-degree burns
- Contraindicated in patients with active vasculitis

Application
- Prepare the wound according to facility policy. If the wound appears healthy and free from necrotic debris, cleaning may not be required.
- Make sure the skin surrounding the wound is dry.
- Position the dressing over the wound site, ensuring that the foam pad covers the wound, and smooth the center portion in place.
- One at a time, peel away the side backing papers while smoothing the adhesive border onto intact skin.

Removal
- Change the dressing when wound fluid is present at the edges of the foam pad. Don't allow exudate to accumulate under the backing. The dressing may be left in place for up to 7 days, depending on exudate.
- Lift one corner and carefully peel dressing back; avoid trauma to skin.
- On fragile or friable skin, use water or normal saline solution to break the adhesive seal.

FOAMS

Versiva Foam Composite Exudate Management Dressing*
ConvaTec

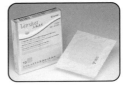

How supplied
Square: $3^1/_2'' \times 3^1/_2''$; A6200
            $5^1/_2'' \times 5^1/_2''$; A6201
            $7^1/_2'' \times 7^1/_2''$; A6202
Rectangular: $7^1/_2'' \times 9^1/_2''$; A6202
Heel: $7.3'' \times 7.7''$; A6202
Sacral: $8.3'' \times 8.7''$; A6202

Action
Versiva is a sterile, adhesive foam composite dressing consisting of a skin-friendly adhesive, a central layer with Hydrofiber technology, a fluid-spreading layer, and a top layer of polyurethane foam-film. The inclusion of the Hydrofiber technology into a foam dressing allows Versiva to decrease the risk of maceration, keep the periwound skin in better condition, cushion more effectively, maintain an optimally moist environment to support wound healing, hold more fluid under compression, and have a thin profile.

Versiva dressing also acts as a barrier to viral and bacterial contamination when intact and without leakage.

Indications
For over-the-counter use, for minor abrasions, lacerations, minor cuts, and minor scalds and burns; under a physician's supervision, for leg ulcers (venous stasis ulcers, arterial ulcers, and leg ulcers of mixed etiology), diabetic ulcers, pressure ulcers and sores (partial- and full-thickness wounds), surgical wounds (left to heal by secondary intention, donor sites, dermatologic excisions), second-degree burns, and traumatic wounds; for use as a secondary dressing with AQUACEL dressing for deep and heavily exuding wounds, or with AQUACEL Ag dressing for wounds at risk of infection

Contraindications
- Not for use on individuals who are sensitive to or who have had an allergic reaction to the dressing or its components

Application
- Before using the dressing, clean the wound with an appropriate wound cleanser or normal saline, and dry the surrounding skin.
- Choose a dressing size to make sure that the absorbent pad is larger than the wound area.
- Remove the release paper from the back, being careful to minimize finger contact with the adhesive surface.
- Hold the dressing over the wound, lining up the center of the dressing with the center of the wound. Place the pad directly over the wound.

FOAMS

- For difficult-to-dress anatomical locations, such as the heel or the sacrum, a supplementary securing device, such as tape, may be required.
- Discard any unused portion of the product after dressing the wound.
- If the immediate product packaging is damaged, don't use the product.
- Protect from light. Store at room temperature (50° to 77°F [10° to 25°C]). Keep dry.

Removal

- Dressing may remain in place up to 7 days. The dressing should be changed when clinically indicated or when strike-through occurs. The wound should be cleaned at each dressing change.
- Press down gently on the skin, and carefully lift one corner of the dressing until it no longer adheres to the skin. Continue until all edges are free. Carefully lift away the dressing.

*See package insert for complete instructions for use.

Hydrocolloids

Action

Hydrocolloids are occlusive or semiocclusive dressings composed of such materials as gelatin, pectin, and carboxymethylcellulose. The composition of the wound contact layer may differ considerably among dressings. These dressings provide a moist healing environment that allows clean wounds to granulate and necrotic wounds to debride autolytically. Some hydrocolloids may leave a residue in the wound, and others may adhere to the skin around the wound. Hydrocolloids are manufactured in various shapes, sizes, adhesive properties, and forms, including wafers, pastes, and powders.

Indications

Hydrocolloid dressings may be used as primary or secondary dressings to manage select pressure ulcers, partial- and full-thickness wounds, wounds with necrosis or slough, and wounds with light to moderate exudate.

Advantages

- Are impermeable to bacteria and other contaminants
- Facilitate autolytic debridement
- Are self-adherent and mold well
- Provide light to moderate absorption
- Minimize skin trauma and disruption of healing
- Allow observation of the healing process, if transparent
- May be used under compression products (compression stockings, wraps, pumps, and Unna's boot)

Disadvantages

- Aren't recommended for wounds with heavy exudate, sinus tracts, or infections; wounds surrounded by fragile skin; or wounds with exposed tendon or bone
- Can make wound assessment difficult, if opaque
- May be dislodged if the wound produces heavy exudate
- Provide an occlusive property that limits gas exchange between the wound and the environment
- May curl at edges
- May injure fragile skin upon removal

HCPCS code overview

The HCPCS codes normally assigned to hydrocolloid wound covers without an adhesive border are:

A6234—pad size < 16 in^2

A6235—pad size > 16 in^2 but < 48 in^2

A6236—pad size > 48 in^2.

The HCPCS codes normally assigned to hydrocolloid wound covers with an adhesive border are:

A6237—pad size < 16 in^2
A6238—pad size > 16 in^2 but < 48 in^2
A6239—pad size > 48 in^2.

The HCPCS codes normally assigned to hydrocolloid wound fillers are:
A6240—paste, per fluid ounce
A6241—dry form, per gram.

CarraSmart Hydrocolloid with Acemannan Hydrogel

Carrington Laboratories, Inc.

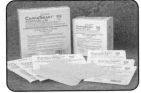

How supplied
Pad: 6″ × 6″; A6235

Action
CarraSmart Hydrocolloid wound dressing is a hydrocolloid with a high moisture vapor transfer rate and Acemannan Hydrogel. The "smart" film backing allows moisture to transpire through the hydrocolloid dressing. The hydrocolloid material reacts with the wound exudate to form a gelatinous mass, which provides for a moist healing environment and reduces the potential for tissue damage during dressing changes.

Indications
To manage minimally to moderately exuding wounds, donor sites, partial- to full-thickness wounds, trauma wounds, postoperative surgical wounds, and dermal lesions; also used as a protective dressing

Contraindications
- Contraindicated for dermal ulcers involving muscle, tendon, or bone
- Contraindicated for ulcers resulting from infection
- Contraindicated in patients with active vasculitis

Application
- Gently clean the wound with a suitable wound cleanser, such as CarraKlenz, UltraKlenz, or MicroKlenz. Dry the surrounding skin.
- Select the correct dressing size to allow 1¼″ (3 cm) overlap at the wound margins; trim as desired.
- Remove the release paper from the dressing, minimizing contact with the adhesive surface.
- Apply dressing with a rolling motion; don't stretch it. When applying to a sacral ulcer, press well down into the anal fold.
- Smooth and press into place.

Removal
- Dressings may be changed up to every 7 days, as indicated.
- Press down on the skin, and carefully lift the dressing edges.

HYDROCOLLOIDS

CombiDERM ACD Absorbent Cover Dressing*
ConvaTec

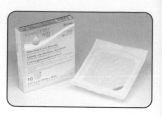

How supplied
Sterile dressing: 4″ × 4″, 5¹⁄₄″ × 5¹⁄₄″,
6″ × 7″; A6237
6″ × 10″, 8″ × 8″,
8″ × 9″; A6238

Action
CombiDERM ACD Absorbent Cover Dressing is a sterile dressing with a hydrocolloid adhesive and an absorbent pad. The absorbent pad wicks exudate and doesn't damage tissue.

Indications
To manage exuding, chronic dermal ulcers, such as pressure ulcers, leg ulcers, and diabetic ulcers, as well as acute wounds, such as abrasions, lacerations, biopsy sites, and open and closed surgical wounds

Contraindications
- Contraindicated for patients with sensitivity to the dressing or its components

Application
- Clean the wound surface and surrounding skin with an appropriate cleansing solution. Dry the surrounding skin thoroughly.
- Debride the wound, if necessary.
- Determine the ideal dressing size, allowing a minimum 1¹⁄₄″ (3 cm) margin beyond the reddened skin.
- If a filler or exudate management product is required, apply AQUACEL Hydrofiber Dressing, KALTOSTAT alginate dressing, or other appropriate dressing.
- Remove CombiDERM ACD release paper, and place the dressing directly over the wound.
- Press and smooth the dressing edges to ensure adherence and a firm seal.

Removal
- Gently press down on the skin, and carefully lift the blue tab on the corner of the dressing. Continue until all edges are free.
- Carefully lift away the dressing.

*See package insert for complete instructions for use.

CombiDERM Non-Adhesive Sterile Dressing*
ConvaTec

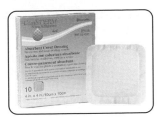

How supplied
Sterile dressing: 3″ × 3″; A6234
5¼″ × 5¼″; A6235
6″ × 10″; A6236

Action
CombiDERM Non-Adhesive is a sterile, nonadhesive wound dressing consisting of absorbent hydrocolloids that provide a moist environment, absorb exudate, and are nondamaging to tissue. The dressing may be used alone or with other primary dressings to manage wound exudate.

Indications
To manage exudate in chronic wounds, such as pressure ulcers, leg ulcers, and diabetic ulcers, as well as acute exuding wounds, such as abrasions, lacerations, biopsy sites, and open and closed surgical wounds

Contraindications
- Contraindicated for patients with sensitivity to the dressing or its components

Application
- Clean the wound site, rinse well, and dry the surrounding skin.
- Choose a dressing that extends 1″ (2.5 cm) beyond the wound.
- Apply the dressing, white side down, directly over the wound.
- Secure the dressing with tape or with a secondary bandage or wrap.
- For highly exuding wounds, it's recommended that CombiDERM Non-Adhesive dressing be used with AQUACEL or KALTOSTAT dressing.

Removal
- Change the dressing when clinically indicated or as the softened area approaches the edge of the dressing. The dressing may be left in place for up to 7 days.
- Carefully lift the dressing away from the wound.

*See package insert for complete instructions for use.

HYDROCOLLOIDS

Comfeel Plus Hydrocolloid Contour Dressing

Comfeel Plus Hydrocolloid Pressure Relief Dressing

Comfeel Plus Hydrocolloid Triangle Dressing

Comfeel Hydrocolloid Paste and Powder
Coloplast Corporation

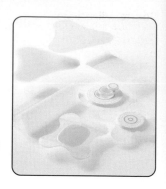

How supplied

Comfeel Plus Hydrocolloid Contour Dressing
Wafer: 24 in^2, 42 in^2; A6238

Comfeel Plus Hydrocolloid Pressure Relief Dressing
Wafer: 3" butterfly, 4" round; A6237
          6" round; A6238

Comfeel Plus Hydrocolloid Triangle Dressing
Wafer: 7" × 8"; A6239

Comfeel Hydrocolloid Paste
Tube: 1.76 oz (50 g); A6240
Single-dose tube: 0.42 oz (12 g); A6240

Comfeel Hydrocolloid Powder
Capsule: 0.21 oz (6 g); A6241

Action
The range of Comfeel hydrocolloid dressings provides an optimal, moist healing environment. Comfeel Hydrocolloid Paste and Comfeel Hydrocolloid Powder are supplements to the chosen wound dressing. Comfeel Hydrocolloid Paste provides filling of the wound cavity, which prevents collapse of undermined wounds. Comfeel Hydrocolloid Powder is highly absorbent and can therefore prolong the wear time of the wound dressing.

Indications
Comfeel Plus Hydrocolloid Contour Dressing to manage pressure ulcers in difficult-to-dress sites; Comfeel Plus Hydrocolloid Pressure Relief Dressing to manage and prevent pressure ulcers; Comfeel Plus Hydrocolloid Triangle Dressing to manage pressure ulcers in the sacral and hard-to-dress areas; Comfeel Hydrocolloid Paste for filling cavity wounds to give the wound extra support and create contact between the wound bed and the dressing; Comfeel Hydrocolloid Paste used with a Comfeel Plus Hydrocolloid dressing to ensure a moist healing environment; Comfeel Hydrocolloid Powder for superficial, highly exuding wounds; all types for diabetic or infected wounds, under physician's supervision

Contraindications

- Contraindicated if a wound becomes infected
- Must be removed before radiation therapy

Application

- Rinse the wound with Sea-Clens or normal saline solution. Gently pat dry the skin around the wound.
- Choose a dressing that allows for $3/8''$ to $1''$ (1 to 2.5 cm) overlap of the wound.

Comfeel Plus Hydrocolloid Contour Dressing

- Remove the protective paper from the center of the dressing, and place the dressing on the wound.
- Remove the protective paper from the wings, and gently press the wings one at a time to ensure that the dressing adheres to the skin.

Comfeel Plus Hydrocolloid Pressure Relief Dressing

- Remove the number of foam rings with orange print to get a foam-free area $3/4''$ to $1''$ (1 to 2.5 cm) larger than the wound.
- Remove the protective paper from the dressing, and roll the dressing on from one side.
- Remove the protective paper from the microporous tape, and gently apply the tape to the skin.

Comfeel Plus Hydrocolloid Triangle Dressing

- Remove the protective paper from the center of the dressing.
- Spread the gluteal fold, place the dressing's narrow end into the deepest depression of the gluteal fold, and secure it in place. Ensure that the wound has $1''$ (2.5 cm) of intact periwound skin and that the dressing adheres to the skin.
- Remove the second protective paper from the dressing, and secure the dressing in place.

Comfeel Hydrocolloid Paste

- Fill the wound with the paste to about one-third of the wound depth.

Comfeel Hydrocolloid Powder

- Gently press the capsule to direct the powder into the wound bed.

Removal

- As Comfeel dressings absorb wound exudate, they turn white or lighten. Change the dressing when the color-change indicator spreads to $3/8''$ (1 cm) from the border. Change Comfeel Hydrocolloid Paste and Powder when changing the wound dressing.
- In case of leakage or nonadherence, change the dressing immediately.
- Although Comfeel dressings are odorproof, the wound itself may have a characteristic odor. This is normal, and the odor should resolve once the wound is rinsed. If the odor persists, contact a physician.

Comfeel Plus Hydrocolloid Ulcer Dressing

Comfeel Hydrocolloid Ulcer Care Dressing

Comfeel Plus Hydrocolloid Clear Dressing

Coloplast Corporation

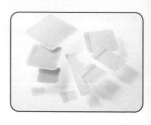

How supplied

Comfeel Plus Hydrocolloid Ulcer Dressing
Wafer: $1^{1}/_{2}'' \times 2^{1}/_{2}''$, $4'' \times 4''$; A6234
         $6'' \times 6''$; A6235
         $8'' \times 8''$; A6236

Comfeel Hydrocolloid Ulcer Care Dressing
Wafer: $1^{1}/_{2}'' \times 2^{1}/_{2}''$, $4'' \times 4''$; A6234
         $6'' \times 6''$; A6235
         $8'' \times 8''$; A6236

Comfeel Plus Hydrocolloid Clear Dressing
Wafer: $2'' \times 2^{3}/_{4}''$, $4'' \times 4''$; A6234
         $3^{1}/_{2}'' \times 5^{1}/_{2}''$, $6'' \times 6''$, $6'' \times 8''$; A6235
         $8'' \times 8''$; A6236

Action

Comfeel hydrocolloid dressings provide an optimal, moist healing environment.

Indications

Primarily to manage minimally to moderately exuding leg ulcers and pressure ulcers; may be used for superficial burns, partial-thickness burns, donor sites, postoperative wounds, and skin abrasions; may also be used for diabetic or infected wounds, under a physician's supervision

Contraindications

- Contraindicated if a wound becomes infected
- Must be removed before radiation therapy

Application

- Rinse the wound with Comfeel Sea-Clens or normal saline solution. Gently pat dry the skin around the wound.
- Choose a dressing that allows for $^{3}/_{8}''$ to $1''$ (1 to 2.5 cm) overlap of the wound.
- Use the handles on the dressing to ensure aseptic application. Remove the protective paper.
- Place the adhesive side to the wound. Remove the handle.

HYDROCOLLOIDS

Removal

- As Comfeel dressings absorb wound exudate, a gel forms. When the gel reaches the upper film surface of the dressing, it turns white or lightens. Change the dressing when the white gel spreads to $^3/_8''$ (1 cm) from the border.
- In case of leakage or nonadherence, change the dressing immediately.
- Although Comfeel dressings are odorproof, the wound itself may have a characteristic odor. This is normal, and the odor should resolve once the wound is rinsed. If the odor persists, contact a physician.

DermaFilm HD
DermaFilm Thin
DermaRite Industries, LLC

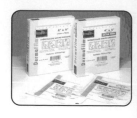

How supplied
DermaFilm HD
Film: 4″ × 4″; A6234
DermaFilm Thin
Film: 4″ × 4″; A6234

Action
DermaFilm is a pressure-sensitive dressing that interacts with wound exudates to form a soft gel. It helps isolate the wound against bacterial and other external contamination. The thin formula allows visibility and maintenance of the wound bed through course treatment.

Indications
To manage pressure ulcers (stages 1, 2, 3, and 4), partial- and full-thickness wounds, clinically infected wounds, minor abrasions, and second-degree burns; also to prevent skin breakdown by providing protection from urine, stool, and other contaminants

Contraindications
- Contraindicated for third-degree burns
- Contraindicated for ulcers involving muscle, tendon, or bone

Application
- Clean the wound area, and dry the periwound skin.
- Choose a dressing that overlaps the wound by at least 1″ (2.5 cm). Apply the dressing without stretching it.
- Press the dressing gently around the perimeter, forming it to the wound site.

Removal
- Change the dressing when the exudate extends to the edges. Dressing may be left in place for up to 7 days.
- Press down on the skin, and carefully lift an edge of the dressing. Continue lifting around the dressing until all edges are free.
- Clean the wound area again.

DERMATELL
GENTELL, Inc.

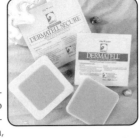

How supplied
Wafer: 4.25″ × 4.25″; A6235

Action
DERMATELL wafers absorb minimal to moderate wound exudate and interact with it to form a soft, protective gel. The dressing promotes autolysis, prevents secondary infection, and reduces pain. It also provides protection from urine, stool, and other contaminants

Indications
To manage venous ulcers in conjunction with compression therapy, pressure ulcers (stages 1, 2, and 3), first- and second-degree burns, and granulating wounds with minimal to moderate exudate

Contraindications
- Contraindicated for heavily exuding wounds, stage 4 pressure ulcers, infected wounds, and third-degree burns

Application
- Clean the wound with a wound cleanser. Gently dry the periwound skin.
- Remove the paper carrier from the dressing, and apply the dressing, allowing 2″ (5 cm) of the wafer to extend beyond the wound margin.
- For proper placement, center the wafer and gently adhere the dressing to the site, especially around the edges.

Removal
- Gently press down on skin, and carefully lift an edge of the dressing. Continue until all edges are free.
- Remember that the wound should be cleaned at each dressing change.

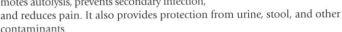

HYDROCOLLOIDS

DuoDERM CGF Border Dressing*

ConvaTec

How supplied

Sterile dressing: 2.5" × 2.5" dressing plus ³/₄"
adhesive border, 4" × 4"
dressing plus ³/₄" adhesive border, 4" × 5" dressing plus
1" adhesive border; A6237
6" × 6" plus 1" adhesive border, 6" × 7" plus 1" adhesive
border; A6238

Action

DuoDERM CGF Border Dressing creates a moist wound environment that
supports the healing process and autolytic debridement and allows for
nontraumatic removal. It helps isolate the wound against bacterial and
other external contamination while remaining intact and without leakage.

Indications

To manage dermal ulcers, diabetic foot ulcers, and leg ulcers; may also be
used on pressure ulcers (stages 1, 2, 3, and 4), full-thickness wounds, minor abrasions, second-degree burns, and donor sites

Contraindications

- Contraindicated for patients with sensitivity to the dressing or its components

Application

- Dressing is sterile; handle appropriately.
- Clean the wound according to facility guidelines, and dry the surrounding
  skin to ensure that it's grease-free.
- Before applying the dressing, remove eschar that's particularly thick or
  fused to the wound margins.
- Choose a dressing size that's at least 1¹/₄" (3 cm) larger than the wound
  margins.
- Remove only the top backing paper.
- Apply the dressing over the wound. Smooth into place, especially at the
  edges of the center adhesive. *Note:* The triangle-shaped dressing can be
  applied in several directions, depending on the location of the ulcer. For
  sacral ulcers, fold the dressing in half lengthwise to make it easy to apply in the sacral fold.
- Fold back the border, and remove the release papers; press the borders
  into place. Additional taping isn't required.
- Obtain a bacterial culture of the site if infection develops, and start appropriate medical treatment as ordered. Continue using the dressing as
  directed by the primary care provider.

HYDROCOLLOIDS

Removal

- Leave the dressing in place for up to 7 days unless it's uncomfortable or leaking, or infection develops.
- Press down on the skin, and carefully lift an edge of the dressing. Continue lifting around the dressing until all edges are free.
- The wound should be cleaned at each dressing change. (It's unnecessary to remove all residual dressing material from the surrounding skin.)

*See package insert for complete instructions for use.

DuoDERM CGF Dressing*
ConvaTec

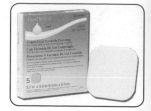

How supplied
Dressing: 4″ × 4″; A6234
              6″ × 6″, 6″ × 8″; A6235
              8″ × 8″, 8″ × 12″; A6236

Action
DuoDERM CGF (Control Gel Formula) Dressing is an adhesive (hydro-colloid) wound contact dressing. The self-adherent dressing absorbs wound fluid and provides a moist environment, which supports the body's heal-ing process and aids in the removal of unnecessary material from the wound (autolytic debridement) without damaging new tissue. The dressing acts as a barrier to the wound against bacterial, viral, and other external cont-amination while intact and without leakage.

Indications
To manage minor abrasions, lacerations, minor cuts, minor scalds and burns, leg ulcers (venous stasis ulcers, arterial ulcers, and leg ulcers of mixed etiology); diabetic ulcers and pressure ulcers (partial- and full-thickness), surgical wounds (postoperative left to heal by secondary intention, donor sites, dermatologic excisions), second-degree burns, and traumatic wounds

Contraindications
- Not for use on individuals who are sensitive to or who have had an al-lergic reaction to the dressing or its components

Application
- Choose a dressing size to ensure that the dressing is 1 1/2″ (3 cm) larger than the wound area.
- Remove the release paper from the back, being careful to minimize fin-ger contact with the adhesive surface.
- Hold the dressing over the wound, and line up the center of the dress-ing with the center of the wound. Place the dressing directly over the wound.
- For difficult-to-dress areas, such as heels or the sacrum, a supplemen-tary securing device, such as tape, may be required.
- Discard any unused portion of the product after dressing the wound.

Removal
- Dressing may remain in place up to 7 days. The dressing should be changed when clinically indicated or when strike-through occurs. The wound should be cleaned at each dressing change.
- Press down gently on the skin, and carefully lift one corner of the dress-ing until it no longer adheres. Continue until all edges are free.

*See package insert for complete instructions for use.

DuoDERM Extra Thin CGF Dressing*

ConvaTec

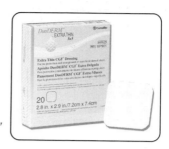

How supplied

DuoDERM Extra Thin CGF Spots:
    $1^{1}/_{4}$" × $1^{1}/_{2}$"; A6234
DuoDERM ExtraThin CGF Dressing:
    2" × 4", 2" × 8", 3" × 3", 4"
    × 4"; A6234
    4" × 6", 6" × 6"; A6235

Action

DuoDERM Extra Thin CGF dressing creates a moist environment that supports the healing process and autolytic debridement, and allows for non-traumatic removal. It acts as a barrier to help isolate the wound against bacterial and other contamination while intact and without leakage. This dressing is particularly suitable for use in areas subject to friction or those requiring contouring, such as elbows or heels.

Indications

To act as a protective dressing and manage superficial, dry to lightly exuding dermal ulcers and postoperative wounds

Contraindications

- Not for use on individuals who are sensitive to or who have had an allergic reaction to the dressings or their components

Application

- Dressing is sterile; handle appropriately.
- Clean the wound and dry the surrounding skin to ensure that it's grease-free.
- Choose a dressing size that extends beyond the wound margin at least $1^{1}/_{4}$" (3 cm).
- Minimize finger contact with the adhesive surface.
- Apply in a rolling motion; avoid stretching.
- Smooth into place, especially around the edges.
- Use tape to secure the edges, if necessary.
- For a heel or elbow, cut a slit about one-third across each side of the dressing to make application easier.
- For a sacral ulcer, press the dressing into the anal fold. Depending on the location and depth of the ulcer, the triangle-shaped dressing can be applied in different directions.
- Obtain a bacterial culture of the wound site if infection develops, and start appropriate medical treatment, as ordered. Continue using the dressing as directed by the physician. Using an occlusive dressing in the

HYDROCOLLOIDS

presence of necrotic material may initially increase wound size and depth when the necrotic debris is cleaned away.

Removal

- Leave the dressing in place for up to 7 days unless it's uncomfortable or leaking or infection develops.
- Press down on the skin, and carefully lift an edge of the dressing. Continue lifting around the dressing until all edges are free.
- The wound should be cleaned at each dressing change. (It's unnecessary to remove all residual dressing material from the surrounding skin.)

*See package insert for complete instructions for use.

DuoDERM Signal Sterile Dressing*

DuoDERM Signal

ConvaTec

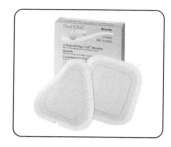

How supplied

Shapes: 4.5" × 7.5" (oval); A6235
8" × 9" (sacral); A6236
7.5" × 7.8" (heel); A6235
6" × 7", 8" × 9"; A6238

Squares: 4" × 4"; A6237
5.5" × 5.5", 8" × 8"; A6238

Action

DuoDERM Signal creates a moist environment that supports healing and autolytic debridement, and allows for nontraumatic dressing removal. An indicator line on the dressing helps to determine when to change the dressing. The dressing acts as a barrier to the wound against bacterial, viral, and other external contamination provided the dressing remains intact and there is no leakage.

Indications

Over-the-counter type used for minor abrasions, lacerations, minor cuts, minor scalds, burns; under a physician's supervision, for leg ulcers (venous stasis ulcers, arterial ulcers, and leg ulcers of mixed etiology), diabetic ulcers and pressure ulcers,sores (partial & full thickness), surgical wounds (postoperative left to heal by secondary intention, donor sites, dermatological excisions), second-degree burns, traumatic wounds

Contraindications

- Not for use on patients who are sensitive to or who have had an allergic reaction to the dressing or its components

Application

- Clean the wound surface and surrounding skin with SAF-Clens AF Dermal Wound Cleanser or normal saline solution, and dry the surrounding skin.
- Debride if necessary.
- Choose a dressing size and shape to ensure that the dressing is 1½" (3 cm) larger than the wound area.
- Hold the dressing by its corner, and pull back the release paper about halfway.
- Apply the dressing from the outside edge toward the wound, completely removing the paper backing.
- Mold the entire dressing gently but firmly into place.

HYDROCOLLOIDS

Removal
- To remove the dressing, gently press down on the skin with one hand.
- Carefully peel up one edge of the dressing with the other hand.
- Continue until all edges are free.

*See package insert for complete instructions for use.

Exuderm OdorShield

Exuderm Satin

Exuderm LP

Exuderm RCD

Exuderm Sacrum

Exuderm Ultra

Medline Industries, Inc.

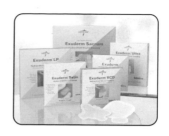

How supplied

Exuderm OdorShield

Wafer:	$2'' \times 2''$, $4'' \times 4''$; A6234
	$6'' \times 6''$; A6235
	$8'' \times 8''$; A6236
Wafer:	$3.6'' \times 4''$; A6234
	$6'' \times 5.6''$; A6235

Exuderm Satin

Wafer:	$2'' \times 2''$, $4'' \times 4''$; A6234
	$6'' \times 6''$; A6235
	$8'' \times 8''$; A6236

Exuderm LP

Wafer:	$4'' \times 4''$; A6234
	$6'' \times 6''$; A6235

Exuderm RCD

Wafer:	$4'' \times 4''$; A6234
	$6'' \times 6''$; A6235
	$8'' \times 8''$; A6236

Exuderm Sacrum

Wafer:	$3^{1}/_{4}'' \times 4''$; A6234
	$6'' \times 6^{1}/_{2}''$; A6235

Exuderm Ultra

Wafer:	$4'' \times 4''$; A6234

Action

Exuderm reacts with wound exudate to create a moist healing environment while absorbing wound exudate. Exuderm OdorShield has a smooth satin backing, tapered edge, no-residue formula plus added odor management via cyclodextrins. Exuderm Satin has a tapered-edge, low-profile, translucent appearance. The smooth satin backing resists rollup. Exuderm LP's low-profile design is used to protect against skin breakdown or to dress superficial wounds. Exuderm Regulated Colloidal Dispersion (RCD) is used

HYDROCOLLOIDS

to manage and absorb exudate with minimal meltdown. Exuderm Sacrum's butterfly design is anatomically shaped to conform to the natural shape of the body and features a hinged center for a flush fit. Exuderm Ultra features a film backing that responds to the exudate level, adjusting the rate of exhaustion to provide an optimally moist wound bed; its low-profile, conformable design resists rollup. All Exuderm dressings provide a protective, occlusive barrier, facilitating granulation or autolytic debridement, if necessary.

Indications

To manage dermal ulcers, leg ulcers, pressure ulcers (stages 2, 3, and 4), partial-thickness wounds, minor abrasions, second-degree burns, donor sites, or wounds with slough or necrosis; Exuderm Sacrum for sacral pressure ulcers (stages 2 to 4) and incontinence-induced denuded areas and for postoperative wounds, superficial wounds, and abrasions; Exuderm LP for wounds with light drainage; Exuderm OdorShield, Exuderm Satin, Exuderm RCD, Exuderm Sacrum, and Exuderm Ultra for wounds with light to moderate drainage

Contraindications

- Contraindicated for third-degree burns

Application

- Clean the application site with normal saline solution or another appropriate cleanser, such as Skintegrity Wound Cleanser. Dry the surrounding area to ensure that it's free from any greasy substance.
- Select the appropriate-sized dressing to allow 1¼" to 1½" (3 to 4 cm) for attachment to healthy periwound skin.

Exuderm Satin, Exuderm LP, Exuderm RCD, and Exuderm Ultra

- Remove the paper carrier from the dressing.
- Center Exuderm over the site, and apply to skin using a rolling motion.
- Smooth the dressing into place, especially around the edges, and hold for 5 seconds to maximize adhesive qualities.
- For traditional hydrocolloids, such as Exuderm RCD, "picture framing" (taping down all sides with a skin-friendly tape, such as Medfix) can help prevent rollup.

Exuderm Sacrum

- Remove one side of the paper carrier from the dressing. Place the dressing's "hinge" into the gluteal fold, and apply the exposed adhesive portion to the buttocks.
- Remove the last part of the protective paper, and apply the second half of the adhesive portion to the skin.
- Inspect the dressing, making sure the edges adhere well.
- Place your hand on top of the dressing for about 1 minute, warming the dressing to body temperature to enhance adherence.

Removal

- Dressing may remain in place for 2 to 7 days, depending on the amount of wound drainage. If the dressing begins to lift or leak, change it immediately.
- An adhesive remover may be used to loosen the dressing.
- Carefully press down on the skin, and lift an edge of the dressing. Continue around the dressing until all edges are free.
- Remember that the wound should be cleaned at each dressing change.

Hydrocol II Hydrocolloid Dressing

Hydrocol II Thin Hydrocolloid Dressing

Mylan Bertek Pharmaceuticals Inc.

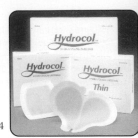

How supplied

Hydrocol II Dressing: 3″ × 3″, 4″ × 4″; A6234
Hydrocol II Sacral Dressing: 6″ × 7″; A6235
Hydrocol II Thin Dressing: 4″ × 4″; A6234

Action

Hydrocol II is a family of sterile hydrocolloid wound dressings formulated to provide a moist environment conducive to wound healing. The wound contact surface of Hydrocol II dressings consists of a layer of hydrocolloid and other polymers. The outer layer is a semipermeable, low-friction polyurethane film.

The hydrocolloid dressing material interacts with the wound exudate to form a soft gel. Hydrocol II absorbs excess exudate to help prevent the over accumulation of fluid. The dressing also protects the wound from exogenous bacteria, urine and feces, and other contamination.

Hydrocol II's unique formulation allows most of the gel—including the absorbed exudate and debris—to come out of the wound with the removal of the dressing. Hydrocol II leaves minimal residue in the wound and may be removed without damaging newly formed tissue.

Indications

To manage dermal wounds, including full-thickness wounds, pressure ulcers (stages 1 through 4), leg ulcers, superficial wounds and abrasions, trauma wounds, and surgical wounds; Hydrocol II manages light to moderately heavy exuding wounds; Hydrocol II Sacral dressing manages sacral ulcers and breakdowns; Hydrocol II Thin manages superficial wounds and abrasions where maximum dressing wear time is desired

Contraindications

- Not indicated for use on third-degree burns
- Contraindicated on individuals with known sensitivity to the dressing or its components

Application

- Prepare the wound area before applying a Hydrocol II dressing. Thoroughly rinse or irrigate the wound area with saline or an appropriate cleansing solution. The periwound area should be clean and dry to ensure optimal adherence.
- A skin prep may be used on the periwound area to increase the adherence and wear time of the dressing.

- While Hydrocol II facilitates autolytic debridement, eschar that is particularly thick or attached to the wound margins should be removed prior to application of the dressing.
- Select a dressing size that allows the dressing to extend beyond the wound margin by at least 1" (2.5 cm) on all sides. Dressings may be overlapped or trimmed with scissors to accommodate the wound.
- Hydrocol II dressings are sterile and should be handled appropriately.

Applying Hydrocol II and Hydrocol II Thin

- Break open the backing paper by folding the dressing back over itself along the cut in the backing.
- Hold the dressing by the side with the smaller release backing. With your other hand, separate the backing paper from the hydrocolloid. Remove the larger backing paper first, pulling it back over the dressing and being careful not to touch the wound contact surface of the dressing.
- With the smaller release backing still on the dressing, center the dressing over the wound site and apply. Avoid touching the wound contact surface of the dressing.
- Remove the remaining backing paper by peeling the backing paper back under itself.
- Smooth out all wrinkles, place your hand over the dressing and apply slight pressure for 30 to 40 seconds to warm the dressing and enhance adherence.

Applying Hydrocol II Sacral

- Fold the dressing down the center crease and back onto itself (backing paper should be facing out). Separate the backing paper from only one side of the dressing and peel off. Be careful not to touch the wound contact surface of the dressing.
- With the dressing still folded, center and place the hinge in the coccygeal fold. Apply slight pressure to the side without the backing paper to obtain adherence.
- Remove the backing paper for the other half of the dressing and secure in place.
- Smoothing out all wrinkles, place hand over the dressing and apply slight pressure for 30 to 40 seconds to warm the dressing and enhance adherence.

Removal

Starting at one corner of the dressing, press down on the skin and carefully peel back the dressing. Continue this process around the dressing until all edges are free of the skin.

Carefully wash or irrigate the wound to remove any residue. Apply a new dressing as described above.

Hydrocol II dressings should be changed after they have been in place for a maximum of 7 days. However, they should be changed immediately when they reach full absorbency or when there is leakage.

HYDROCOLLOIDS

MPM Excel Hydrocolloid Wound Dressing

MPM Medical, Inc.

How supplied

Pad: 2″ × 2″, 3.6″ × 4″, 4″ × 5″,
       6″ × 6.5″

Action

MPM Excel Hydrocolloid Wound Dressings are thin and transparent with a foam top, allowing the wound to be viewed through the dressing. They protect the wound from the outside environment and assist the body in healing by maintaining a moist environment.

Indications

To manage pressure ulcers (stages 1, 2, and 3) and leg ulcers

Contraindications

- Contraindicated for infected wounds
- Contraindicated for stage 4 wounds
- Contraindicated for third-degree burns

Application

- Select a dressing that overlaps the wound by 1″ (2.5 cm).
- Clean the wound, and dry the periwound skin.
- Apply the dressing directly over the wound. The dressing is self-adherent.

Removal

- Change the dressing every 2 to 5 days, when exudate begins to leak from the edges.
- Lift one corner, and then gently remove entire dressing.

PrimaCol Bordered Hydrocolloid Dressing
Derma Sciences, Inc.

How supplied
Wafer: 2″ × 2″, 4″ × 4″, 6″ × 6″, 8″ × 8″

Action
PrimaCol Bordered Hydrocolloid Dressing provides a moist healing environment and protects the wound from outside contaminants. In contact with wound fluid, it produces a soft mass, allowing nontraumatic removal. PrimaCol Bordered Hydrocolloids don't require a secondary dressing.

Indications
To manage minimally to moderately exuding partial-thickness wounds

Contraindications
- Contraindicated for third-degree burns

Application
- Clean the wound with PrimaDerm Dermal Cleanser or normal saline solution. Dry the skin adjacent to the wound.
- Choose a dressing that allows the hydrocolloid pad to extend 1″ (2.5 cm) beyond the wound margins.
- Place the dressing directly on the wound without stretching the dressing.
- Smooth the film border to ensure secure adherence.

Removal
- Carefully lift an edge of the dressing, and continue lifting around the entire perimeter of the dressing until all of the adhesive edge is free.

PrimaCol Hydrocolloid Dressing
Derma Sciences, Inc.

How supplied
Wafer: 4" × 4", 6" × 6", 8" × 8"

Action
PrimaCol Hydrocolloid Dressing provides a moist healing environment and protects the wound from outside contaminants. In contact with wound fluid, it produces a soft mass, allowing nontraumatic removal.

Indications
To manage minimally to moderately exuding partial- and full-thickness wounds

Contraindications
- Contraindicated for third-degree burns

Application
- Clean the wound with PrimaDerm Dermal Cleanser or normal saline solution. Dry the skin adjacent to the wound.
- Choose a dressing that extends 1" (2.5 cm) beyond the wound margins.
- Place the dressing directly on the wound without stretching the dressing.

Removal
- Carefully lift an edge of the dressing, and continue lifting around the entire perimeter of the dressing until all of the adhesive edge is free.

PrimaCol Specialty Hydrocolloid Dressing
Derma Sciences, Inc.

How supplied
Wafer: Heel, elbow, and sacrum

Action
PrimaCol Specialty Hydrocolloid Dressing provides a moist healing environment and protects the wound from outside contaminants. In contact with wound fluid, it produces a soft mass, allowing nontraumatic removal. PrimaCol Specialty Hydrocolloids are designed for difficult-to-dress areas, such as the sacrum, the heels, and the elbows.

Indications
To manage minimally to moderately exuding, partial-thickness wounds; also used for difficult-to-dress areas, such as bony prominences

Contraindications
- Contraindicated for third-degree burns

Application
- Clean the wound with PrimaDerm Dermal Cleanser or normal saline solution. Dry the skin adjacent to the wound.
- Choose a dressing that allows the hydrocolloid pad to extend 1″ (2.5 cm) beyond the wound margins.
- Place the dressing directly on the wound without stretching the dressing.
- Smooth the film border to ensure secure adherence.

Removal
- Carefully lift an edge of the dressing, and continue lifting around the entire perimeter of the dressing until all of the adhesive edge is free

HYDROCOLLOIDS

PrimaCol Thin Hydrocolloid Dressing
Derma Sciences, Inc.

How supplied
Wafer: 2″ × 2″, 4″ × 4″, 6″ × 6″

Action
PrimaCol Thin Hydrocolloid Dressing provides a moist healing environment and protects the wound from outside contaminants. In contact with wound fluid, it produces a soft mass, allowing nontraumatic removal. PrimaCol Thin is a transparent hydrocolloid, which facilitates wound inspection.

Indications
To manage superficial and minimally exuding partial-thickness wounds; also used for difficult-to-dress areas, such as bony prominences

Contraindications
- Contraindicated for third-degree burns

Application
- Clean the wound with PrimaDerm Dermal Cleanser or saline solution. Dry the skin adjacent to the wound.
- Choose a dressing that extends 1″ (2.5 cm) beyond the wound margins.
- Place the dressing directly on the wound without stretching the dressing.

Removal
- Carefully lift an edge of the dressing, and continue lifting around the entire perimeter of the dressing until all of the adhesive edge is free.

Procol Hydrocolloid Dressing
DeRoyal

How supplied
Wafer: 2″ × 2″, 4″ × 4″; A6237
           6″ × 6″; A6238

Action
Procol is a self-adherent, hydrocolloid wound dressing that creates a moist environment conducive to local wound healing. It protects against wound dehydration, acts as a bacterial barrier, and helps to control wound drainage. Procol's matrix formulation helps reduce the residue left in the wound and also helps avoid damaging newly formed tissue during dressing changes.

Indications
For use as a primary or secondary dressing to manage dermal ulcers, superficial wounds, lacerations, abrasions, first- and second-degree burns, donor sites, and postoperative wounds

Contraindications
■ Contraindicated for third-degree burns

Application
■ Clean the wound site with normal saline solution.
■ If necessary, cut Procol Hydrocolloid Dressing to the desired size.
■ Remove the dressing's release liner, and apply the exposed side to the wound.
■ Because the dressing adheres to the skin around the wound, extra tape isn't necessary.

Removal
■ Gently lift edges, and peel the dressing off.

HYDROCOLLOIDS

RepliCare Hydrocolloid Dressing
RepliCare Thin Hydrocolloid Dressing
RepliCare Ultra Advanced Hydrocolloid Alginate Dressing
Smith & Nephew, Inc.
Wound Management

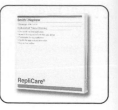

How supplied
RepliCare
Wafer: 1¹/₂″ × 2¹/₂″, 4″ × 4″; A6234
          6″ × 6″; A6235
          8″ × 8″; A6236

RepliCare Thin
Wafer: 2″ × 2³/₄″; A6234
          3¹/₂″ × 5¹/₂″, 6″ × 8″; A6235

RepliCare Ultra
Wafer: 4″ × 4″; A6234
          6″ × 6″; A6235
          8″ × 8″; A6236
Sacral dressing: 7″ × 8″; A6235

Action
These products support the creation and maintenance of a moist wound environment, which has been established as the optimal environment for management of the wound. They provide physical separation between the wound and external environments to help prevent bacterial contamination of the wound.

RepliCare
RepliCare is a hydrocolloid dressing that contains a dense concentration of absorbent material in a thin dressing for superior absorption in the management of exuding wounds. RepliCare's cohesive properties keep the wound free from dressing residue. With the one-handed application system, the product won't stick to gloves. RepliCare has a waterproof film exterior that helps prevent bacterial contamination. The top film can be wiped clean easily.

RepliCare Thin
RepliCare Thin is a hydrocolloid dressing made from a polyurethane film with a thin layer of absorbent colloid. RepliCare Thin maintains a moist wound environment that assists in promoting autolytic debridement while managing low levels of exudate.

RepliCare Ultra

RepliCare Ultra is an advanced hydrocolloid dressing with alginate, which offers superior exudate management and increased absorption capability. RepliCare Ultra's improved design provides better evaporation through an adaptable polyurethane top film that regulates moisture vapor transmission rate. This allows excess moisture to evaporate while maintaining the proper moist wound environment. The top film is waterproof, easy to clean, and aids in the prevention of bacterial contamination. Unique microthin edges and enhanced adhesive offer better adherence, reduced leakage potential, and reduced chance of edge roll. RepliCare Ultra can remain in place for up to 7 days for convenience, fewer dressing changes, and a reduction in nursing costs. In addition, it's offered in a sacral design to conform to the difficult to dress sacral region.

Indications

RepliCare

For exudate absorption and management of partial- to full-thickness wounds such as ulcers (venous, arterial, diabetic); pressure sores; donor sites; surgical incisions and excisions; and first- and second-degree burns

RepliCare Thin

For exudate absorption and management of partial- to full-thickness wounds such as ulcers (venous, arterial, diabetic); pressure sores; donor sites; surgical incisions and excisions; and first- and second-degree burns

RepliCare Ultra

Under a physician's supervision, for stage 1 through stage 4 wounds with light to moderate exudate, such as pressure ulcers, leg ulcers, superficial and partial-thickness burns, superficial wounds, donor sites, and skin abrasions

Contraindications

Replicare

■ Contraindicated for use on third-degree or full thickness burns

Replicare Thin

■ Contraindicated for use on third-degree burns

Replicare Ultra

■ Not to be continued if any signs of irritation (reddening, inflammation), maceration (overhydration of the skin), hypergranulation (excess tissue), or sensitivity (allergic reactions) appear; consult a health care professional
■ Not to be used if packaging is open or damaged
■ Not to be reused
■ Not for use on ulcers resulting from infection, such as tuberculosis, syphilis, and deep fungal infections; lesions in patients with acute vas-

culitis, such as periarteritis nodosa, systemic lupus erythematosus, and cryoglobulinemia; or third-degree burns
- Must be removed before radiation therapy

Application

RepliCare
- Cleanse the wound with saline solution or an appropriate wound cleanser. Cleanse and dry the periwound skin. If the periwound skin is particularly friable, it may be protected from trauma by applying Skin-Prep.
- Choose a dressing large enough to cover the wound with 1″ (2.5 cm) of overlap on all sides of the wound. Remove the printed backing paper, exposing the adhesive surface.
- Center the dressing over the wound, and press the edges firmly to the surrounding skin. Remove the small plastic application tab from the underside of the dressing, and press all the sides firmly to the skin.

RepliCare Thin
- Cleanse the wound with saline solution or an appropriate wound cleanser. Cleanse and dry the periwound skin. If the periwound skin is particularly friable, it may be protected from trauma by applying Skin-Prep.
- Choose a dressing large enough to cover the wound with 1″ of overlap on all sides of the wound. Remove the printed backing paper, exposing the adhesive surface.
- Center the dressing over the wound, and press the edges firmly to the surrounding skin. Remove the small plastic application tab from the underside of the dressing, and press all the sides firmly to the skin.

RepliCare Ultra
The following are designed to act as general guidelines and should only be used under the supervision of a health care professional.
- Cleanse the wound using sterile saline or a recommended commercial brand of wound cleanser such as Dermal Wound Cleanser. Gently pat dry the skin around the wound. Skin-Prep is recommended to protect the periwound skin.
- Choose a dressing that allows for $^{1}/_{2}$″ to 1″ (1.25 to 2.5 cm) overlap of the wound.
- Remove the protective paper, exposing the adhesive surface. Use the clear, plastic handle to ensure aseptic application.
- Place the adhesive side to the wound, and remove the handle.
- During the body's normal healing process, unnecessary material is removed from the wound, which will make the wound appear larger after the first few dressing changes. If the wound continues to get larger after the first few dressing changes, discontinue use and consult a health care professional.

HYDROCOLLOIDS

Removal

RepliCare, RepliCare Thin

- Change the dressing every 4 days or when transparent or leaking.
- Support the dressing with one hand while using the other hand to pull the edges laterally (parallel to the skin surface) away from the center.

RepliCare Ultra

- As RepliCare Ultra absorbs wound exudate, a gel is formed. When the gel reaches the upper film surface of the dressing, the dressing becomes white or opaque. Maximum absorbency is reached when the dressing becomes opaque and the exudate extends $1/2''$ (1.25 cm) from the edges of the dressing.
- To remove the RepliCare Ultra dressing, lift one corner of the dressing and gently pull the dressing away from the wound. To aid in removal of the dressing, Remove Adhesive Remover may be used.
- Gently cleanse the wound with tap water, sterile saline, or recommended commercial brand wound cleanser such as Dermal Wound Cleanser.
- Follow package instructions for applying a fresh dressing.

Restore Extra Thin Hydrocolloid Dressing*

Hollister Wound Care, LLC

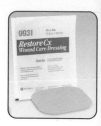

How supplied

Sheet: 4″ × 4″; A6234
6″ × 8″; A6235
8″ × 8″; A6236

Action

Restore Extra Thin is a sterile, occlusive dressing. The flexible outer layer helps isolate the wound against bacterial and viral human immunodeficiency virus (HIV-1) and hepatitis B virus (HBV) contaminants and other external contamination such as urine and feces while the dressing remains intact without leakage. The self-adhesive dressing helps maintain a moist environment for wound healing. Disposable wound measuring guide included.

Indications

To protect skin from friction injury and to manage superficial wounds with minimal or no exudate

Contraindications

- Not for use on patients with active vasculitis or ulcers involving muscle, tendon, or bone
- Contraindicated on patients with deep systemic infections
- Contraindicated on patients with signs of active local infection at the wound site (erythema, cellulitis, or purulent discharge)

Application

- To ensure attachment to healthy skin, the dressing should extend at least 1″ (2.5 cm) beyond the wound edge. Dressings may be overlapped or cut to accommodate the wound site.
- Remove the printed release paper from the patient side of the dressing. Center the dressing over the wound site. Press the dressing to the skin and smooth it to remove all wrinkles.

Removal

- Carefully lift an edge of the dressing, and peel away from the skin. The dressing should be left in place until one or more of the following occurs: leakage of exudate, loosening of the edges of the dressing, tenderness or signs of infection, 7 days have elapsed, or there is no longer a clinical need for the dressing.

*See package insert for complete instructions for use.

HYDROCOLLOIDS

Restore Hydrocolloid Dressing*
Hollister Wound Care, LLC

How supplied
Sheet: 4″ × 4″; A6234
          6″ × 8″; A6235
          8″ × 8″; A6236

Action
Restore Hydrocolloid dressings are sterile, occlusive dressings with foam backing. The heat-activated, self-adhesive inner layer maintains a moist environment while absorbing excess wound exudate. Restore Hydrocolloid Dressing is ideal for low friction areas with moderate exudate. Includes disposable wound measuring guide.

Indications
For use on light to moderately exuding dermal ulcers and partial-thickness wounds; also for venous stasis ulcers, superficial wounds, pressure ulcers (stages 1 and 2), arterial ulcers, diabetic ulcers, surgical incisions, and traumatic wounds

Contraindications
■ Not for use on patients with active vasculitis, infection, or stage 3 or 4 pressure ulcers

Application
■ To ensure attachment to healthy skin, the dressing should extend at least 1″ (2.5 cm) beyond the wound edge. Dressings may be overlapped or cut to accommodate the wound site.
■ Remove the release paper from the dressing. Center the dressing over the wound, being careful to minimize touching the adhesive side. Press the dressing in place. Initial tack may be improved by warming the dressing with your hands prior to application or after dressing is in place.

Removal
■ Carefully lift an edge of the dressing while pressing down on the skin adjacent to the edge. Continue this procedure around the wound until all of the edges are free of the skin. Gently lift the dressing off the wound. Gently rinse or irrigate the wound as needed, remove excess moisture, and apply a new dressing.
*See package insert for complete instructions for use.

HYDROCOLLOIDS

Restore Hydrocolloid Dressing with Foam
Hollister Wound Care, LLC

How supplied
Dressing: 4″ × 4″ without tapered edges; A6234
6″ × 8″ without tapered edges; A6235
8″ × 8″ without tapered edges; A6236
4″ × 4″ with tapered edges; A6234
6″ × 6″ with tapered edges, 6″ × 8″ with tapered edges; A6235
8″ × 8″ with tapered edges; A6236
With tapered edges, triangle-shaped 17 in², with tapered edges, triangle-shaped 26.5 in²; A6235

Action
Restore Hydrocolloid Dressings are sterile, occlusive dressings. The flexible outer layer helps isolate the wound against bacterial and human immunodeficiency virus (HIV-1) and hepatitis B virus (HBV) contaminants and other external contamination such as urine and feces while the dressing remains intact without leakage. The self-adhesive inner layer maintains a moist wound environment while absorbing excess wound exudate to prevent fluid pooling. Disposable wound measuring guide included.

Indications
For use on dermal ulcers including full-thickness wounds, diabetic ulcers, pressure ulcers, leg ulcer management, superficial wounds, second-degree burns, and donor sites; partial- and full-thickness wounds; moist to moderately exudative wounds

Contraindications
■ Not for use on third-degree burns

Application
■ Rinse or irrigate the wound area. The skin should be clean and dry for secure application. To ensure attachment to healthy skin, the dressing should extend at least 1″ (2.5 cm) beyond the wound edge. Dressings may be overlapped or cut to accommodate the size of the wound.
■ Partially remove the release paper from the dressing, exposing the center of the dressing. Do not remove the paper completely at this point.
■ Center the adhesive side of the dressing over the wound site. Be careful not to touch the adhesive side of the dressing (side applied to the wound).
■ Remove the remaining pieces of the release paper from the dressing, and press the dressing margins to the skin.
■ If clinical signs of infection are present, appropriate medical treatment should be initiated. Management of the wound with Restore Hydrocolloid Dressings may be continued at the discretion of the clinician.

HYDROCOLLOIDS

Removal

- Carefully lift an edge of the dressing while pressing gently down on the skin.
- Continue this procedure around the wound bed until all edges of the dressing are free. Wash the wound area to remove any residual materials. Remove excess moisture, and apply a new dressing. The dressing should be left in place (not more than 7 days) unless it is uncomfortable, leaking, or there are clinical signs of infection.

*See package insert for complete instructions for use.

3M Tegaderm Hydrocolloid Dressing

3M Tegaderm THIN Hydrocolloid Dressing

3M Health Care

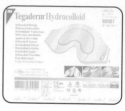

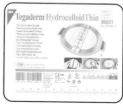

How supplied

3M Tegaderm Hydrocolloid Dressing

Oval wafer: $2^3/4'' \times 3^1/2''$; A6237
              $4'' \times 4^3/4''$; A6238
              $5^1/2'' \times 6^3/4''$; A6238

Square wafer: $4'' \times 4''$; A6234
              $6'' \times 6''$; A6235

Sacral wafer: $6^3/4'' \times 6^{11}/16''$; A6238

3M Tegaderm THIN Hydrocolloid Dressing

Oval wafer: $2^3/4'' \times 3^1/2''$; A6237
              $4'' \times 4^3/4''$; A6238
              $5^1/2'' \times 6^3/4''$; A6238

Square wafer: $4'' \times 4''$; A6234

Action

3M Tegaderm hydrocolloid dressings support wound management in two ways. First, the inner layer of hydrocolloid adhesive rapidly absorbs exudate—providing significantly higher absorbency during the first 48 hours than the leading competitive hydrocolloid. In addition to excellent absorbency, the breathable outer film layer provides a consistently high rate of moisture vapor transmission, reducing the potential for skin maceration. Together, these features ensure an optimal moist wound environment, minimize the chance for damage to healthy periwound skin, and provide cost-effective wear time for up to 7 days. The dressings also offer protection from the contaminants: The outer film barrier protects the wound and surrounding skin from contaminants and body fluids.

Indications

To manage partial-thickness dermal ulcers, superficial wounds, abrasions, first- and second-degree burns, and donor sites; full-thickness dermal ulcers; leg ulcers; and to protect at-risk, undamaged skin or skin beginning to show signs of damage from friction or shear

Contraindications

- None provided by the manufacturer

Application

- Clip excess hair at the wound site, thoroughly clean the wound and surrounding skin, and allow the skin to dry.

- If the patient's skin is easily damaged or drainage is expected to go beyond the wound edge, a skin protectant or a skin barrier film may be applied.
- Select a dressing that extends 1″ (2.5 cm) beyond the wound edge.

Oval dressing

- Remove the paper liner from the dressing by lifting and pulling one of the square end tabs marked "1," exposing the adhesive surface. Minimize contact with the border or the adhesive side of the dressing.
- Center the dressing over the wound. Then, gently press the adhesive side against the wound. Press from the center outward, and avoid stretching the dressing or the skin.
- Smooth the film edges to ensure good adherence.
- Remove the top delivery film by lifting one of the center tabs marked "2," and pulling it toward the edge of the dressing. Smooth down the dressing edges as you remove the film. Remove the other side of the top film in the same way.
- Gently tear off the square end tabs marked "1" at the perforations in a downward direction and discard. Avoid lifting the film edge while removing the tabs. Secure the entire film edge by pressing firmly.

Square dressing

- Remove the top liner from the back of the dressing. 3M Tegaderm THIN Hydrocolloid Dressing may be cut to size before removing its top liner.
- Peel the dressing from its paper liner, minimizing contact with the dressing adhesive surface.
- Center the dressing over the wound, and gently press the adhesive side against the wound. Press from the center outward, and avoid stretching the dressing or the skin.
- Apply tape firmly around the edges of the dressing.

Sacral dressing

- Before removing the printed liner, fold the dressing in half.
- Hold the tabs together, and remove the printed liner on one half of the dressing until the adhesive is exposed.
- Continue to remove the printed liner from the other half until the adhesive surface is completely exposed.
- While still holding both tabs, position the dressing over the wound, tilting the dressing toward the anal area. Spread the buttocks to get better placement. Secure the dressing notch in the anal region first to minimize risk of incontinence contamination or wrinkling.
- Gently press the adhesive side of the dressing down from the center outward. Avoid stretching the dressing or the skin.
- Remove the dressing frame, starting at the top and pulling down. Don't lift the film edge. Reinforce and smooth the dressing from the center outward.
- Repeat until all sections of the frame are removed.

HYDROCOLLOIDS

Removal

- The dressing should be changed if it's leaking, falling off, or has been on the wound for 7 days.
- Carefully lift the dressing edges from the skin. For easy removal, apply tape to the edge of the dressing, and use the tape to lift.
- Continue lifting the edges until all are free from the skin surface.
- Remove the dressing slowly, folding it over itself. Pull carefully in the direction of hair growth.
- Note that it isn't unusual for wounds to have an odor. This may be noticed when the dressing is removed or when leakage occurs. The odor should disappear after the wound is cleaned.

Triad Hydrophilic Wound Dressing
Coloplast Corporation

How supplied
Tube: 2.5 oz, 6 oz; A6240

Action
Triad Hydrophilic Wound Dressing is a zinc oxide–based hydrophilic paste that gently adheres to moist, exuding wounds and spreads evenly over areas inaccessible to conventional dressings. It's noncytotoxic and promotes autolytic debridement.

Indications
To manage pressure ulcers (stages 2, 3, and 4), venous stasis ulcers, partial- and full-thickness wounds, superficial wounds, scrapes, and first- and second-degree burns; may be used on tunneling wounds; wounds with minimal, moderate, or heavy drainage; wounds with serosanguineous drainage; and red, yellow, or black wounds

Contraindications
- Contraindicated for third-degree burns
- Contraindicated for infected wounds

Application
- Clean the wound using a wound cleanser or normal saline solution.
- Fill the wound bed with the dressing, and apply a lighter layer on the periwound area. Cover this with a secondary dressing.
- For an open skin tear, apply a thin layer of dressing over it, then cover it with petroleum-impregnated gauze or a nonadherent dressing, and secure.
- For necrotic tissue, cover all the tissue and periwound skin with a thin layer of the dressing. Use a cover dressing if desired.

Removal
- If the dressing has dried out, spray with a wound cleanser or normal saline solution. Then, cover with gauze moistened with cleanser or normal saline solution, and allow it to remain for 2 to 3 minutes before removing the dressing.
- If the dressing is moist, spray with a wound cleanser or normal saline solution. Then, gently remove the dressing.

HYDROCOLLOIDS

Ultec Hydrocolloid Dressing
Ultec Pro Alginate Hydrocolloid Dressing
Tyco Healthcare/Kendall

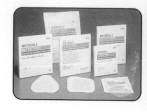

How supplied
Ultec Hydrocolloid Dressing
Wafer: 4″ × 4″; A6234
           6″ × 6″, 6″ × 8″; A6235
           8″ × 8″; A6236

Ultec Pro Alginate Hydrocolloid Dressing
Wafer: 4″ × 4″, 6″ × 6″, 8″ × 8″, 2$\frac{1}{2}$″ × 3$\frac{1}{2}$″ with adhesive island,
           4″ × 4″, 4″ × 5″ sacral (both with adhesive island); A6237
           6″ × 6″, 6″ × 7″ sacral (both with adhesive island); A6238

Action
Ultec Hydrocolloid Dressings are pressure-sensitive adhesive dressings that absorb exudate and interact with it to form a soft gel. The gel helps form and maintain a seal against bacterial contamination, which allows the dressings to remain in place for up to 7 days and to minimize potential contamination from urine and feces. Ultec Pro Alginate Hydrocolloid Dressing's alginate/hydrocolloid formulation also helps prevent exudate from macerating periwound skin.

Indications
To manage a wide range of wound types, to relieve pressure at potential ulcer sites, and to prevent skin breakdown; may be used on pressure ulcers (stages 1, 2, 3, and 4); partial- and full-thickness wounds; infected and noninfected wounds; wounds with minimal drainage; wounds with serosanguineous drainage; surgical sites; and red, yellow, or black wounds; may also be used as a secondary dressing over hydrocolloid fillers

Contraindications
- Contraindicated for ulcers involving muscle, tendon, or bone

Application
- Clean the wound site.
- Choose a dressing that overlaps the wound by at least 1″ (2.5 cm), and apply it using a clean technique. Avoid stretching the dressing.
- Press the dressing gently, forming it to the wound area and to any skin folds or creases.

Removal
- Change the dressing weekly. Change it more often if exudate leaks or if the occlusive seal breaks.
- Lift and slowly pull in the direction of hair growth.
- If removal is difficult, soak the edges with sterile water.

Hydrogels

ACTION

Hydrogels are water- or glycerin-based amorphous gels, impregnated gauzes, or sheet dressings. Because of their high water content, some can't absorb large amounts of exudate. Hydrogels help maintain a moist healing environment, promote granulation and epithelialization, and facilitate autolytic debridement.

INDICATIONS

Hydrogel dressings may be used as primary dressings (amorphous and impregnated gauzes) or as primary or secondary dressings (sheets). They may also be used to manage partial- and full-thickness wounds, deep wounds (amorphous, impregnated gauzes), wounds with necrosis or slough, minor burns, and tissue damaged by radiation.

ADVANTAGES

- Are soothing and reduce pain
- Rehydrate the wound bed
- Facilitate autolytic debridement
- Fill in dead space (amorphous, impregnated gauzes)
- Provide minimal to moderate absorption
- Are applied and removed easily from the wound
- Can be used when infection is present

DISADVANTAGES

- Aren't usually recommended for wounds with heavy exudate
- Dehydrate easily if not covered
- Some require secondary dressing
- Some may be difficult to secure
- Some may cause maceration

HCPCS CODE OVERVIEW

The HCPCS codes normally assigned to hydrogel wound covers without an adhesive border are:

A6242—pad size < 16 in^2

A6243—pad size > 16 in^2 but ≤ 48 in^2

A6244—pad size > 48 in^2.

The HCPCS codes normally assigned to hydrogel wound covers with an adhesive border are:

A6245—pad size < 16 in^2

A6246—pad size > 16 in^2 but ≤ 48 in^2

A6247—pad size > 48 in^2.

The HCPCS code normally assigned to hydrogel wound fillers is:

A6248—gel, per fluid ounce

The HCPCS codes normally assigned to gauze dressings impregnated with hydrogel without an adhesive border are:

A6231—pad size < 16 in^2

A6232—pad size > 16 in^2 but ≤ 48 in^2

A6233—pad size > 48 in^2.

AmeriDerm Wound Gel Dressing with Vitamin E and Aloe Vera

AmeriDerm Laboratories, Ltd.

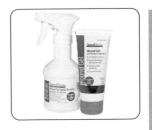

How supplied

Tube: 3 oz; A6248
Spray bottle: 8 oz; A6248

Action

AmeriDerm Wound Gel is a greaseless hydrogel dressing used for the maintenance of a moist healing environment.

Indications

For dressing and management of stasis ulcers, pressure ulcers (stages 1, 2, 3, and 4), first- and second-degree burns, cuts and abrasions, skin irritations, postoperative incisions, and skin conditions associated with peristomal care

Contraindications

- Not for use in those with sensitivity to the gel or its components

Application

- Flush wound with AmeriDerm Wound Cleanser.
- Apply AmeriDerm Wound Gel liberally to cover involved areas. Apply as often as necessary. If gauze is used as a wound covering, moisten first with AmeriDerm Wound Cleanser.

Removal

- Flush with AmeriDerm Wound Cleanser.

HYDROGELS

AmeriGel Hydrogel Saturated Gauze Dressing
Amerx Health Care Corp.

How Supplied
Pad: 2″ × 2″; A6231

Action
AmeriGel Gauze Dressing contains Oakin (an oak extract), meadowsweet extract, zinc acetate, polyethylene glycol 400 and 3350, and water, impregnated into a nonwoven gauze sponge and individually foil wrapped. Broad-spectrum antimicrobial-antifungal (bactericidal) against 51 microbes, including MRSA and VRE. AmeriGel maintains a moist wound environment, assists in debriding, and provides an antimicrobial barrier at the wound site.

Indications
Stages 1 to 4 pressure ulcers, lower-extremity ulcerations of mixed vascular etiologies, diabetic skin ulcers, first- and second-degree burns, postsurgical incisions

Contraindications
- Contraindicated in patients who are sensitive or allergic to any ingredient

Application
- Irrigate wound with saline and blot dry.
- Place the AmeriGel gauze pad over the wound so that it covers the wound bed and overlaps onto the periwound skin.
- Cover with appropriate secondary dressing.

Removal
- Remove dressings and irrigate with saline daily.

AmeriGel Wound Dressing
Amerx Health Care Corp.

How supplied
Tube: 1 oz; A6248

Action
AmeriGel Wound Dressing contains
Oakin (an oak extract), meadowsweet extract, zinc acetate, polyethylene
glycol 400 and 3350, and water. Broad-spectrum antimicrobial-antifungal
(bactericidal) against 51 microbes, including MRSA and VRE. AmeriGel
maintains a moist wound environment, assists in debriding and provides
an antimicrobial barrier at the wound site.

Indications
Stages 1 to 4 pressure ulcers, lower-extremity ulcerations of mixed vascular etiologies, diabetic skin ulcers, first- and second-degree burns, postsurgical incisions

Contraindications
- Contraindicated in patients who are sensitive or allergic to any ingredient

Application
- Irrigate wound with saline and blot dry.
- Apply a thin layer of AmeriGel to the wound bed and overlap onto the
  periwound skin.
- Cover with appropriate secondary dressing.

Removal
- Remove secondary dressing and irrigate with saline daily.

HYDROGELS

HYDROGELS

Aquaflo
Tyco Healthcare/Kendall

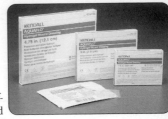

How supplied
Disk: 3", 4³/₄"

Action
Aquaflo hydrogel wound dressings offer superior fluid management and
can be used on mildly to moderately
exuding wounds. These dressings maintain an optimal moist healing environment.

Indications
To manage partial- and full-thickness wounds, dermal ulcers (stages 1, 2
and 3), diabetic leg ulcers, donor sites, first- and second-degree burns, and
incisions

Contraindications
■ Contraindicated for heavily draining wounds

Application
■ Clean the wound with normal saline solution or an appropriate wound
  cleanser.
■ Cut the dressing to shape, if desired.
■ Apply the dressing and secure it.

Removal
■ Gently lift edge and peel dressing away.

Aquasite Amorphous Hydrogel
Derma Sciences, Inc.

How supplied
Amorphous hydrogel: 1 fl oz

Action
Aquasite Amorphous Hydrogels are clear, preserved hydrogels used to fill wound space and provide a moist healing environment. These products are capable of absorbing small to moderate amounts of exudate and provide a soothing, cooling, pain-reducing effect. A secondary dressing is required to secure the dressing in place.

Indications
For use on partial- and full-thickness wounds with minimal to moderate drainage

Contraindications
- Contraindicated for third-degree burns

Application
- Clean the wound with PrimaDerm Dermal Cleanser or saline solution.
- Dry the skin adjacent to the wound.
- Squeeze the desired amount of Aquasite Amorphous Hydrogel into the wound bed.
- Cover with an appropriate secondary dressing.

Removal
- Remove the secondary dressing.
- Remove remaining Aquasite Amorphous Hydrogel.
- Clean the wound according to facility policy.

Aquasite Impregnated Gauze Hydrogel
Derma Sciences, Inc.

How supplied
Gauze: $2'' \times 2''$, $4'' \times 4''$, $4'' \times 8''$

Action
Aquasite Impregnated Gauze Hydrogels are sterile hydrogels impregnated into 100% cotton sponges. These products are used to fill wound space and provide a moist healing environment. They're capable of absorbing small to moderate amounts of exudate, and they provide a soothing, cooling, pain-reducing effect. A secondary dressing is required to secure the dressing in place.

Indications
For use on partial- and full-thickness wounds with minimal to moderate drainage

Contraindications
- Contraindicated for third-degree burns

Application
- Clean the wound with PrimaDerm Dermal Cleanser or saline solution Dry the skin adjacent to the wound.
- Place Aquasite Impregnated Gauze Hydrogel into the wound bed. Pack deeper wounds loosely to avoid excess pressure on delicate wound tissue.
- Cover with an appropriate secondary dressing.

Removal
- Remove the secondary dressing.
- Remove the gauze and remaining hydrogel.
- Clean the wound according to facility policy.

Aquasite Impregnated Non-Woven Hydrogel
Derma Sciences, Inc.

How supplied
Gauze: $2'' \times 2''$, $4'' \times 4''$, $4'' \times 8''$

Action
Aquasite Impregnated Non-Woven Hydrogel, a sterile hydrogel impregnated into a special nonwoven sponge, is used to fill wound space and provide a moist healing environment. It's capable of absorbing small to moderate amounts of exudate, and it provides a soothing, cooling, pain-reducing effect. A secondary dressing is required to secure the dressing in place.

Indications
For use on partial- and full-thickness wounds with minimal to moderate drainage

Contraindications
- Contraindicated for third-degree burns

Application
- Clean the wound with PrimaDerm Dermal Cleanser or saline solution. Dry the skin adjacent to the wound.
- Place Aquasite Impregnated Non-Woven Hydrogel into the wound bed. Pack deeper wounds loosely to avoid excess pressure on delicate wound tissue.
- Cover with an appropriate secondary dressing.

Removal
- Remove the secondary dressing.
- Remove the gauze and remaining hydrogel.
- Clean the wound according to facility policy.

HYDROGELS

Aquasite Sheet Hydrogel
Derma Sciences, Inc.

How supplied
Sheet: 2″ × 2″, 2″ × 3″, 4″ × 4″, 6″ × 8″, 12″ × 12″, 12″ × 24″

Action
Aquasite Sheet Hydrogels are clear sheets of sterile hydrogel used to provide a moist healing environment and absorb small to moderate amounts of exudate. The products provide a soothing, cooling, pain-reducing effect. A secondary dressing is required to secure the dressing in place.

Indications
For use on partial- and full-thickness wounds with minimal to moderate drainage

Contraindications
- Contraindicated for third-degree burns
- Contraindicated for deep, tunneling wounds

Application
- Clean the wound with PrimaDerm Dermal Cleanser or saline solution Dry the skin adjacent to the wound.
- Choose a dressing that extends at least 1″ (2.5 cm) beyond the wound margins.
- Position Aquasite Sheet Hydrogel directly on the wound.
- Secure with an appropriate secondary dressing.

Removal
- Remove the secondary dressing.
- Remove the Aquasite Sheet Hydrogel.

Aquasorb Hydrogel Wound Dressing
DeRoyal

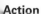

How supplied
Sheet: $2\frac{1}{2}'' \times 2\frac{1}{2}''$; $3\frac{3}{4}'' \times 3\frac{3}{4}''$; A6242
         $3\frac{3}{4}'' \times 4\frac{1}{2}''$; $3\frac{3}{4}'' \times 6''$; A6243
         $7\frac{1}{2}'' \times 7\frac{1}{2}''$; A6244
Sheet with border: $2\frac{1}{2}'' \times 2\frac{1}{2}''$ gel, $\frac{5}{8}''$ film or tape
         border; A6245
         $3\frac{3}{4}'' \times 4\frac{1}{4}''$ gel, $1\frac{1}{2}''$ film or tape border; A6246

Action
Aquasorb Hydrogel Wound Dressings are nonadherent, transparent dressings that incorporate a gel matrix with a semipermeable film. They allow for moisture vapor transmission, which provides a moist healing environment and protects against wound dehydration. The products act as a bacterial barrier, absorb drainage from the wound, and provide a cool, pain-relieving cover.

Indications
For use as primary dressings to manage leg ulcers, pressure ulcers (stages 1, 2, 3, and 4), superficial wounds, lacerations, cuts, abrasions, donor sites, and first- and second-degree burns; also on partial- and full-thickness wounds, infected and noninfected wounds, wounds with moderate to heavy drainage, and red, yellow, or black wounds

Contraindications
- Contraindicated for third-degree burns

Application
- Clean excess exudate from the wound.
- Cut the sheet to the desired size, if necessary.
- Remove the release liner, and apply the dressing to the wound.
- Secure the dressing, if necessary.

Removal
- Leave the dressing in place for up to 7 days, unless patient discomfort, exudate leakage, or infection occurs.
- Lift the edge of the dressing carefully, and then peel off.

CarraDres Clear Hydrogel Sheet
Carrington Laboratories, Inc.

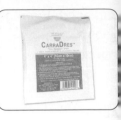

How supplied
Sheet: 4" × 4"; A6242

Action
CarraDres Clear Hydrogel Sheets consist of
89.5% water combined with a crosslinked poly-
ethylene matrix in sterile hydrogel polymer sheets especially formulated
for managing partial- and full-thickness wounds. The hydrophilic dressings absorb at least three times their weight in water, serum, and blood.
The products have a high specific heat to provide a cooling effect; the sheets
may be refrigerated for maximum cooling.

Indications
To dress and manage pressure ulcers (stages 1, 2, 3, and 4), venous stasis
ulcers, first- and second-degree burns, cuts, abrasions, skin irritations, radiation dermatitis, diabetic ulcers, foot ulcers, postsurgical incisions, and
skin conditions associated with peristomal care. May also be used on par-
tial- and full-thickness wounds, tunneling wounds, infected and noninfected wounds, wounds with moderate exudate, wounds with serosanguineous drainage, and red, yellow, or black wounds.

Contraindications
- None known

Application
- Flush the wound with a suitable cleanser, such as CarraKlenz, UltraK-
  lenz, or MicroKlenz.
- Remove dressing's blue backing, and apply moist side of the dressing to
  the wound bed.
- Cover with a secondary dressing, such as CarraFilm or CarraSmart Film.

Removal
- Change dressing according to the wound condition and amount of ex-
  udate or as directed by the physician.
- The dressing may remain in place 3 to 5 days.
- Gently lift to remove.

CarraGauze Pads with Acemannan Hydrogel

Carrington Laboratories, Inc.

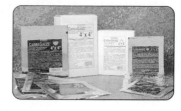

How supplied
Pad: 2″ × 2″, 4″ × 4″; A6231

Action
CarraGauze Pads are impregnated with Carrasyn Gel Wound Dressing containing Acemannan Hydrogel. They provide a primary cover or filler for wounds, absorb exudate, and create a moist healing environment.

Indications
To manage pressure ulcers (stages 1, 2, 3, and 4), stasis ulcers, first- and second-degree burns, cuts, abrasions, skin conditions associated with peristomal skin, diabetic ulcers, foot ulcers, radiation dermatitis, postoperative incisions, and trauma wounds

Contraindications
■ Contraindicated in patients with known hypersensitivity to Acemannan Hydrogel or other components of the dressing

Application
■ Flush wound with a suitable cleanser, such as CarraKlenz, UltraKlenz, or MicroKlenz.
■ Pack the wound loosely with CarraGauze Pads.
■ Cover with a secondary dressing of CarraFilm, CarraSmart Film, or gauze. If using gauze and the wound bed is dry, moisten the gauze.

Removal
Change all hydrogel dressings as often as needed, usually daily.
Remove the secondary dressing.
Gently remove the gauze pad or strip from the wound bed.

CarraSmart Gel Wound Dressing with Acemannan Hydrogel

Carrington Laboratories, Inc.

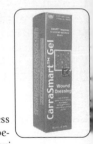

How supplied
Tube: 3 oz

Action
CarraSmart Gel is a nonadherent, smooth, colorless wound dressing containing Acemannan Hydrogel, especially formulated to create and maintain the moist environment vital to wound healing. The gel has the unique property of donating moisture to dry wounds and absorbing moisture from wet wounds; it also relieves pain by cooling, coating, and protecting the wound.

Indications
To manage pressure ulcers (stages 1, 2, 3, and 4), stasis ulcers, foot ulcers, first- and second-degree burns, minor cuts and abrasions, and skin conditions associated with peristomal care

Contraindications
- None known

Application
- Clean the wound with a suitable cleanser, such as CarraKlenz, Ultra Klenz, or MicroKlenz, by spraying the affected area.
- Gently dry the surrounding skin with soft gauze. No rinsing is required
- Apply a $^1/_8$" to $^1/_4$" (0.3 to 0.5 cm) thick layer of CarraSmart Gel to areas of ulceration.
- Cover with an appropriate nonadherent secondary dressing.

Removal
- Change dressing according to the wound condition and amount of exudate or as directed by the physician.
- Rinse away any remaining gel with gentle irrigation.

Carrasyn Gel Wound Dressing with Acemannan Hydrogel

Carrasyn Spray Gel Wound Dressing with Acemannan Hydrogel

Carrasyn V with Acemannan Hydrogel
Carrington Laboratories, Inc.

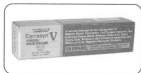

How supplied
Carrasyn Gel Wound Dressing
Tube: 1 oz, 3 oz; A6248

Carrasyn Spray Gel Wound Dressing
Bottle: 8 oz; A6248

Carrasyn V
Tube: 3 oz; A6248

Action
All three products provide the moist environment necessary for healing and autolytic debridement. All three are nonoily hydrogels containing Acemannan Hydrogel. Carrasyn V is a thicker, more viscous version of Carrasyn Gel Wound Dressing.

Indications
All three products manage pressure ulcers (stages 1, 2, 3, and 4), venous stasis ulcers, first- and second-degree burns, cuts, abrasions, skin irritations, and skin conditions associated with peristomal care. They may also be used on partial- and full-thickness wounds, tunneling wounds, infected and noninfected wounds, wounds with serosanguineous drainage, and red, yellow, or black wounds. Carrasyn Spray Gel Wound Dressing may be used on wounds with moderate drainage. Carrasyn Gel Wound Dressing and Carrasyn V also manage radiation dermatitis, diabetic ulcers, foot ulcers, postsurgical incisions, and wounds with low exudate

Contraindications
- Contraindicated in patients with known sensitivity to aloe vera extract or to Acemannan Hydrogel

Application
- Flush the wound with a suitable wound cleanser, such as CarraKlenz, UltraKlenz, or MicroKlenz.

Carrasyn Gel Wound Dressing and Carrasyn V (when a thicker formulation of gel is desired)

- Apply a generous amount of gel to the wound area in a layer about ¼″ (0.5 cm) thick.
- If using gauze as a secondary dressing, moisten it first.
- If using CarraSmart Film Transparent Dressing as the secondary dressing, dry the periwound tissue first. Use a skin barrier wipe on any intact skin under the film.

Carrasyn Spray Gel Wound Dressing

- Adjust the nozzle setting on the bottle to either spray or stream.
- Apply a generous amount of gel, about ¼″ (0.5 cm) thick, to the wound and wound margins.
- Apply spray gel as often as needed, usually daily.
- If using gauze as a cover dressing, moisten it first.

Removal

- Change all hydrogel dressings as often as needed, usually daily.
- Flush wound with normal saline solution or an appropriate wound cleanser, such as CarraKlenz, UltraKlenz, or MicroKlenz.

ClearSite Hydrogel Wound Dressing
ClearSite Hydrogel Bandage Roll
Conmed Corporation

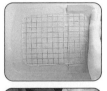
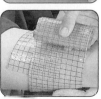

How supplied

ClearSite Hydrogel Wound Dressing

Bordered dressing:	3″ × 4″, 5″ × 5″; A6245
	7½″ × 9½″; A6246
Borderless dressing:	2″ × 3″, 4″ × 4″; A6242
	4½″ × 5″; A6243
	8″ × 8″, 5″ × 11½″, 4″ × 48″;
	A6244
Island dressing:	1¾″ × 2½″, 3″ × 4″, 5″× 5″
	A6245
	5″ × 6″, 4½″ × 9½″; A6246
	8½″ × 9½″; A6247

ClearSite Hydrogel Bandage Roll

Bandage roll:	4′ × 48″; A6244

Action

Wound Dressing with ClearSite and Bandage Roll with ClearSite contain an absorbent, hydration balanced hydrogel. Both products promote a moist healing environment and allow continuous wound assessment and charting through transparent dressing and its 1½″ (1 cm) grid pattern.

Indications

To prevent and manage pressure ulcers (stages 1, 2, 3, and 4), partial- and full-thickness wounds, uninfected wounds, first- and second-degree burns, dermal leg ulcers, skin tears, and venous stasis ulcers

Contraindications

- Contraindicated for infected wounds
- Contraindicated for use during laser procedures, but may be used as intended after the procedure is completed
- Contraindicated for third-degree burns

Application

- Consult a physician before using these products.
- Cleanse and rinse the wound according to facility policy.
- Dry the wound and surrounding areas because lotions, salves, and moisture will render auxiliary adhesive tapes ineffective.
- Use scissors to trim the borderless Wound Dressing with ClearSite, if necessary, while the dressing is still on the release liner.

ClearSite Hydrogel Wound Dressing (bordered, borderless, and island)
- Remove the larger section of the release liner by flexing the dressing and grasping the exposed edge at the split.
- Keep the smaller, unexposed part elevated, and gently position the exposed portion of the gel surface into place on the wound.
- Carefully peel the remaining liner from the dressing, avoiding contact with the exposed gel surface and the wound, and then press remaining dressing into place.
- Tape or wrap the dressing to maintain position.

ClearSite Hydrogel Bandage Roll
- Grasp the dressing's leading edge, and unroll a convenient starting length.
- Wrap the limb, starting the leading edge at an undamaged site. Unroll the dressing as needed.
- Cut dressing to desired length.
- Tape or overwrap the dressing to maintain position.

Removal
- Press down, support the skin surrounding the dressing, and carefully lift an edge of the tape.
- Continue slowly around the wound margins until all tape edges are free from the skin surface.
- Lift tape and dressing carefully from the wound.

HYDROGELS

Comfort-Aid
Southwest Technologies, Inc.

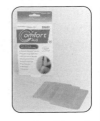

How supplied
Sheet with adhesive border: overall size, 3″ × 4″
(7.5 cm × 10 cm); gel size,
1.5″ × 2.5″

Action
Comfort-Aid is designed to provide effective management of a wide variety of wounds and to protect the skin and newly formed tissue. The gel's high glycerin content facilitates the natural wound-healing process. Glycerin is a main component in every fat molecule and is a natural moisturizing agent. Comfort-Aid provides cool, soothing relief when applied to an open wound. It will not dry out and is bacteriostatic and fungistatic.

Indications
To manage first- and second-degree burns, cuts, abrasions, rashes, radiation skin reactions, surgical incisions, foot and leg ulcers, pressure ulcers (stages 1, 2, 3, and 4), partial- and full-thickness wounds, wounds with moderate drainage, wounds with serosanguineous drainage, and red, yellow, or black wounds

Contraindications
- Contraindicated for highly exuding wounds that may require packing with additional dressing or other highly absorbent material
- Use caution when applying to an infected wound

Application
- Clean the wound with normal saline solution or an appropriate wound cleanser.
- Remove the sterile gel dressing from the package.
- Remove protective cover to expose gel and adhesive.
- Apply the dressing to the wound, being sure that the gel fully covers the wound area.
- Gently press the adhesive border to assure a watertight seal.
- Change dressing as needed (if leaking occurs and/or the dressing becomes highly saturated with exudate).
- Consult physician if signs of infection occur (such as redness, swelling or fever).

Removal
- Change the dressing when it's saturated with exudate.

Curafil Gel Wound Dressing and Impregnated Strips
Tyco Healthcare/Kendall

How supplied
Tube: ½ oz, 1 oz, 3 oz;
  A6248
Impregnated pad: 2″ × 2″, 4″ × 4″, 4″ × 8″, 1″ × 36″

Action
Curafil Gel Wound Dressing and Impregnated Strips help maintain a moist healing environment, promote granulation and epithelialization, and facilitate autolytic debridement.

Indications
To manage pressure ulcers (stages 2, 3, and 4), partial- and full-thickness wounds, tunneling wounds, uninfected wounds, wounds with light drainage, and red, yellow, or black wounds

Contraindications
- None provided by the manufacturer

Application
- Apply hydrogel dressing or hydrogel gauze to wound, gently filling in dead space.
- Secure in place with hydrogel wafer or transparent dressing.

Removal
- Gently remove dressing.
- For gel dressing, flush out remaining gel with cleanser or saline solution.

Curagel
Tyco Healthcare/Kendall

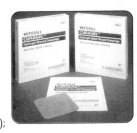

How supplied
Borderless dressing: 2″ × 3″, 4″ × 4″; A6242
8″ × 8″; A6244
Island dressing: 3″ × 4″ (2″ × 3″ pad),
5″ × 5″ (4″ × 4″ pad),
8½″ × 9½″ (8″ × 8″ pad);
A6245

Action
Curagel hydrogel dressings offer balanced hydration in a soothing, clear gel. The polyurethane layer maintains dressing integrity and controls fluid management.

Indications
To manage partial- and full-thickness wounds, dermal ulcers (stages 1, 2, and 3), diabetic leg ulcers, donor sites, abrasions, and first- and second-degree burns

Contraindications
■ Contraindicated for heavily draining wounds

Application
■ Clean the wound.
■ Select the appropriate size dressing.
■ Allow 1″ (2.5 cm) overlap around wound margins for best fit. If necessary, cut the dressing
■ Secure the dressing.

Removal
■ Change the dressing every 3 to 5 days.

CURASOL Gel Wound Dressing

Healthpoint, Ltd.

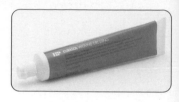

How supplied
Nonsterile tube: 1 oz, 3 oz;
                        A6248
Impregnated gauze: 4″ × 4″

Action
CURASOL Gel Wound Dressing is a clear, viscous hydrogel that protects the wound from foreign contaminants and provides a moist healing environment.

Indications
To manage pressure ulcers (stages 1, 2, 3, and 4), stasis ulcers, diabetic ulcers, foot ulcers, postoperative wounds, first- and second-degree burns, cuts, abrasions, and minor irritations of the skin

Contraindications
None provided by the manufacturer

Application
- Clean the wound with ALLCLENZ Wound Cleanser.
- Apply ⅛″ to ¼″ (0.3 to 0.5 cm) of CURASOL Gel onto the wound bed. If using CURASOL Gel Wound Dressing, loosely pack it into the wound.
- Cover with a secondary dressing.

Removal
- Remove the secondary dressing.
- Flush CURASOL Gel from the wound bed with ALLCLENZ Wound Cleanser during each dressing change.

DermaGel Hydrogel Sheet
Medline Industries, Inc.

How supplied
Sheet: 4" × 4"; A6242

Action
DermaGel Hydrogel Sheet is a bacteriostatic
and fungistatic semiocclusive hydrogel dress-
ing that is soft and flexible and creates a moist healing environment. It
won't liquefy into the wound, and it absorbs about five times its own weight
in exudate.

Indications
To manage leg ulcers, pressure ulcers (stages 1, 2, 3, and 4), superficial
wounds, lacerations, cuts, abrasions, donor sites, partial- and full-thickness
wounds, infected and noninfected wounds, and wounds with light to moderate drainage

Contraindications
■ Contraindicated for deep, tunneling wounds

Application
■ Clean the application site with normal saline solution or an appropriate wound cleanser, such as Skintegrity Wound Cleanser. Dry the surrounding area to ensure that it's free from greasy substances.
■ Select the appropriate size dressing for the wound. Be sure it will cover
the entire wound area.
■ Remove the clear plastic cover from the dressing, and apply the pad to
the wound. Leave the cloth backing in place.
■ Tape the edges of the dressing to keep it in place, or use an elastic net to
secure it without adhesive.
■ If waterproofing is desired, cover with a transparent film.

Removal
■ Change the dressing every 2 to 5 days, depending on the amount of
drainage.
■ Carefully press down on the skin, and lift an edge of the dressing. Con-
tinue around the dressing until all edges are free.
■ Remember to clean the wound with each dressing change.

Dermagran Hydrophilic Wound Dressing

Derma Sciences, Inc.

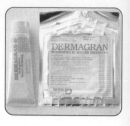

How supplied
Tube: 3 oz (amorphous); A6248
Sterile impregnated gauze: 2" × 2", 4" × 4"; A6231
              4" × 8"; A6232

Action
Dermagran Hydrophilic Wound Dressing contains a zinc-nutrient formulation and provides a primary cover or filler, absorbs mild exudate, and creates a mildly acidic environment that's conducive to wound healing.

Indications
To manage skin ulcers (diabetic, venous stasis), pressure ulcers (stages 1, 2, 3, and 4), surgical incisions, and superficial injuries such as partial-thickness burns, superficial lacerations, cuts, or abrasions

Contraindications
- None provided by the manufacturer

Application
- Clean the wound.
- Choose an appropriate size Dermagran Hydrophilic Wound Dressing.
- Place dressing directly into the wound.
- Cover with an appropriate dressing, and secure in place.

Removal
- Change dressing once daily or as directed by the physician.
- Remove the dressing, and clean the wound.

Dermagran Zinc-Saline Hydrogel
Derma Sciences, Inc.

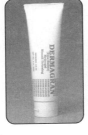

How supplied
Tube: 3 oz; A6248

Action
Dermagran Zinc-Saline Hydrogel is an amorphous hydrogel that contains zinc-nutrient formulation and balanced pH technology. It provides a primary cover or filler for wound deficiencies that absorbs wound exudate and creates a moist environment for granulation tissue formation.

Indications
To manage pressure ulcers (stages 1, 2, 3, and 4), venous stasis ulcers, partial-thickness thermal burns, surgical incisions, skin irritations, abrasions, and conditions associated with peristomal care

Contraindications
- None provided by the manufacturer

Application
- Obtain surgical consult, or consider sharp debridement of necrotic tissue.
- Clean the wound, and then wick out excessive moisture using a gauze sponge.
- Apply a generous layer of Dermagran Zinc Saline Hydrogel to entire wound bed.
- Cover with an appropriate secondary dressing, such as DermaSite or DermaFilm.

Removal
- Change the dressing once daily or as directed by the physician.
- Remove the dressing.
- Clean the area with Dermagran Wound Cleanser or other appropriate wound cleanser.

DermaSyn

DermaGauze

DermaRite Industries, LLC

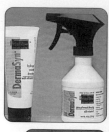

How supplied

DermaSyn
Tube: 3 oz; A6248
Spray: 8 oz; A6248

DermaGauze
Sterile pad: 2″ × 2″, 4″ × 4″; A6231

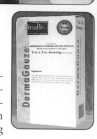

Action

DermaSyn hydrogel dressings and DermaGauze hydrogel-impregnated gauze dressings provide a primary cover or filler for wounds and promote a moist healing environment. Their primary purpose is to fill in dead space associated with sinus tracts and undermining or deep wounds.

Indications

To manage partial-thickness dermal wounds, including pressure ulcers, venous ulcers, diabetic ulcers, and arterial ulcers. Used for tunneling wounds, infected and noninfected wounds, and wounds with minimal or moderate drainage

Contraindications

- Contraindicated for third-degree burns

Application

- Clean the wound.
- Using either the tube or the spray, apply a layer of DermaSyn hydrogel directly into the wound bed. For deep wounds and packing material, use DermaGauze and pack it loosely into the wound.
- Cover with an appropriate secondary dressing.

Removal

- Remove the secondary dressing.
- During each dressing change, irrigate the wound bed with DermaKlenz.

New Product

DiaB Daily Care Gel Hydrogel Wound Dressing

Carrington Laboratories, Inc.

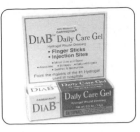

How supplied
Tube: ¹/₂ oz

Action
DiaB Gel is a hydrogel wound dressing for routine use on fingersticks, minor cuts, and injectios sites. It can also be used on burns and abrasions.

Indications
To treat fingersticks, injections sites, minor cuts, abrasions, and callused fingers

Contraindications
■ None known

Application
■ Cleanse the area with a suitable cleanser such as DiaB Klenz.
■ Apply a small amount of DiaB Daily Care Gel to the affected area.
■ Repeat as needed.

Removal
■ Cleanse the area with a suitable cleanser such as DiaB Klenz.

DiaB Gel with Acemannan Hydrogel

Carrington Laboratories, Inc.

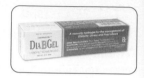

How supplied
Tube:　　3 oz

Action
DiaB Gel is a hydrogel wound dressing containing acemannan hydrogel in a nonoily preparation, especially targeted for diabetic foot ulcers.

Indications
To manage diabetic ulcers

Contraindications
- Contraindicated for patients with known hypersensitivity to aceman-nan hydrogel or any components of the dressing.

Application
- Clean the wound with a suitable cleanser, such as DiaB Klenz, by spray-ing the affected area.
- Gently dry the surrounding skin with soft gauze. No rinsing is required.
- Follow with a layer of DiaB Gel $1/8''$ to $1/4''$ (0.3 to 0.5 cm) thick on ul-cerated areas.
- Cover with an appropriate nonadherent secondary dressing.

Removal
- Change dressing according to the wound condition and amount of ex-udate or as directed by the physician.
- Rinse away any remaining gel with gentle irrigation.

Elasto-Gel
Elasto-Gel Plus
Southwest Technologies, Inc.

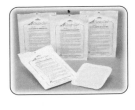

How supplied
Elasto-Gel
Sheet without tape:

> 2" × 3" (5 cm × 7.5 cm; A6242
> 4" × 4" (10 cm × 10 cm); A6242
> 5" × 5" (12.7 cm × 12.7 cm); A6243
> 6" × 8" (15 cm × 20 cm); A6243
> 8" × 16" (20 cm × 40 cm); A6244
> 12" × 12" (30 cm × 30 cm); A6244

Elasto-Gel Plus
Sheet with tape:

> 4" × 4" (10 cm × 10 cm) island; A6246
> 4" × 4" (10 cm × 10 cm) tape not affixed; A6242, bill tape separately
> 2" × 3" (5 cm × 7.5 cm) tape not affixed; A6242, bill tape separately
> 8" × 8" (20 cm × 20 cm) horseshoe-shaped tape affixed; A6247

Action
Elasto-Gel absorbs exudate and seals, protects, and cushions the wound. It permits water vapor transmission and is bacteriostatic and fungistatic. It also reduces odor, acts as a thermal barrier, and reduces pressure.

Indications
To manage first- and second-degree burns, cuts, abrasions, rash, radiation skin reactions, surgical incisions, foot and leg ulcers, pressure ulcers (stages 1, 2, 3, and 4), partial- and full-thickness wounds, wounds with moderate drainage, wounds with serosanguineous drainage, and red, yellow, or black wounds. Used to prevent skin breakdown and to pad tracheostomy and pressure ulcer sites. Also used under casts and splints and on heels and elbows

Contraindications
- Contraindicated for highly exuding wounds that may require packing
- Consult the physician before applying to an infected wound

Application
- Clean wound with normal saline solution or suitable wound cleanser.
- Select the appropriate size dressing or cut one to the desired size or shape. It should extend 1" to 2" (2.5 cm to 5 cm) beyond the wound opening. Leave the clear plastic film on the gel while cutting.

- Remove the clear plastic film, and apply the exposed gel directly on the wound. Don't remove the white fabric backing.
- Secure dressing with tape, elastic or gauze wrap, or stretch netting.
- If the dressing is exposed to moisture, protect it from contamination with a waterproof covering, such as the tape supplied with the dressing.

Removal

- Change the dressing when it's saturated with exudate.

Elta Hydrogel Impregnated Gauze
Swiss-American Products, Inc.

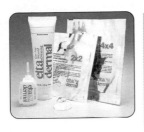

How supplied
Sterile foil pouch: 2" × 2", 4" × 4"; A6231
4" × 8"; A6232
8" × 8"; A6233

Action
Elta Hydrogel Impregnated Gauze maintains a moist healing environment for 24 hours and absorbs moderate exudate. The dressings are kept in place by their viscous glycerin base.

Indications
For use on dry to moderately exudative wounds (stages 1, 2, 3, and 4); may also be helpful in tunneling wounds

Contraindications
■ None provided by the manufacturer

Application
■ Apply dressing appropriate to the size of the wound bed.
■ Cover with an appropriate dressing.

Removal
■ Gently lift the dressing away from the wound.
■ Clean the wound with saline solution or wound cleanser.

Elta Hydrovase Wound Gel
Swiss-American Products, Inc.

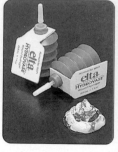

How supplied
Bellows bottle: 1 oz; A6248

Action
Elta Hydrovase Wound Gel with Protease Technology controls moisture delivery by maintaining a moist wound environment without macerating the wound. Elta's protease formulas, enhanced with Pro-N9, destroy proteins that inhibit healing while preserving beneficial cytokines in damaged tissue. The product contains 10% glycerin for moisture retention, and its high viscosity allows it to stay in place. Absorbs dry to moderate exudate.

Indications
To keep the wound bed moist for 24 hours

Contraindications
- None provided by the manufacturer

Application
- Apply $\frac{1}{4}$" (0.5 cm) layer of gel to wound bed.
- Cover with an appropriate dressing.

Removal
- Gently lift the dressing away from the wound site.
- Spray the wound with wound cleanser to lift away necrotic tissue, and clean the wound.

Elta Wound Gel

Swiss-American Products, Inc.

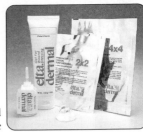

How supplied

Bellows bottle: 1 oz; A6248
Squeeze tube: 4 oz; A6248

Action

Elta Wound Gel maintains a moist wound environment for 24 hours. It's kept in place by its viscous glycerin base.

Indications

For use on dry to moderately exudative stage 1, 2, 3, and 4 wounds

Contraindications

- None provided by the manufacturer

Application

- Apply $\frac{1}{4}''$ (0.5 cm) layer of gel to wound bed.
- Cover with an appropriate dressing.

Removal

- Gently lift the dressing away from the wound site.
- Spray the wound with wound cleanser to lift away necrotic tissue, and clean the wound.

FlexiGel Hydrogel Sheet Dressing
Smith & Nephew, Inc.
Wound Management

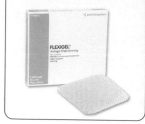

How supplied
Sheet   2" × 2", 4" × 4"; A6242
4" × 8"; A6243

Action
FlexiGel Hydrogel creates and maintains a moist wound environment, which has been established as the optimal environment for the management of the wound. It provides physical separation between the wound and external environments to assist in preventing bacterial contamination of the wound. It's made with a polyacrylaride matrix with embedded hydrophilic polysaccharide particles, is moisture vapor permeable, absorbs up to five times its own weight, creates a cooling, soothing effect on superficial wounds, and is transparent for easy monitoring. Either side of dressing can be used.

Indications
For exudate absorption and the management of partial- to full-thickness wounds, such as ulcers (venous, arterial, diabetic); pressure sores; donor sites; surgical incisions; surgical excisions; and first- and second-degree burns

Contraindications
- Contraindicated for third-degree burns

Application
- Cleanse wound.
- Apply a skin preparation to the periwound skin.
- Apply FlexiGel Sheet dressing (cut to fit wound, if necessary).
- Secondary dressing is required. Roll gauze or OpSite film may be used.
  Note: A film dressing will decrease evaporation, holding more moisture over the wound bed. A gauze dressing allows for evaporation over wounds that are very moist.

Removal
- Change every 3 to 5 days based on drainage.

Gentell Hydrogel

GENTELL, Inc.

How supplied

Impregnated
12-ply gauze pads: 2″ × 2″; 4″ × 4″; A6231
Spray gel: 8-oz adjustable spray; A6248
Tube: 4 oz; A6248

Action

Gentell Hydrogel is an aloe vera–based hydrogel that protects the wound bed and promotes the moist environment essential to the natural healing process.

Indications

To manage pressure ulcers (stages 2, 3, and 4), venous ulcers, first- and second-degree burns, and nondraining wounds

Contraindications

■ None provided by the manufacturer

Application

■ Clean the wound with an appropriate cleanser.
■ Choose and apply the appropriate size Gentell Hydrogel dressing.
■ Cover with a secondary dressing, such as Gentell Bordered Gauze.

Removal

■ Change the dressing every 24 hours or as indicated.

HYDROGELS

Gentell HydrogelAG
Gentell

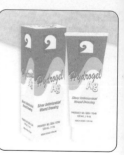

How supplied
Tube (hydrogel with silver): 4 oz; A6248

Action
Gentell HydrogelAG is an antimicrobial wound gel that combines the unique properties of silver sulfadiazine and an aloe vera–based hydrogel. Silver sulfadiazine decreases the bacterial load of both gram-positive and gram-negative bacteria, inhibits bacteria that are resistant to other antimicrobials without harming healthy tissue, and is an effective antifungal.

Indications
To manage full- and partial-thickness wounds with no or minimal drainage, first- and second-degree burns, venous ulcers, pressure ulcers (stages 1, 2, 3, and 4), skin graft donor sites, postoperative incisions, avulsions (skin tears), wound dehiscence, abrasions, and lacerations

Contraindications
- Contraindicated in patients sensitive to sulfonamides or silver sulfadiazine
- Contraindicated for use during pregnancy
- Rare adverse effect: induction of hemolysis in patients with glucose-6-phosphate dehydrogenase deficiency
- Causes a transient leukopenia in some patients

Application
- Remove all dressing material.
- Cleanse the wound with Gentell Wound Cleanser.
- Gently pat dry the entire area surrounding the wound.
- Apply ⅛" layer of Gentell HydrogelAG to the entire surface of the wound using an appropriate, clean applicator or gauze to cover the wound bed sufficiently and evenly.

Removal
- Change the dressing every 24 hours or as indicated.

Product name	Manufacturer/Distributor
Medlite Transparent Tape	Derma Sciences, Inc.
Mefix Self-Adhesive Fabric Tape	Derma Sciences, Inc.
*Mepitac Soft Silicone Tape	Derma Sciences, Inc.
Sta-Fix Tape	Derma Sciences, Inc.
TENDERSKIN	Derma Sciences, Inc.
Ultraclear Transparent Tape	Tyco Healthcare/Kendall
Ultrafix Adhesive Dressing	Derma Sciences, Inc.
Ultrapore Paper Tape	Medline Industries, Inc.
Ultraproof Waterproof Tape	Mölnlycke Health Care
Ultrasilk Cloth Tape	Mölnlycke Health Care
WET-PRUF	Southwest Technologies, Inc.
Woundstrip Wound Closure Strips	Tyco Healthcare/Kendall

Wound cleansers

Wound cleansers are an essential step in wound management. These solutions are used to remove debris or foreign materials from the wound. Each cleanser listed provides the health care professional with proactive products for positive outcomes.

The HCPCS code normally assigned wound cleansers is:
A6260– any type, any size.

Product name	Manufacturer/Distributor
*AlexaCare Skin and Wound Cleanser	AciesHealth, Inc.
ALLCLENZ Wound Cleanser	Healthpoint, Ltd.
Amerigel Wound Wash	Amerx Health Care Corp.
CarraKlenz Wound and Skin Cleanser	Carrington Laboratories, Inc.
ClinsWound Wound Cleanser	SAGE Pharmaceuticals
Comfeel Sea-Clens	Coloplast Corporation
CONSTANT-CLENS	Tyco Healthcare/Kendall
Dermagran Wound Cleanser with Zinc	Derma Sciences, Inc.
DermaKlenz	DermaRite Industries
Dermal Wound Cleanser	Smith & Nephew, Inc. Wound Management
DermaMed	DermaRite Industries
DiaB Klenz Wound Cleanser	Carrington Laboratories, Inc.
Gentell Wound Cleanser	Gentell, Inc.
Hypertonic Seasalt Dermal Solution	Derma Sciences, Inc.
Medi-Tech Wound Cleanser	Medi-Tech International Corporation

*Denotes new product

Product name	**Manufacturer/Distributor**
MicroKlenz Antimicrobial, Deodorizing Wound Cleanser	Carrington Laboratories, Inc.
MPM Antimicrobial Wound Cleanser	MPM Medical, Inc.
*MPM Silvermed Antimicrobial Wound Cleanser	MPM Medical, Inc.
MPM Wound and Skin Cleanser	MPM Medical, Inc.
PrimaDerm Dermal Cleanser – Preservative Free	Derma Sciences, Inc.
PrimaDerm Dermal Cleanser - Preserved	Derma Sciences, Inc.
RadiaKlenz	Carrington Laboratories, Inc.
Restore Wound Cleanser	Hollister Wound Care, LLC
SAF-Clens AF Dermal Wound Cleanser	ConvaTec
Sea-Clens Wound Cleanser	Coloplast Corporation
SeptiCare	SAGE Pharmaceuticals
Skintegrity Wound Cleanser	Medline Industries, Inc.
UltraKlenz Wound Cleanser	Carrington Laboratories, Inc.

*Denotes new product

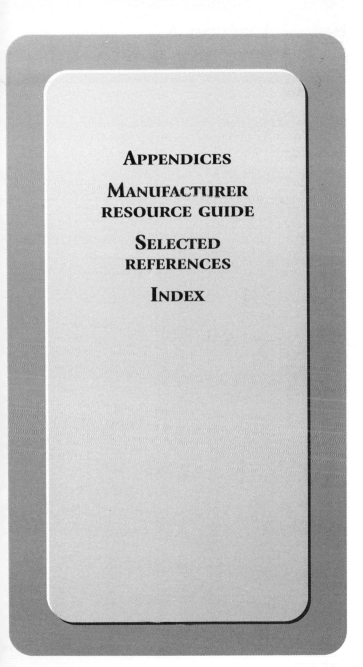

APPENDICES

MANUFACTURER
RESOURCE GUIDE

SELECTED
REFERENCES

INDEX

APPENDIX A
BODY MASS INDEX

The body mass index (BMI) is the relationship between height and weigh Use this chart as an indicator for determining optimal weight for health an as a resource to assess obesity.

HEIGHT (inches)

WEIGHT (lbs)	58	59	60	61	62	63	64	65	66	67	68	69	70	71	72	73	74	75	76
	4'10"	4'11"	5'0"	5'1"	5'2"	5'3"	5'4"	5'5"	5'6"	5'7"	5'8"	5'9"	5'10"	5'11"	6'0"	6'1"	6'2"	6'3"	6'4"
100	21	20	20	19	18	18	17	17	16	16	15	15	14	14	14	13	13	13	13
105	22	21	21	20	19	19	18	18	17	16	16	16	15	15	14	14	14	13	13
110	23	22	22	21	20	20	19	18	18	17	17	16	16	15	15	15	14	14	13
115	24	23	23	22	21	20	20	19	19	18	18	17	17	16	16	15	15	14	14
120	25	24	23	23	22	21	21	20	19	19	18	18	17	17	16	16	15	15	15
125	26	25	24	24	23	22	22	21	20	20	19	18	18	17	17	16	16	15	15
130	27	26	25	25	24	23	22	22	21	20	20	19	19	18	18	17	17	16	16
135	28	27	26	26	25	24	23	23	22	21	21	20	19	19	18	18	17	17	16
140	29	28	27	27	26	25	24	23	23	22	21	21	20	20	19	19	18	18	17
145	30	29	28	27	27	26	25	24	23	23	22	21	21	20	20	19	19	18	18
150	31	30	29	28	27	27	26	26	24	24	23	22	22	21	20	20	19	19	18
155	32	31	30	29	28	28	27	26	25	24	24	23	22	22	21	20	20	19	19
160	34	32	31	30	29	28	27	26	25	24	24	23	22	22	21	21	20	20	20
165	35	33	32	31	30	29	28	28	27	26	25	24	24	23	22	22	21	21	20
170	36	34	33	32	31	30	29	28	27	27	26	25	24	24	23	22	22	21	21
175	37	35	34	33	32	31	30	29	28	27	27	26	25	24	24	23	23	22	21
180	38	36	35	34	33	32	31	30	29	28	27	27	26	25	24	24	23	23	22
185	39	37	36	35	34	33	32	31	30	29	28	27	27	26	25	24	24	23	23
190	40	38	37	36	35	34	33	32	31	30	29	28	27	27	26	25	24	24	23
195	41	39	38	37	36	35	34	33	32	31	30	29	28	27	27	26	25	24	24
200	42	40	39	38	37	36	34	33	32	31	30	30	29	28	27	26	26	25	24
205	43	41	40	39	38	36	35	34	33	32	31	30	29	29	28	27	26	26	25
210	44	43	41	40	38	37	36	35	34	33	32	31	30	29	29	28	27	26	26
215	45	44	42	41	39	38	37	36	35	34	33	32	31	30	29	28	28	27	26
220	46	45	43	42	40	39	38	37	36	35	34	33	32	31	30	29	28	28	27
225	47	46	44	43	41	40	39	38	36	35	34	33	32	31	31	30	29	28	27
230	48	47	45	44	42	41	40	38	37	36	35	34	33	32	31	30	30	29	28
235	49	48	46	44	43	42	40	39	38	37	36	35	34	33	32	31	30	29	29
240	50	49	47	45	44	43	41	40	39	38	37	36	35	34	33	32	31	30	29
245	51	50	48	46	45	43	42	41	40	38	37	36	35	34	33	32	32	31	30
250	52	51	49	47	46	44	43	42	40	39	38	37	36	35	34	33	32	31	30

HEIGHT (inches)

	58	59	60	61	62	63	64	65	66	67	68	69	70	71	72	73	74	75	76
	4'10"	4'11"	5'0"	5'1"	5'2"	5'3"	5'4"	5'5"	5'6"	5'7"	5'8"	5'9"	5'10"	5'11"	6'0"	6'1"	6'2"	6'3"	6'4"
255	53	52	50	48	47	45	44	43	41	40	39	38	37	36	35	34	33	32	31
260	54	53	51	49	48	46	45	43	42	41	40	38	37	36	35	34	33	33	32
265	56	54	52	50	49	47	46	44	43	42	40	39	38	37	36	35	34	33	32
270	57	55	53	51	49	48	46	45	44	42	41	40	39	38	37	36	35	34	33
275	58	56	54	52	50	49	47	46	44	43	42	41	40	38	37	36	35	34	34
280	59	57	55	53	51	50	48	47	45	44	43	41	40	39	38	37	36	35	34
285	60	58	56	54	52	51	49	48	46	45	43	42	41	40	39	38	37	36	35
290	61	59	57	55	53	51	50	48	47	46	44	43	42	41	39	38	37	36	35
295	62	60	58	56	54	52	51	49	48	46	45	44	42	41	40	39	38	37	36
300	63	61	59	57	55	53	52	50	49	47	46	44	43	42	41	40	39	38	37

KEY:

Underweight	Healthy weight	Hefty	Overweight	Obese

Excerpted from Hess, C.T. *Clinical Wound Manager Manual Series for the Wound Care Department.* © Wound Care Strategies, Inc., 2001.

APPENDIX B
WAGNER ULCER GRADE CLASSIFICATION

This system classifies foot ulcers.

GRADE	CHARACTERISTICS
0	■ Preulcer lesion ■ Healed ulcer ■ Presence of bony deformity
1	■ Superficial ulcer without subcutaneous tissue involvement
2	■ Penetration through the subcutaneous tissue; may expose bone, tendon, ligament, or joint capsule
3	■ Osteitis, abscess, or osteomyelitis
4	■ Gangrene of a digit
5	■ Gangrene requiring foot amputation

Reprinted from Glugla, M., and Mulder, G.D., "The Diabetic Foot: Medical Management of Foot Ulcers," in *Chronic Wound Care.* Edited by Krasner, D. King of Prussia, Pa.: Health Management Publications, Inc., 1990, with permission of the publisher.

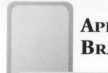

APPENDIX C
BRADEN SCALE

To use this scale, assess the patient for each category, assign a score of 1 to 4, and then calculate the total score. If the patient's score is 16 or less, consider him at high risk for pressure ulcer development.

SENSORY PERCEPTION
Ability to respond appropriately to pressure-related discomfort

1. Completely limited
Patient is unresponsive to painful stimuli (doesn't moan, flinch, or grasp) or has limited ability to feel pain over most of body surface due to diminished level of consciousness or sedation.

2. Very limited
Patient responds only to painful st... can't communicate discomfort exce... by moaning or restlessness, or has... sensory impairment that limits the... ity to feel pain or discomfort over h... of body.

MOISTURE
Degree to which skin is exposed to moisture

1. Constantly moist
Skin is moistened almost constantly by perspiration, urine, and so on. Dampness is detected every time patient is moved or turned.

2. Moist
Skin is usually but not always mois... linen change is required at least o... each shift.

ACTIVITY
Degree of physical activity

1. Bedbound
Patient is confined to bed.

2. Chairbound
Patient's ability to walk is severely... ited or nonexistent. Patient can't b... his own weight or must be assiste... into a chair or wheelchair.

MOBILITY
Ability to change and control body position

1. Completely immobile
Patient doesn't make even slight changes in body or extremity position without assistance.

2. Very limited
Patient makes occasional slight changes in body or extremity posit... but is unable to make frequent or s... nificant changes independently.

NUTRITION
Usual food intake pattern

1. Very poor
Patient never eats a complete meal and rarely eats more than one-third of any food offered. Patient eats two servings or less of protein (meat or dairy products) per day, takes fluids poorly, doesn't take a liquid dietary supplement, or is NPO or maintained on clear liquids or I.V. fluids for more than 5 days.

2. Probably inadequate
Patient rarely eats a complete mea... and generally eats only about one-... of any food offered. Patient eats th... servings of protein (meat or dairy p... ucts) per day, occasionally will tak... dietary supplement, or receives les... than an optimum amount of liquid... or tube feeding.

FRICTION AND SHEAR

1. Problem
Patient requires moderate to maximum assistance in moving. Complete lifting without sliding against sheets is impossible and he frequently slides down in the bed or chair, requiring repositioning with maximum assistance. Spasticity, contractures, or agitation lead to almost constant friction.

2. Potential problem
Patient moves feebly or requires m... mum assistance. During a move, sk... slides to some extent against shee... the chair, restraints, or other device... Patient maintains relatively good p... tion in a chair or bed most of the ti... but occasionally slides down.

	DATE OF ASSESSMENT				
3. Slightly limited Patient responds to verbal commands but can't always communicate discomfort or need to be turned or has some sensory impairment that limits his ability to feel pain or discomfort in one or two extremities.	**4. No impairment** Patient responds to verbal commands and has no sensory deficit that would limit his ability to feel or voice pain or discomfort.				
3. Occasionally moist Skin is occasionally moist, and an extra linen change is required approximately once per day.	**4. Rarely moist** Skin is usually dry and linen requires changing only at routine intervals.				
3. Walks occasionally Patient walks occasionally during the day but only for very short distances, with or without assistance. Patient spends most of each shift in a bed or chair.	**4. Walks frequently** Patient walks outside the room at least twice per day and inside the room at least once every 2 hours during waking hours.				
3. Slightly limited Patient independently makes frequent though slight changes in body or extremity position.	**4. No limitations** Patient makes major and frequent changes in position without assistance.				
3. Adequate Patient eats over one-half of most meals and eats a total of four servings of protein (meat or dairy products) each day. Occasionally, patient will refuse a meal but will usually take a supplement if offered or is on a tube feeding or total parenteral nutrition regimen.	**4. Excellent** Patient eats most of every meal and never refuses a meal. Patient usually eats a total of four or more servings of protein (meat or dairy products) daily. Patient occasionally eats between meals and doesn't require supplementation				
3. No apparent problem Patient moves in a bed or chair independently and has sufficient muscle strength to lift up completely during the move. Patient maintains good position in a bed or chair at all times.					
	TOTAL SCORE				

APPENDIX D
TREATMENT ALGORITHM FOR PRESSURE ULCERS

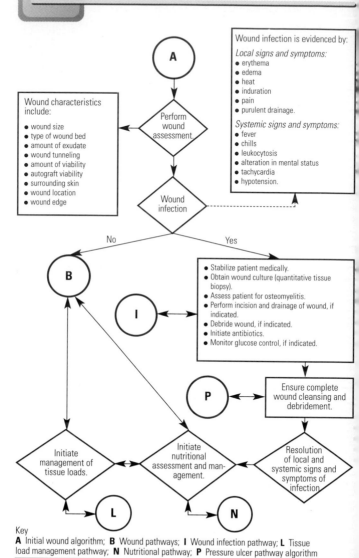

Wound infection is evidenced by:

Local signs and symptoms:
- erythema
- edema
- heat
- induration
- pain
- purulent drainage.

Systemic signs and symptoms:
- fever
- chills
- leukocytosis
- alteration in mental status
- tachycardia
- hypotension.

Wound characteristics include:
- wound size
- type of wound bed
- amount of exudate
- wound tunneling
- amount of viability
- autograft viability
- surrounding skin
- wound location
- wound edge

A

Perform wound assessment.

Wound infection

No — Yes

B

I
- Stabilize patient medically.
- Obtain wound culture (quantitative tissue biopsy).
- Assess patient for osteomyelitis.
- Perform incision and drainage of wound, if indicated.
- Debride wound, if indicated.
- Initiate antibiotics.
- Monitor glucose control, if indicated.

P
Ensure complete wound cleansing and debridement.

Initiate management of tissue loads.

Initiate nutritional assessment and management.

Resolution of local and systemic signs and symptoms of infection

L   **N**

Key
A Initial wound algorithm; **B** Wound pathways; **I** Wound infection pathway; **L** Tissue load management pathway; **N** Nutritional pathway; **P** Pressure ulcer pathway algorithm

Hess, C.T., *Clinical Wound Manager Manual Series for the Wound Care Department.* © Wound Care Strategies, Inc., 2004.

Appendix E
Treatment algorithm for arterial ulcers

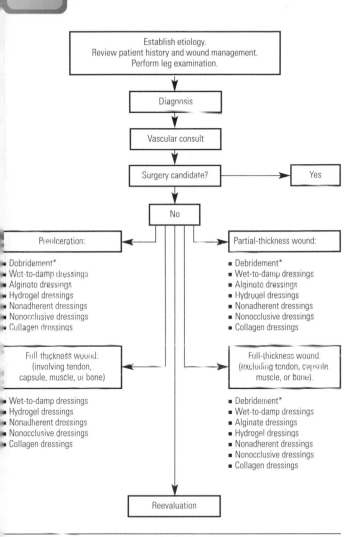

Establish etiology.
Review patient history and wound management.
Perform leg examination.

↓

Diagnosis

↓

Vascular consult

↓

Surgery candidate? → Yes

↓

No

Preulceration:

- Debridement*
- Wet-to-damp dressings
- Alginate dressings
- Hydrogel dressings
- Nonadherent dressings
- Nonocclusive dressings
- Collagen dressings

Partial-thickness wound:

- Debridement*
- Wet-to-damp dressings
- Alginate dressings
- Hydrogel dressings
- Nonadherent dressings
- Nonocclusive dressings
- Collagen dressings

Full-thickness wound:
(involving tendon, capsule, muscle, or bone)

- Wet-to-damp dressings
- Hydrogel dressings
- Nonadherent dressings
- Nonocclusive dressings
- Collagen dressings

Full-thickness wound:
(excluding tendon, capsule, muscle, or bone).

- Debridement*
- Wet-to-damp dressings
- Alginate dressings
- Hydrogel dressings
- Nonadherent dressings
- Nonocclusive dressings
- Collagen dressings

↓

Reevaluation

---

* Debride only arterial ulcers with necrotic tissue. Be careful not to disturb the already compromised arteries.
Adapted with permission from *Advances in Skin & Wound Care* 14(3):147, May/June 2001.

APPENDIX F
TREATMENT ALGORITHM FOR VENOUS ULCERS

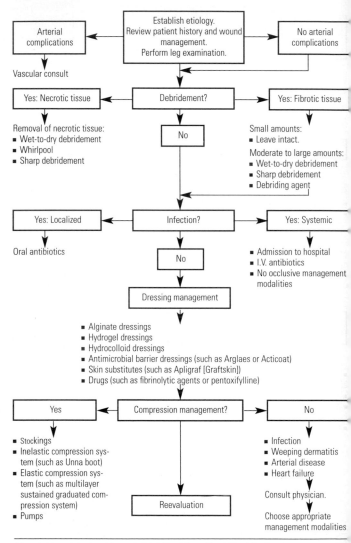

	Establish etiology. Review patient history and wound management. Perform leg examination.	
Arterial complications		No arterial complications
Vascular consult		

Debridement?

Yes: Necrotic tissue

Removal of necrotic tissue:
- Wet-to-dry debridement
- Whirlpool
- Sharp debridement

No

Yes: Fibrotic tissue

Small amounts:
- Leave intact.

Moderate to large amounts:
- Wet-to-dry debridement
- Sharp debridement
- Debriding agent

Infection?

Yes: Localized

Oral antibiotics

No

Yes: Systemic

- Admission to hospital
- I.V. antibiotics
- No occlusive management modalities

Dressing management

- Alginate dressings
- Hydrogel dressings
- Hydrocolloid dressings
- Antimicrobial barrier dressings (such as Arglaes or Acticoat)
- Skin substitutes (such as Apligraf [Graftskin])
- Drugs (such as fibrinolytic agents or pentoxifylline)

Compression management?

Yes

- Stockings
- Inelastic compression system (such as Unna boot)
- Elastic compression system (such as multilayer sustained graduated compression system)
- Pumps

No

- Infection
- Weeping dermatitis
- Arterial disease
- Heart failure

Consult physician.

Choose appropriate management modalities

Reevaluation

Adapted with permission from *Advances in Skin & Wound Care* 14(3):147, May/June 2001.

APPENDIX G
TREATMENT ALGORITHM FOR DIABETIC ULCERS

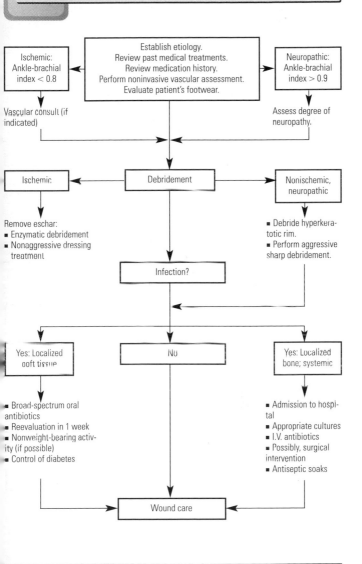

Establish etiology.
Review past medical treatments.
Review medication history.
Perform noninvasive vascular assessment.
Evaluate patient's footwear.

Ischemic:
Ankle-brachial index < 0.8

Neuropathic:
Ankle-brachial index > 0.9

Vascular consult (if indicated)

Assess degree of neuropathy.

Ischemic

Debridement

Nonischemic, neuropathic

Remove eschar:
■ Enzymatic debridement
■ Nonaggressive dressing treatment

■ Debride hyperkeratotic rim.
■ Perform aggressive sharp debridement.

Infection?

Yes: Localized soft tissue

No

Yes: Localized bone; systemic

■ Broad-spectrum oral antibiotics
■ Reevaluation in 1 week
■ Nonweight-bearing activity (if possible)
■ Control of diabetes

■ Admission to hospital
■ Appropriate cultures
■ I.V. antibiotics
■ Possibly, surgical intervention
■ Antiseptic soaks

Wound care

Adapted with permission from *Advances in Skin & Wound Care* 13(1):35, January/February 2000.

577

APPENDIX H
TREATMENT ALGORITHM FOR
DIABETIC ULCER WOUND CARE

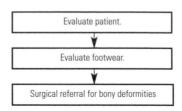

Evaluate patient.

↓

Evaluate footwear.

↓

Surgical referral for bony deformities

Grade 0

- Padding and accommodative devices
- Callus debridement

Grade 1

- Follow Grade 1 protocol.
- Topical silver sulfadiazine on highly contaminated wounds
- Nonocclusive dressing
- Weekly evaluation until healed
- Plantar surface — gauze dressing
- Dorsal surface — occlusive or nonocclusive dressing
- Growth factor (rhPDGF-BB) when ankle-brachial index (ABI) is > 0.45

Grade 2

- Follow Grade 1 protocol.
- Rule out osteomyelitis (X-ray, bone scan, bone biopsy)
- Nonweight-bearing activity
- Surgical consult
- Plantar surface — gauze, amorphous hydrogel, alginate, or foam dressing
- Dorsal surface — occlusive dressing
- Topical antimicrobial cream, ointment, or amorphous hydrogel
- Growth factor (rhPDGF-BB) when ABI is < 0.45

Grade 3

- Follow Grade 1 protocol.
- Rule out osteomyelitis (X-ray, bone scan, bone biopsy)
- Plantar surface — gauze, amorphous hydrogel, alginate, or foam dressing
- Dorsal surface — nonocclusive dressing
- Topical antimicrobial cream, ointment, or amorphous hydrogel

Grades 4 and 5

- Surgical consult and intervention

Adapted with permission from *Advances in Skin & Wound Care* 13(1):35, January/February 2000.

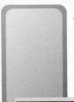

APPENDIX I
LABORATORY TESTS TO RULE OUT ATYPICAL CAUSES OF LEG ULCERS

Chemistries

Kidney (BUN, creatinine)
Liver (liver enzymes, hepatitis panel)
Electrolytes
Glucose
Fasting lipids
Hemoglobin A1c
Amylase/lipase
Iron
Folate
Ferritin
Parathyroid hormone
Calcium
Phosphorus
Magnesium
Transferrin
Albumin
Prealbumin
Vitamins/minerals
Aldolase
Creatine kinase

Immunologic tests

(autoimmune disorders, vasculitis)
ASO
Antinuclear antibodies
Rheumatoid factor
Quantitative immunoglobulins
Protein electrophoresis (SPEP, IPEP)
Complement (CH50, C3, C4)
a-ANCA, p-ANCA
Indirect immunofluorescence
Antiphospholipid antibodies (lupus anticoagulant, IgG or IgM anticardiolipin antibodies)

Hematologic tests

CBC with differential
Sedimentation rate
C-reactive protein
Antithrombin III
Protein C
Protein S
Factor V Leiden
Peripheral blood smear
Homocyteine
Hemoglobin electrophoresis
Cryoglobulins/cryofibrinogens
Glucose 6 phosphate dehydrogenase
Complement
Fibrinogen/FDP/D-dimers
PT/PTT

Tissue biopsy

For differential diagnosis of inflammatory, microthrombotic, and bullous disorders, such as:
Nonatherosclerotic ischemic ulcers (vasculitis, vasculopathy)
Inflammatory conditions
Malignancies
Infections
Autoimmune bullous disorders
Atherosclerotic ischemic ulcers
Venous ulcers
Neuropathic ulcers
Medication-induced wounds
Pressure ulcers
Traumatic wounds
Note: Location is crucial to accurate diagnosis. Biopsy newest lesions along the advancing edge of the abnormal area, including a rim of normal tissue; consider several biopsies in different areas of the wound.

APPENDIX J
ANKLE-BRACHIAL INDEX USE IN PATIENTS WITH DIABETES

Peripheral arterial disease (PAD) in the lower extremities signals widespread arterial disease and a high risk of stroke, myocardial infarction, and death. Because many patients with diabetes also have PAD, the American Diabetes Association now recommends testing for PAD in any patient with diabetes who is over age 50.[1] Patients with diabetes who are younger than age 50 should be screened for PAD if they have risk factors for PAD, such as smoking, hypertension, hyperlipidemia, or diabetes for more than 10 years.[1]

The recommended test is the ankle-brachial index (ABI), which measures the ratio of systolic blood pressure in the ankle and the arm. The ABI can be used to detect decreased blood pressure distal to sites of artery narrowing. If the results are normal, the ADA recommends that patients be rechecked every 5 years.[1]

However, the ABI is not a foolproof way to assess patients with diabetes. These patients may have falsely elevated ABIs because their disease process causes calcification that decreases compressibility of the arteries. Clinicians must, therefore, pay close attention to the patient's physical condition. A patient with cold and/or hairless lower extremities, for example, may have PAD regardless of a normal ABI. If the physical examination warrants, the patient may need a toe-brachial index to determine arterial perfusion in the feet and toes.

When measuring the ABI, use a handheld, 5 to 10 MHz Doppler ultrasound device[1] and follow the steps listed here to detect the brachial and ankle pulses.

1. Gather the following equipment:
   - mercury or aneroid sphygmomanometer with cuff
   - handheld Doppler device with vascular probe
   - conductivity gel compatible with the Doppler device
   - gauze or tissues.

2. Have the patient lie in the supine position for at least 5 minutes. Remove the patient's shoes and socks. Apply the blood pressure cuff to the arm and palpate for the brachial pulse. Apply conductivity gel over the brachial artery.

3. Turn on the Doppler device and place the tip of the probe into the top of the gel at a 45-degree angle. Listen for a whooshing sound, which indicates the brachial pulse.

Calculating the ABI

To determine the ABI, divide each ankle systolic pressure (A) by the higher brachial pressure (B) to calculate the ankle-brachial index (ABI). For example:

	Left		**Right**
	140	(A)	128
divided by	144	(B)	144
equals	0.97	(AB)	0.89

According to the ADA,[1] diagnostic criteria for PAD based on the ABI are as follows.
- Normal: 0.91-1.30
- Mild obstruction: 0.70-0.90
- Moderate obstruction: 0.40-0.69
- Severe obstruction: less than 0.40
- Poorly compressible (due to medial arterial calcification): > 1.3

4. Pump up the cuff to the point at which the sound is no longer heard, then to 20 mm Hg above that point. Slowly release the air and listen again for the whooshing sound. The point at which the sound is first heard indicates systolic blood pressure. Repeat the procedure in the other arm and record the higher reading.

5. Locate the posterior tibial pulse at the medial aspect of the patient's ankle. With the same technique used on the arms, assess and record systolic pressures in both ankles. Use the gauze or tissue to clean the gel from the patient's skin. Calculate the ABI for each ankle and document the results and the sites in the medical record. (See *Calculating the ABI*.)

Adapted with permission from Sloan, H., and Wills, E.M. "Ankle-Brachial Index: Calculating Your Patient's Vascular Risk," *Nursing99* 29(10):58-9, October 1999.

Reference: 1. American Diabetes Association. "Peripheral Arterial Disease in People with Diabetes. *Diabetes Care* 26:3333-41, 2003.

AciesHealth, Inc.
103 South Spring Street
Bellefonte, PA 16823
www.acieshealth.com

AFASSCO
P.O. Box 1767
Carson City, NV 89702
www.afassco.com

Ameriderm Laboratories
Ltd
13 Kentucky Ave
Paterson, NJ 07503
www.ameriderm.com

Amerx Health Care Corpo-
ration
Procyon Corporation
1300 S. Highland Ave.
Clearwater, FL 33756-6519
www.amerigel.com

Argentum Medical, LLC
240 81st Street
Willowbrook, IL 60527
www.silverlon.com

Bio Med Sciences, Inc.
7584 Morris Court, Suite
218
Allentown, PA 18106
www.silon.com

Brennen Medical, Inc.
1290 Hammond Road
Saint Paul, Minnesota
55110-5867
www.brennenmedical.com

Carrington Laboratories
2001 Walnut Hill Lane
Irvin, TX 75038
www.carringtonlabs.com
www.woundcare.com

Coloplast Corporation
220 South Sixth Street,
Suite 900
Minneapolis, MN 55402
www.us.coloplast.com

Conmed Corporation
525 French Road
Utica, NY 13502
www.conmed.com

Convatec
A Bristol-Myers Squibb
Company
100 Headquarters Drive
Skillman, NJ 08558
www.convatec.com
www.aquacel.com

DermaRite Industries, LLC
3 East 26th Street
Patterson, NJ 07513
www.DermaRite.com

Derma Sciences, Inc.
214 Carnegie Center, Suite
100
Princeton, NJ 08540
www.dermasciences.com

DeRoyal
200 DeBusk Lane
Powell, TN 37849
www.deroyal.com

Ethex Corporation
10888 Metro Court
St. Louis, MO 63043
www.ethex.com

Ferris Manufacturing Cor-
poration
16W300 83rd Street
Burr Ridge, IL 60527
www.ferriscares.com

Gentell, Inc.
3600 Boundbrook Ave.
Trevose, PA 19053
www.gentell.com

Healthpoint, Ltd.
3909 Hulen Street
Fort Worth, TX 76107
www.healthpoint.com

Hollister, Inc.
2000 Hollister Drive
Libertyville, IL 60048
www.hollister.com

Hydrofera, LLC
322 Main Street
Willimantic, CT 06226
www.hydrofera.com

The Hymed Group
1890 Bucknell Drive
Bethlehem, PA 18015
www.hymed.com

Johnson & Johnson
Wound Management
A division of Ethicon, Inc.
P.O. Box 151
Sommerville, NJ 08876
www.advancedwound-
care.com

Kinetic Concepts, Inc.
8023 Vantage Drive
San Antonio, TX 78230
www.kci1.com

Lescarden, Inc.
420 Lexington Avenue
Suite 212
New York, NY 10170
www.catrix.com

Medi-Tech International
Corporation
26 Court Street
Brooklyn, NY 11242
www.medi-techintl.com

Medline Industries, Inc.
One Medline Place
Mundelein, IL 60060
www.medline.com/wound
care

Molnlycke Health Care US,
LLC
Apax Partners
5550 Peachtree Parkway,
Suite 500
Norcross, GA 30092
www.molnlycke.com

MPM Medical, Inc.
RBC Life Sciences
2301 Crown Court
Irving,TX 75038
www.mpmmedicalinc.com

Mylan Bertek Pharmaceuti-
cals, Inc.
12720 Dairy Ashford
Sugar Land, TX 77478
www.udllabs.com

OrthoNeutrogena
Johnson & Johnson
5760 West 96th Street
Los Angeles, CA 90045
www.biafine.com

Regenesis Biomedical, Inc.
1435 N. Hayden Road
Scottsdale, AZ 82527
www.regenesisbiomed-
ical.com

Rejuveness Pharmaceuti-
cals
480 Broadway LL10
Saratoga Springs, NY
12866
www.rejuveness.com

SAGE Pharmaceuticals,
Inc.
5408 Interstate Drive
Shreveport, LA 71109

Smith & Nephew Wound
Management
11775 Starkey Road
Largo, FL 33773
www.snwmd.com

Southwest Technologies,
Inc.
1746 Levee Road
N. Kansas City, MO 64116
www.elastogel.com

Swiss-American Products
4641 Nall Road
Dallas, TX 75244
www.elta.net

3M Health Care
Bldg. 275-4W-02
St. Paul, MN 55144-1000
www.3M.com/healthcare

Tyco Healthcare/Kendall
15 Hampshire Street
Mansfield, MA 02048
www.kendallhq.com

Winfield Laboratories, Inc.
P.O. Box 832297
Richardson, TX 75083-
2297
www.winfieldlabs.com

Wound Care Innovations
2589 State Road
Fort Lauderdale, FL 33313
www.celleraterx.com

Xylos Corporation
838 Town Center Drive
Langhorne, PA 19047
www.xcellwoundcare.com

SELECTED REFERENCES

Abu-Rumman, P.L., et al. "Use of Clinical Laboratory Parameters to Evaluate Wound Healing Potential in Diabetes Mellitus," *Journal of the American Podiatric Medical Association* 92(1):38-47, January 2002.

Armstrong, D.G., et al. "Maggot Debridement Therapy: A Primer." *Journal of the American Podiatric Medical Association* 92(7):398-401, July 2002.

Bergstrom, N., et al. Treatment of Pressure Ulcers. Clinical Practice Guideline, No. 15. AHCPR Publication No. 95-0652. Rockville, MD: Agency for Health Care Policy and Research; December 1994.

Bowler, P.G. The 10(5) bacterial growth guideline: reassessing its clinical relevance in wound healing. *Ostomy/Wound Management* 49(1):44-53, January 2003.

Burton, C.S. Venous leg ulcers. *American Journal of Surgery* 167(suppl):37S-41S, 1994:

Centers for Disease Control and Prevention. *National Diabetes Fact Sheet: General Information and National Estimates on Diabetes in the United States, 2000.* Atlanta: U.S. Department of Health and Human Services, Centers for Disease Control and Prevention, 2002.

Centers for Medicare and Medicaid Services: *State Operations Manual.* Available online at http://www.cms.hhs.gov/Manuals/iom/itemdetail.asp?filterType=none&filterByDID=-99&sortByDID=1&sortOrder=ascending&itemID=CMS0190 27&intNumPerPage=10

Falanga, V. "Classifications for wound bed preparation and stimulation of chronic wounds," *Wound Repair and Regeneration* 8:347-52, 2000.

Falanga, V. *Cutaneous Wound Healing.* London: Martin Dunitz Ltd., 2001.

Falanga, V. "Wound bed preparation and the role of enzymes: a case for multiple actions of therapeutic agents," *Wounds* 14:47-57, 2002.

Falanga, V, and Eaglstein, W.H. "The trap hypothesis of venous ulceration," *Lancet* 341(8851):1006-1008, May 1993.

Harriet, W., et al. "Guidelines for the Treatment of Arterial Insufficiency Ulcers," *Wound Repair and Regeneration.* 14(6):693-710, 2006.

Hess, C.T. "Algorithms and Pathways Manual," *TriAssess Software* and *Clinical Wound Manager Manual Series.* Harrisburg, Pa.: Wound Care Strategies, Inc., 2006.

International Working Group on the Diabetic Foot. "Practical Guidelines." Available at http://www.iwgdf.org/index.php?option=com_content&task=view&id=27&Itemid=29
Au: previous URL didn't work; replaced with this one—OK?

Whitney, J., et al. "Guidelines for the Treatment of Pressure Ulcers," *Wound Repair and Regeneration* 14(6):663-679, 2006.

Kaleta, J.L., et al. "The Diagnosis of Osteomyelitis in Diabetes Using Erythrocyte Sedimentation Rate: A Pilot Study," *Journal of the American Podiatric Medical Association* 91(9):445-50, October 2001.

Katz, D. *Nutrition in Clinical Practice.* Philadelphia: Lippincott Williams & Wilkins, 2001.

Kirsner, R.S. "Wound Healing." In Bolognia, J.L, et al., editors. *Dermatology.* New York: Mosby, 2003.

Kloth, L.C., and McCulloch, J. *Wound Healing Alternatives in Management.* Philadelphia: F.A. Davis, 2002.

Ladwig, G.P., et al. "Ratios of Activated Matrix Metalloproteinase-9 to Tissue

Inhibitor of Matrix Metalloproteinase-1 in Wound Fluids Are Inversely Correlated With Healing of Pressure Ulcers," *Wound Repair and Regeneration* 10:26-37, 2002.

Mann, J., and Truswell, A.S. *Essentials of Human Nutrition.* Oxford: Oxford University Press, 2002.

Martin, C., et al. "Guidelines for the Treatment of Venous Ulcers," *Wound Repair and Regeneration* 14 (6), 649-62, 2006.

Martin, C., et al. "Guidelines for the Best Care of Chronic Wounds," *Wound Repair and Regeneration* 14(6).647-8, 2006.

Mulder, G.D., and Vande Berg, J.S. "Cellular Senescence and Matrix Metalloproteinase Activity in Chronic Wounds Relevance to Debridement and New Technologies," *Journal of the American Podiatric Medical Association* 92(1):34-7, January 2002.

National Patient Safety Foundation. Public opinion of patient safety issues: research findings; 1997. Available online at http://www.npsf.org/download/1997survey.pdf; accessed June 11, 2004.

Panel on the Prediction and Prevention of Pressure Ulcers in Adults. "Pressure Ulcers in Adults: Prediction and Prevention." Clinical Practice Guideline, No. 3. AHCPR Publication No. 92-0047. Rockville, Md.: Agency for Health Care Policy and Research; May 1992.

Pressure Ulcers in America: "Prevalence, Incidence, and Implications for the Future. An Executive Summary of the National Pressure Ulcer Advisory Panel Monograph," *Advances in Skin and Wound Care* 14:208-15, 2001.

Robson, M.C. "Wound Infection. A Failure of Wound Healing Caused by an Imbalance of Bacteria," *Surgical Clinics of North America* 77(3):637-50, May 1997.

Steed, D.L., et al. "Guidelines for the Treatment of Diabetic Ulcers," *Wound Repair and Regeneration* 14(6):680-692, 2006.

Veves, A., et al. "Graftskin, a Human Skin Equivalent, Is Effective in the Management of Noninfected Neuropathic Diabetic Foot Ulcers: A Prospective Randomized Multicenter Clinical Trial," *Diabetes Care* 24:290-5, 2001.

Visse, R., and Nagase, H. "Matrix Metalloproteinases and Tissue Inhibitors of Metalloproteinases: Structure, Function, and Biochemistry," *Circulation Research* 92(8):827-39, May 2003.

Weenig, R.H., et al. "Skin ulcers misdiagnosed as pyoderma gangrenosum," *New England Journal of Medicine* 347(18); 1412-1418, 2002.

Wissing, U.E., et al. "Can Individualized Nutritional Support Improve Healing in Therapy-Resistant Leg Ulcers?" *Journal of Wound Care* 11(1):15-20, January 2002.

Wound, Ostomy & Continence Nurses Society. *Guideline for Management of Patients with Lower-Extremity Neuropathic Disease.* Glenview, Ill.: Wound, Ostomy & Continence Nurses Society, 2004.

Wound, Ostomy & Continence Nurses Society. *Guideline for Management of Patients with Lower-Extremity Venous Disease.* Glenview, Ill.: Wound, Ostomy & Continence Nurses Society, 2005.

Wound, Ostomy & Continence Nurses Society. *Guideline for Management of Patients with Lower-Extremity Arterial Disease.* Glenview, Ill.: Wound, Ostomy & Continence Nurses Society, 2002.

Wound, Ostomy & Continence Nurses Society. *Guideline for Prevention and Management of Pressure Ulcers.* Glenview, Ill.: Wound, Ostomy & Continence Nurses Society, 2003.

WrongDiagnosis.com. "How Common Is Misdiagnosis?" Available online at http://www.wrongdiagnosis.com. Accessed July 6, 2004.

Zacur, H., and Kirsner, R.S. "Debridement: Rationale and Therapeutic Options," *Wounds* 14(7 Suppl E):2E-7E, 2002.

INDEX

---

i refers to an illustration; t refers to a table; **boldface** indicates color pages.

---

i refers to an illustration; t refers to a table; **boldface** indicates color pages.

---

i refers to an illustration; t refers to a table; **boldface** indicates color pages.

---

i refers to an illustration; t refers to a table; **boldface** indicates color pages.

---

i refers to an illustration; t refers to a table; **boldface** indicates color pages.

refers to an illustration; t refers to a table; **boldface** indicates color pages.

---

i refers to an illustration; t refers to a table; **boldface** indicates color pages.

Hypergel
Mölnlycke Health Care

How supplied
Tube: 5 g, 15 g; A6248

Action
Hypergel is a water-based hypertonic saline gel that softens and debrides necrotic tissue (eschar). The 20% sodium chloride gel hydrates and creates a hypertonic environment, thus promoting autolytic debridement.

Indications
To soften and remove dry and moist necrotic eschar on pressure ulcers (stages 3 and 4), partial- and full-thickness wounds, tunneling wounds, noninfected wounds, wounds with minimal drainage (if eschar is still present), wounds with serosanguineous or purulent drainage (if eschar is still present), and black wounds. Treatment is discontinued when the wound is covered with less than 25% eschar.

Contraindications
- Not recommended for ulcers with no devitalized (dead) tissue
- Not recommended for wounds that have compromised arterial blood supply

Application
- Gently irrigate or flush the wound with normal saline solution, if necessary, and blot excess saline solution with absorbent gauze.
- Unscrew and remove cap and distance ring. Reapply the cap to the tube, and twist it firmly back on to break the seal of the tube.
- Unscrew the cap and apply a light coating (dime thickness) to the dry necrotic eschar. Avoid applying it to intact skin. (*Note:* Hypergel isn't a wound filler; it's designed to coat the wound surface.)
- Pack deep wounds with suitable material.
- Cover with Alldress or other cover dressing.

Removal
- Change the dressing every 24 hours or when drainage is visible through the cover dressing.

HYDROGELS

IntraSite Gel Hydrogel Wound Dressing
Smith & Nephew, Inc.
Wound Management

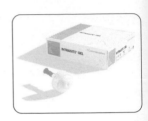

How supplied
Applipaks: 8 g, 15 g, 25 g; A6248

Action
IntraSite Gel is an amorphous hydrogel that gently rehydrates necrotic tissue, facilitating autolytic debridement, while being able to loosen and absorb slough and exudate. It can also be used to provide the optimum moist wound management environment during the later stages of wound closure. It's nonadherent and doesn't harm viable tissue or the skin surrounding the wound. This makes IntraSite Gel ideal for every stage in the wound management process.

Indications
IntraSite Gel is used to create a moist wound environment for the treatment of conditions such as minor burns, superficial lacerations, cuts and abrasions (partial-thickness wounds), and skin tears. Under the direction of a health care professional, IntraSite Gel is used to create a moist wound environment for the management of venous ulcers (leg ulcers), surgical incisions, diabetic foot ulcers, and pressure ulcers (including stage 4). IntraSite creates a moist wound environment, which assists in autolytic debridement of wounds covered with necrotic tissues

Contraindications
- Contraindicated in patients who are sensitive to IntraSite Gel or any of its ingredients
- Should be used with care in the vicinity of the eyes and in deep wounds with narrow openings (for example, fistulas) where removal of the gel may be difficult
- For external use only; not to be taken internally

Application
- Prepare the wound site. Remove the secondary dressing. Irrigate the wound with sterile saline solution to clean the site.
- Prepare the pack. Remove the blue protective cap from the nozzle. Swab the snap-off tip and nozzle of the pack with a suitable antiseptic swab. Snap the patterned tip off the nozzle.
- Introduce IntraSite Gel into the wound. Keeping the nozzle tip clear of the wound surface, gently press the bowl of the pack to dispense gel into the wound. Smooth IntraSite Gel over the surface of the wound to a depth of about 5 mm (0.2"). Discard any unused gel.

- Dress the wound. Cover with a secondary dressing of choice, for example:
  - Necrotic stage: Site Flexigrid Moisture Vapour Permeable Adhesive Film Dressing
  - Sloughy stage: Allevyn Hydrocellular Hydrophillic Wound Dressing/Melolin Low-Adherent Absorbent Dressing
  - Granulating stage: Allevyn/Melolin/OpSite Flexigrid

Removal

- IntraSite Gel can be removed from the wound by rinsing with sterile saline solution.
- On necrotic and sloughy wounds, it's recommended that the dressing be changed at least every 3 days.
- On clean granulating wounds, the frequency of dressing changes depends on the clinical condition of the wound and the amount of exudate produced.

MacroPro Wound Gel with Oat Beta-Glucan

Brennen Medical, LLC

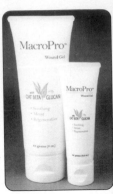

How supplied

Tube: 25 g (.9 oz), 85 g (3 oz); A6248

Action

MacroPro Wound Gel is a soothing, viscous gel composed of a natural complex carbohydrate derived from oats. It creates a moist healing environment that supports autolytic debridement of wounds with scattered areas of necrosis and slough.

Indications

To help manage superficial and partial-thickness burns; pressure ulcers (stages 1, 2, 3, and 4); venous, diabetic, and arterial ulcers; donor graft sites; superficial through full-thickness wounds such as surgical wounds, minor abrasions, and lacerations; and skin irritations

Contraindications

- Contraindicated in patients with a known allergy to plants such as gum oat

Application

- Clean the wound with sterile water, normal saline, or according to facility guidelines. Dry the surrounding skin.
- Apply MacroPro Wound Gel sufficiently to cover entire area of the wound up to a depth of ¼" (6 mm).
- Cover gel and wound with an appropriate secondary dressing.
- Secure secondary dressing in place with tape or a net dressing retainer.
- Carefully monitor wound progress.
- MacroPro Gel applications may be repeated every 24 to 48 hours when used on sloughy, necrotic wounds, or within 7 days when used on clean, granulating wounds.

Removal

- Remove secondary dressing and discard.
- Gently clean the wound.
- Repeat application of MacroPro Wound Gel as needed.

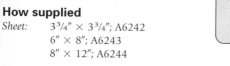

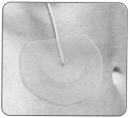

New Product

MPM CoolMagic Sheet Hydrogel Dressing
MPM Medical, Inc.

HYDROGELS

How supplied
Sheet: 3³/₄" × 3³/₄"; A6242
6" × 8"; A6243
8" × 12"; A6244

Action
MPM CoolMagic is a semiocclusive sterile hydrogel polymer sheet consisting of 90% water and 10% crosslinked polyethelene oxide matrix. Hydrophyllic and absorptive, absorbing three times its weight, MPM CoolMagic is excellent for reducing pain from burns and skin reactions to radiation.

Indications
For use on partial-thickness wounds, such as pressure ulcers, vascular and diabetic ulcers, abrasions, skin tears, and first- and second-degree burns

Contraindications
■ Contraindicated for use on third degree burns, infected wounds, and full-thickness wounds

Application
■ Clean the wound with MPM Wound and Skin Cleanser or saline solution, and dry.
■ Remove red backing by gripping extended edge and pulling back.
■ Apply exposed hydrogel to wound bed, allowing for overlap on intact skin.
■ MPM CoolMagic Dressing may be left in place for up to 3 days.

Removal
■ Carefully remove dressing and clean with MPM Wound and Skin Cleanser.
■ Reapply in accordance with your protocol.

MPM Excel Gel
MPM Hydrogel
MPM Medical, Inc.

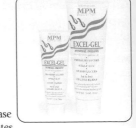

How supplied
Tube: 1 oz, 3 oz; A6248

Action
MPM Excel Gel has an aloe vera and glycerin base that maintains a moist environment, promotes healing, and facilitates autolytic debridement.

Indications
To manage pressure ulcers (stages 2, 3, and 4), venous stasis ulcers, partial- and full-thickness wounds, superficial wounds, first- and second-degree burns, and tunneling wounds

Contraindications
- Not recommended for draining wounds

Application
- Clean wound with MPM Wound Cleanser or normal saline solution.
- Apply MPM Excel Gel to the wound in a layer ⅛″ to ¼″ (0.3 to 0.5 cm) thick.
- Cover with a secondary dressing.

Removal
- Change dressing daily.
- Flush the wound with MPM Wound Cleanser or normal saline solution
- Gently remove the dressing.

HYDROGELS

MPM GelPad Hydrogel Saturated Dressing

MPM Medical, Inc.

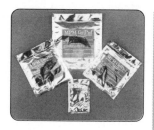

How supplied

Sterile pad: 2″ × 2″, 4″ × 4″; A6231
8″ × 4″; A6232
10″ × 6″; A6233

Action

MPM GelPad Hydrogel Saturated Dressing is saturated with stabilized aloe vera hydrogel and provides a primary cover for wounds. It creates a moist environment that facilitates wound healing and autolytic debridement.

Indications

To manage pressure ulcers (stages 1, 2, 3, and 4), partial- and full-thickness wounds, first- and second-degree burns, tunneling wounds, infected and noninfected wounds, and red, yellow, or black wounds; excellent for wound packing

Contraindications

■ Not recommended for draining wounds

Application

■ Clean the wound with MPM Wound Cleanser or normal saline solution.
■ Apply the dressing to the wound, or loosely pack the wound with the dressing.
■ Secure with an appropriate secondary dressing.

Removal

■ Change the dressing daily.
■ Remove the secondary dressing.
■ Flush the wound with MPM Wound Cleanser or normal saline solution

MPM Regenecare with Lidocaine (2%)

MPM Medical, Inc.

How supplied
Tube: 3 oz; A6248

Action
MPM Regenecare is the first wound gel containing lidocaine, collagen, aloe vera, and vitamin E that maintains a moist environment, promotes healing, facilitates autolytic debridement, and reduces wound pain.

Indications
To manage pressure ulcers (stages 2, 3, and 4), venous stasis ulcers, partial- and full-thickness wounds, secreting dermal lesions, superficial wounds, first- and second-degree burns, and tunneling wounds

Contraindications
- None provided by the manufacturer

Application
- Clean the wound with MPM Wound Cleanser or normal saline solution.
- Apply MPM Regenecare with lidocaine to the wound in a layer ¼" (0.5 cm) thick.
- Cover with a secondary dressing.

Removal
- Change hydrogel dressing daily.
- Remove the dressing.
- Flush the wound with MPM Wound Cleanser or normal saline solution.

New Product

MPM Silvermed Antimicrobial Hydrogel
MPM Medical, Inc.

How supplied
Amorphous Hydrogel tube: 1.5 oz, 3 oz; A6248

Action
MPM Silvermed Hydrogel is an amorphous gel wound dressing designed for use in moist wound care management. Stabilized silver microparticles are immediately activated on contact with wounds to continuously release ionic silver to help reduce infection by bacteriostatic and bacteriocidal action on clinically relevant pathogens. Bioavailable silver binds to and reduces the activity of matrix metalloproteinase (MMPs).

Indications
Under the care of health care professional, appropriate for use in the management of partial- to full-thickness wounds with light to moderate exudate, such as pressure ulcers, diabetic and leg ulcers, skin abrasions, lacerations and tears, first- and second-degree burns, surgical wounds, and grafted wound and donor sites

Contraindications
- Contraindicated in patients who are sensitive to components of the gel

Application
- Cleanse wound with MPM Silvermed Wound Cleanser.
- Spread MPM Silvermed Hydrogel throughout the wound to about ¼" thickness
- Cover with nonadherent dressing, preferably waterproof with good vapor transmission rate.

Removal
- Carefully remove secondary dressing.
- Moisten dressing for removal if necessary.
- Cleanse wound with MPM Silvermed Wound Cleanser, and reapply MPM Silvermed Hydrogel according to your facility's protocol.

HYDROGELS

MPM Silvermed Saturated Gauze
MPM Medical, Inc.

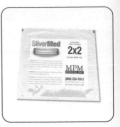

How supplied
Saturated gauze dressing: 2" × 2"; A6231
4" × 4"; A6232

Action
MPM Silvermed products provide sustained antimicrobial barrier activity to reduce infection and promote an effective wound healing environment. Bioavailable silver binds to matrix metalloproteinase (MMPs) and facilitates the healing of difficult-to-heal wounds. This product is excellent for packing infected wounds and for treating chronic deep wounds.

Indications
Under a physician's care, for the management of partial- to full-thickness wounds with light to moderate exudate, such as pressure ulcers, diabetic foot and leg ulcers, skin abrasions, lacerations and tears, first- and second-degree burns, surgical wounds, and grafted and donor sites

Contraindications
- Contraindicated for patients who are hypersensitive to components of the gel

Application
- Cleanse the wound with MPM Silvermed Wound Cleanser.
- Pack wound with MPM Silvermed Saturated Gauze Dressing, and cover with an appropriate nonadherent dressing.
- Repeat as often as required to keep wound moist and free of contamination.

Removal
- Carefully remove secondary dressing and MPM Silvermed Saturated Gauze Dressing from the wound.
- Moisten with MPM Silvermed Wound Cleanser if necessary.
- Cleanse wound with MPM Silvermed Wound Cleanser.
- Reapply MPM Silvermed Saturated Gauze Dressing, and cover with appropriate wound cover.

Normlgel 0.9% Isotonic Saline Gel

Mölnlycke Health Care

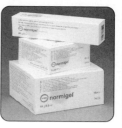

How supplied

Tube: 5 g, 15 g (single dose); A6248

Action

Normlgel is a moisture-donating gel that helps maintain an optimum environment for healing.

Indications

May be used in granulating and open wounds with light to moderate exudate including pressure ulcers, diabetic ulcers, superficial first- and second-degree burns, lower-extremity ulcers, open surgical wounds, and wounds covered with dry fibrin

Contraindications

- None provided by the manufacturer

Application

- Irrigate or flush the wound gently with normal saline or nonirritating solution, if necessary. Gently blot excess moisture with absorbent gauze.
- Unscrew and remove cap and distance ring. Reapply the cap to the tube, and twist it firmly back on to break the seal of the tube.
- Unscrew the cap and apply a thin coat of the gel to the wound, being careful not to apply the gel over the periwound skin.
- If the wound is deep, pack it lightly with gauze impregnated with Normlgel.
- Apply a cover dressing, such as Alldress or Mepilex Border. Avoid covering with gauze because this will promote wound drying.

Removal

- Change cover dressing every 48 hours or when drainage is visible through the dressing.

PanoPlex Hydrogel Wound Dressing
PanoGauze Non-Woven Hydrogel Dressing
Sage Pharmaceuticals, Inc.

How supplied
PanoPlex Hydrogel Wound Dressing
Syringe: 1 oz
Tube: 3 1/2 oz

PanoGauze Non-Woven Hydrogel Dressing
Impregnated gauze pad: 2" × 2", 4" × 4", 4" × 8", 6" × 10"

Action
PanoPlex Hydrogel Wound Dressing and PanoGauze Non-Woven Hydrogel Dressing help create and maintain a moist healing environment and prevent contaminants from entering the wound area.

Indications
To manage pressure ulcers (stages 1, 2, 3, and 4), dermal ulcers, first- and second-degree burns, postoperative incisions, skin conditions associated with peristomal care, and partial- and full-thickness wounds; may also be used on tunneling wounds, infected and noninfected wounds, and red, yellow, or black wounds

Contraindications
- None provided by the manufacturer

Application
- Clean the wound thoroughly with a suitable wound cleanser, such as ClinsWound or SeptiCare.
- Apply dressing generously onto the wound.
- Cover with appropriate dressing.

Removal
- Change dressing as needed.
- Remove PanoPlex Hydrogel Wound Dressing or PanoGauze Non-Woven Hydrogel Dressing with a wound cleanser, such as ClinsWound or SeptiCare.

Purilon Gel
Coloplast Corporation

How supplied
Accordion pack: 8 g, 15 g, 25 g; A6248

Action
Purilon Gel is a sterile, clear, cohesive, amorphous hydrogel with hydrating and absorbing properties that provide fast and effective autolytic debridement of necrotic tissue, while maintaining a moist wound environment.

Indications
To treat necrotic and sloughy wounds, such as leg ulcers and pressure ulcers; may be used throughout the healing process to provide a moist healing environment in all types of wounds; may also be used with medical supervision on infected wounds

Contraindications
- Contraindicated for third-degree burns

Application
- Clean the wound with Sea-Clens wound cleanser or normal saline solution. Gently dry the skin around the wound.
- Remove the label from the accordion pack by pulling the corner, as indicated on the package. Swab the nozzle below the snap-off tip with a suitable antiseptic; remove the tip.
- Gently press the base of the accordion pack to apply Purilon Gel to the wound, in a layer no higher than the periwound skin.
- Cover with a secondary dressing.

Removal
- For necrotic and sloughy wounds, change Purilon Gel at least every 3 days. For clean wounds, change Purilon Gel according to the amount of exudate.
- To remove the gel from the wound, rinse with a wound cleanser or normal saline solution.

New Product

RadiaDres Gel Sheet
Carrington Laboratories, Inc.

How supplied
Sheet: 4″ × 4″

Action
RadiaDres Gel Sheet is a wound dressing consisting of a hydrogel with a matrix to form a solid gel sheet for radiation-related skin reactions. It facilitates the formation of a moist wound healing environment while preventing bacteria and foreign matter from entering the wound. The Radia Dres Gel Sheet may be refrigerated for maximum cooling effect.

Indications
For management of pressure ulcers (stages 1, 2, 3, and 4), partial-thickness draining and nondraining wounds, first- and second-degree burns, radiation reactions, and noninfected wounds

Contraindications
- Contraindicated for infected wounds

Application
- Before application, thoroughly cleanse the wound with an appropriate wound cleanser such as RadiaKlenz Dermal Wound Cleanser. Gently dry the skin surrounding the wound.
- Peel open package and remove RadiaDres Gel Sheet using a clean technique.
- Grab the tabbed edges of the pink polyethylene film backing to remove. Discard the backing.
- Apply uncovered hydrogel side to wound. RadiaDres Gel Sheet may overlap intact skin if desired.
- The dressing may be trimmed or overlapped, if preferred, to more closely approximate the wound size and shape.

Removal
- To remove, carefully lift an edge of the dressing while gently pressing against the skin.
- Change as often as necessary until the wound is healed. May be left on up to 3 days.
- Before applying a new dressing, cleanse the wound with a suitable cleanser such as RadiaKlenz Dermal Wound Cleanser.

RadiaGel with Acemannan Hydrogel

Carrington Laboratories, Inc.

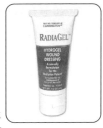

How supplied
Tube: $^{1}/_{2}$ oz, 3 oz

Action
RadiaGel is a hydrogel wound dressing containing acemannan hydrogel in a nonoily preparation, especially formulated for the management of radiation dermatitis.

Indications
To condition the skin before radiation therapy and to manage skin reactions after radiation therapy; may also be used to manage radiation-induced dermatitis

Contraindications
- Contraindicated in patients who are hypersensitive to acemannan hydrogel or other components of the dressing

Application

Pretherapy
- Clean the skin with a suitable cleanser, such as RadiaKlenz.
- Massage a small amount of RadiaGel into the skin 2 or 3 times daily to condition the skin. Begin as far in advance of therapy as possible.

During therapy
- Continue to massage a small amount of RadiaGel into the skin 3 or 4 times daily throughout the entire treatment period.
- Clean the affected area with a suitable cleanser, such as RadiaKlenz, by spraying it onto the desired area.
- Gently pat affected area with a soft gauze. No rinsing is required.
- Follow with the appropriate topical preparation, such as a thin layer of RadiaGel to intact skin, or a $^{1}/_{8}$" to $^{1}/_{4}$" (0.3 to 0.5 cm) layer of gel to areas of ulceration.
- Cover with appropriate nonadhering dressing, such as RadiaDres Gel Sheet. Remove the red film backing from the sheet, and gently press it in place over the area of ulceration or reaction.

Removal
- Change dressing according to the wound condition and amount of exudate or as directed by the physician.
- Gently lift RadiaDres Gel Sheet to remove.
- Rinse away any remaining gel with gentle irrigation.

Restore Hydrogel Dressing*
Hollister Wound Care, LLC

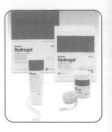

How supplied
Amorphous/tube: 3 oz; A6248
Impregnated gauze sponge, sterile: 4″ × 4″; A6231
Impregnated gauze strip, sterile: 2″ × 3.5 yards; A6266

Action
Amorphous Restore Hydrogel Dressing maintains a moist healing environment. Restore Hydrogel Impregnated Gauze Sponges and Packing Strips fill in dead space associated with sinus tracts and undermining or deep wounds.

Indications
For maintenance of a moist environment in pressure ulcers, stasis ulcers, first- and second-degree burns, skin tears, cuts, and abrasions

Contraindications
- For external use only
- Not for contact with eyes

Application
- Cleanse wound if indicated.

Amorphous Restore Hydrogel Dressing
- Apply to the wound to a minimum depth of ¼″ (5 mm). Cover with a secondary dressing and secure.

Restore Hydrogel Impregnated Gauze Sponges and Strips
- Apply sponge or strip to the wound. Cover with a secondary dressing, and secure with tape or other appropriate material.

Removal
- Remove tape securing the secondary dressing to the skin, and lift away the dressing. Gently remove Restore Hydrogel Gauze Sponge or Packing Strip. Cleanse wound, if indicated, before applying new dressing.
- Change the dressing every 24 to 72 hours or as required to maintain a moist environment.
- If condition worsens or doesn't improve within 7 days, consult a physician.

*See package insert for complete instructions for use.

SAF-Gel Hydrating Dermal Wound Dressing*
ConvaTec

How supplied
Tube: 3 oz; A6248

Action
SAF-Gel Hydrating Dermal Wound Dressing is an alginate-containing wound gel designed to create an optimal moist environment to support the wound healing process.

Indications
To manage chronic wounds, pressure ulcers (stages 1, 2, 3, and 4), stasis ulcers, first- and second-degree burns, cuts, abrasions, and skin tears

Contraindications
- None provided by the manufacturer.

Application
- Clean the wound with normal saline solution or an appropriate cleansing solution, such as SAF-Clens AF Dermal Wound Cleanser, Chronic Wound Cleanser, or Shur-Clens Skin Wound Cleansing Solution.
- Apply ⅛" to ¼" (0.3 to 0.5 cm) layer of SAF-Clens AF Dermal Wound Cleanser Hydrating Dermal Wound Dressing to cover the entire wound surface.
- Cover with an appropriate secondary dressing.

Removal
- Change the dressing daily or when the wound begins to dry out.

*See package insert for complete instructions for use.

Skintegrity Amorphous Hydrogel
Skintegrity Hydrogel Impregnated Gauze
Medline Industries, Inc.

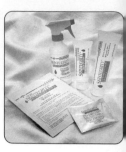

How supplied
Bellows bottle: 1 oz; A6248
Tube: 4 oz; A6248
Impregnated gauze: 2" × 2", 4" × 4"; A6231

Action
Skintegrity Hydrogel dressings are greaseless and maintain a moist healing environment. Skintegrity Hydrogel Impregnated Gauze is a compression-saturated gauze sponge, which ensures thorough hydration. A special formulation balances viscosity and hydration, added aloe vera aids healing, and the greaseless formulation irrigates easily from the wound bed.

Indications
To manage pressure ulcers (stages 2, 3, and 4), partial- or full-thickness wounds, venous stasis ulcers, first- and second-degree burns, cuts, abrasions, skin irritations, postoperative incisions, infected and noninfected wounds, and wounds with no drainage or light drainage

Contraindications
- Contraindicated in patients who are hypersensitive to components of the gel

Application
- Clean the wound with normal saline solution or appropriate wound cleanser, such as Skintegrity Wound Cleanser.
- Dry the periwound skin.

Skintegrity Amorphous Hydrogel
- Apply a generous layer of hydrogel to all wound surfaces.
- Cover with an appropriate secondary dressing, such as Stratasorb composite dressing or bordered gauze.
- Repeat every 72 hours or as necessary to maintain a moist wound bed.

Skintegrity Hydrogel Impregnated Gauze
- Unfold the hydrogel gauze pad and loosely pack it in the wound bed, filling any undermining and tunneling areas.
- Cover with an appropriate secondary dressing, such as Stratasorb composite dressing or bordered gauze.
- Change the dressing every 72 hours or as necessary to maintain a moist wound bed.

Removal

- Carefully remove the secondary dressing and irrigate the wound bed with normal saline solution or appropriate wound cleanser, such as Skintegrity Wound Cleanser. Dry the periwound skin.
- If the dressing has dried to the wound edge or the base of the wound, moisten with Skintegrity Wound Cleanser or normal saline solution until it loosens, then remove it.

HYDROGELS

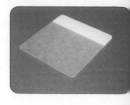

New Product

Skintegrity Hydrogel Sheet
Medline Industries, Inc.

How supplied
Sheet: 6″ × 8″; A6243

Action
Skintegrity Hydrogel Sheet is a moist, soothing, cooling, water-rich hydrogel sheet that is soft and flexible and creates a moist healing environment. The dressing is occlusive, water-retentive, and translucent (permitting wound monitoring). It can absorb light drainage.

Indications
To manage leg ulcers, pressure ulcers (stages 1, 2, 3, and 4), superficial wounds, lacerations, cuts, abrasions, donor sites, partial- and full-thickness wounds, infected and noninfected wounds, and wounds with no drainage to light drainage

Contraindications
- Contraindicated for deep, tunneling wounds

Application
- Clean the application site with normal saline solution or an appropriate wound cleanser, such as Skintegrity Wound Cleanser. Dry the surrounding area to ensure that it's free from greasy substances.
- Select the appropriate size dressing for the wound. Be sure it will cover the entire wound area.
- Remove the clear plastic cover from the dressing, and apply the pad to the wound. Leave the remaining backing in place if appropriate.
- Tape the edges of the dressing to keep it in place, or use an elastic net to secure it without adhesive.
- If waterproofing is desired, cover with a transparent film.

Removal
- Change the dressing every 2 to 5 days, depending on the amount of drainage.
- Carefully press down on the skin, and lift an edge of the dressing. Continue around the dressing until all edges are free.

SoloSite Wound Gel
SoloSite Gel Conformable Wound Dressing
Smith & Nephew, Inc.
Wound Management

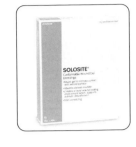

How supplied
SoloSite Wound Gel
Tube: 3 oz; A6248
Push-button applicators: 2 oz, 7 oz; A6248

SoloSite Gel Conformable Wound Dressing
Gel pad: 2″ × 2″, 4″ × 4″; A6231

Action
SoloSite Wound Gel
SoloSite is a hydrogel wound dressing with preservatives. It can donate moisture to rehydrate nonviable tissue. It absorbs exudate while retaining its structure in the wound. It rehydrates and helps deslough dry escar, absorbs exudate, and assists autolytic debridement. It is nonirritating, nonsensitizing, gentle to fragile granulation tissue.

SoloSite Gel Conformable Wound Dressing
SoloSite Gel Conformable is designed to keep the gel in intimate contact with the wound bed. It's ideal for packing into and around the sides of the wound. While wound gels alone tend to pool at the base of deeper wounds, leaving portions of the wound bed uncovered, SoloSite Gel Conformable maintains close contact of the wound surface and the gel It keeps gel in intimate contact with wound surface, absorbs excess exudate, creates a moist wound healing environment, which may promote desloughing, meets USP requirements for cytotoxicity, and is nonsensitizing.

Indications
Used to create a moist wound environment for the treatment of minor conditions such as minor burns, superficial lacerations, cuts and abrasions (partial-thickness wounds), and skin tears; under the direction of a health care professional, used to create a moist wound environment for the management of venous ulcers (leg ulcers), surgical incisions, diabetic foot ulcers, and pressure ulcers (including stage IV); creates a moist wound environment, which assists in autolytic debridement of wounds covered with necrotic tissues

Contraindications
SoloSite Wound Gel
- For external use only
- If condition worsens or doesn't improve within 7 days, consult a physician

SoloSite Gel Conformable Wound Dressing
- Contraindicated for the management of full-thickness burns

Application
SoloSite Wound Gel
- Cleanse the wound with saline or an appropriate wound cleanser.
- Apply Solosite Gel to cover the wound bed $1/4''$ (5 mm) thick and cover with a gauze, foam, or transparent film dressing.

SoloSite Gel Conformable Wound Dressing
- Gently and thoroughly cleanse the wound area of necrotic (damaged) tissue or dressing residue with sterile saline or other appropriate wound cleanser.
- Remove pouch from outer packaging.
- Tear open pouch using notched opening.
- Remove dressing from pouch and carefully unfold dressing.
- Carefully place dressing in the wound so that the entire wound bed is covered.
- Don't overlay the dressing on the healthy skin surrounding the wound because this could lead to maceration (overhydration) of the healthy skin.
- Secure the dressing in place by placing a secondary dressing of the following type over the total wound area:
  - A transparent film such as OpSite or OpSite FLEXIGRID, especially where the wound is necrotic (full of damaged tissue) or sloughy (full of wound fluid)
  - A nonwoven, nonsensitizing (nonallergic) dressing such as CovRSite or retention tape such as Hypafix where there is little wound drainage
  - Gauze held in place with a conforming bandage, a net bandage, or a cohesive bandage such as Coban, where there are skin tears and an adhesive secondary dressing is inappropriate.
- If you're unsure of which secondary dressing to use, consult a health care professional.

Removal
- Change the dressing each day or as directed by the physician.

Spand-Gel

Medi-Tech International
Corp.

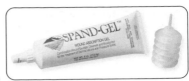

How supplied

Bellows bottle (sterile): 1 oz; A6248
Tube (sterile):   3 oz; A6248

Action

Spand-Gel is a hydrogel-and-glycerin–based, primary wound absorption
dressing filler. It provides a moist healing environment and encourages the
regeneration of epithelial defects. It allows full development of the body's
own resistance-and-repair mechanism, and it can be adapted to the requirements of successful trauma treatment. Furthermore, because it's water-
soluble, it won't disturb the traumatized area when the gel is irrigated.

Indications

For management of stages 1, 2, 3, and 4 dermal ulcers, partial- and full-
thickness wounds, venous stasis ulcers, diabetic foot ulcers, first- and second-
degree burns, tunneled wounds, postsurgical incisions, and wounds with
moderate exudate

Contraindications

- None provided by the manufacturer

Application

- Irrigate wound with Medi-Tech Wound Cleanser.
- Apply gel about half the size of the wound area or cavity.
- Moisten gauze if secondary dressing is required.
- Retain dressing with suitable size of Spandage, latex-free, elastic, tubu-
  lar, open-netted dressing retainer
- Change Spand-Gel 2 or 3 times daily, depending on the amount of ex-
  udate. If there is no accumulation of exudate, change the gel daily.

Removal

- Irrigate the wound with normal saline or Medi-Tech Wound Cleanser.

HYDROGELS

Spand-Gel Dressing Sheets with Diamond Aloe Vera
Medi-Tech International Corp.

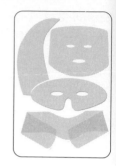

How supplied
Sterile sheet: 4″ × 4″; A6242
                     3″ × 8″, 5″ × 9″, 6″ × 8″; A6243
Full-face mask: A6244
Half-face mask: A6243
Breast wrap: A6243
Neck wrap: A6244

Action
Spand-Gel is a primary wound dressing that provides a cool, moist healing environment; absorbs wound exudate three times its weight; and provides a barrier from exogenous bacteria and fluids. It conforms readily to all wound configurations.

Indications
To manage first- and second-degree burns, thermal burns, donor graft sites, radiation-induced reaction sites, excoriation caused by dermatologic procedures, postoperative incisions, dermal ulcers (stages 1, 2, and 3), moderately exuding wounds, and laser resurfacing sites

Contraindications
- Contraindicated in infected wounds, unless dressing is used with an appropriate topical antibiotic

Application
- For best results, refrigerate Spand-Gel for at least 30 minutes before applying it.
- Clean the wound with Medi-Tech Wound Cleanser.
- Remove Spand-Gel from sterile foil pouch.
- Place the side of the dressing, from which the polyethylene film has been removed, into the wound.
- Apply the appropriate size of latex-free MT Spandage elastic, open-netted, secondary dressing retainer.
- Change dressings if excess exudate or desquamation accumulates. The dressing maybe changed as frequently as every 2 days.
- Moisten dressing with water or saline solution 3 or 4 times daily.

Removal
- Remove appropriate MT Spandage secondary dressing.
- Carefully lift off the Spand-Gel primary dressing.
- If the dressing appears or feels dry, moisten, remove, and redress, if necessary.

TenderWet Gel Pad

Medline Industries, Inc.

How supplied

*TenderWet System and TenderWet Cavity
System, preactivated with Ringer
solution:* 1.6" or 2.2" rounds, or
3" × 3" or 4" × 5" squares;
A6242
3" × 8" rectangle (cavity-style
only); A6243

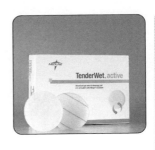

Action

TenderWet is a multilayer wound dressing pad whose central component
is an absorbent polymer gel. The covering layer is composed of a hydrophobic, knitted fabric that allows wound exudate to pass through to
the absorptive gel layer while helping to prevent the dressing from adhering to the wound. The gel holds a significant amount of TenderWet (Ringer)
solution, providing a moist healing environment. The solution is released
into the wound bed while the wound exudate is absorbed, providing an
autolytic debriding process that helps remove necrotic tissue and debris
while allowing tissue granulation to occur.

The side of the TenderWet dressing with green stripes has a water-repellent
layer, making this dressing appropriate for flat wounds or wounds with superficial depth.

The cavity dressings have a symmetrical structure without a water repellent
layer. Both sides function equally, making it particularly suitable for packing deeper wounds.

Indications

To manage dry, light to moderately exuding, and partial and full-thickness
wounds, such as minor burns, superficial injuries, lacerations, cuts, abrasions, incisions or surgical wounds, and skin tears; also for chronic wounds,
such as pressure ulcers (stages 2, 3, and 4), lower-extremity ulcers, venous
ulcers, arterial ulcers, diabetic ulcers, and ulcers of mixed etiology; may
also be used on infected wounds

Contraindications

- Contraindicated for third-degree burns unless otherwise advised by the
physician

Application

- Remove dressing from foil pouch and apply the white side of the TenderWet dressing to the entire surface of the wound. Make sure that the
green stripes (on topper style) face away from the patient.
- Pack deeper wounds with TenderWet Cavity, which doesn't feature a water-repellent layer; it then can be covered with regular TenderWet if man
aging high levels of exudate.

Note: TenderWet must cover the edge of the wound. The white, soft tissue that forms around the wound edges is sometimes mistaken for maceration of the epidermis; in fact, it's a layer of squames or corneocytes. These harmless cells are nonviable and are usually sloughed off when bathing, scratching, or changing clothes.

■ Secure TenderWet by using a roll gauze, such as Sof-Form Conforming Gauze, or a six-ply roll bandage, such as Bulkee II. Or use a self-adherent cohesive bandage; an elastic net for adhesive-sensitive patients; a dressing retention tape, such as Medfix; a bordered gauze; or a waterproof, composite island dressing, such as Stratasorb.

■ If the dressing dries out, rewet using Ringer solution.

Removal

■ Change TenderWet within 24 hours. Depending on drainage, TenderWet Cavity dressings may need to be changed twice daily.

■ Gently remove the secondary dressing and lift TenderWet out of the wound bed.

Note: Don't reuse TenderWet; product is intended for single use only. Don't mechanically damage the TenderWet covering layer.

3M Tegaderm Hydrogel Wound Filler
3M Health Care

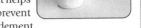

How supplied
Tube: 15 g, 25 g; A6248

Action
3M Tegaderm Hydrogel Wound Filler is a clear, non-adherent, viscous wound dressing. The product helps provide a moist healing environment, helps prevent wound desiccation, assists with autolytic debridement by hydrating devitalized tissue, and fills dead space in full-thickness wounds.

Indications
3M Tegaderm Hydrogel wound filler products are indicated for the management of nondraining to minimally draining dermal wounds including pressure ulcers, venous ulcers, arterial ulcers, diabetic ulcers, dehisced surgical wounds, superficial partial-thickness burns, skin tears, abrasions, radiation, dermatitis, and malignant lesions; may be used with gauze to lightly pack tunneling or undermined chronic wounds

Contraindications
- Contraindicated for third-degree burns
- Contraindicated in patients who have sensitivity to any ingredient in the product
- If infection develops, consult the physician and implement appropriate medical treatment

Application
- Clean skin and wound thoroughly.
- Protect periwound skin, as appropriate, using a barrier film.
- Apply enough wound filler to cover the wound base and necrotic tissue, or saturate a sterile gauze pad with wound filler and place it in the wound.
- Cover with an appropriate secondary dressing.

Removal
- Gently lift off cover dressing and discard.
- Remove saturated gauze or irrigate gel from the wound. Monitor periwound skin for maceration.

HYDROGELS

TOE-AID Toe and Nail Dressing

Southwest Technologies, Inc.

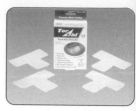

How supplied

Tape: 1.25" square affixed to a T-shape tape; A6245

Action

Because of its high glycerin content, TOE-AID assists in the natural wound-healing process. The soft gel pad provides a protective cushion to the injury, is highly absorbent, won't dry out, and is bacteriostatic and fungistatic. TOE-AID absorbent dressing is a uniquely formulated glycerin gel pad attached to a hypoallergenic, water-resistant, adhesive T-shaped tape.

Indications

To manage toe conditions ranging from toenail removal to toenail fungus and other toe injuries

Contraindications

- Contraindicated for highly exuding wounds that may require packing with additional dressing or other highly absorbent material
- Use cautiously on an infected wound. Consult a physician before use.

Application

- Prepare the wound site by cleaning the wound, as needed.

After toenail removal or on an open wound

- Fold the dressing under the toe first, and then overlap the tape to make a waterproof seal.
- Wrap one side of the dressing down around the toe, and then repeat with the other side of the dressing.
- Don't get the gel wet.

On intact skin or directly on toenail

- Make a waterproof seal to protect the gel from getting wet. The product may be worn in the shower if the tape is properly secured.

Removal

- Change the dressing if leaking occurs or the dressing becomes highly saturated with exudate. When applied to intact skin or directly to the toenail, the dressing may be left in place for up to 7 days.

TransiGel Conformable Wound Dressing
Smith & Nephew, Inc. Wound Management

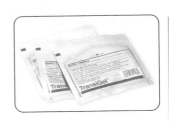

How supplied
Dressing: 2″ × 2″, 4″ × 4″; A6231
4″ × 8″; A6232

Action
TransiGel is a sterile dressing, manufactured using woven gauze impregnated with a water-soluble wound gel. It keeps gel in close contact with wound surface, absorbs excess exudate, helps rehydrate necrotic tissue, loosens slough, is noncytotoxic, assists autolytic debridement, and provides gentle effective debriding.

Indications
TransiGel is used to create a moist wound environment for the treatment of minor conditions such as minor burns, superficial laceration, cuts and abrasions (partial-thickness wounds), skin tears; under the direction of a health care professional, TransiGel is used to create a moist wound environment for the management of venous ulcers (leg ulcers), surgical incisions, diabetic foot ulcers, pressure ulcers (including stage 4); creates a moist wound environment, which assists in autolytic debridement of wounds covered with necrotic tissues

Contraindications
- Contraindicated for third-degree burns

Application
- Completely cover the wound surface with the dressing.
- Hold in place with an appropriate secondary dressing.

Removal
- Change the dressing each day or as directed by the physician.

HYDROGELS

Ultrex Gel Wound Dressing with Acemannan Hydrogel
Carrington Laboratories, Inc.

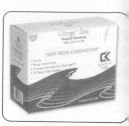

How supplied
Tube: 8 g, 15 g

Action
Ultrex Gel is a sterile, preservative-free, color-less wound dressing containing acemannan hydrogel. It's specifically formulated to maintain the moist environment essential to wound healing in patients with painful wounds or sensitivities to other topical dressings.

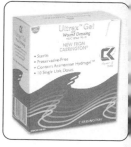

Indications
To manage pressure ulcers (stages 1, 2, 3, and 4), stasis ulcers, foot ulcers, first- and second-degree burns, postsurgical incisions, and skin conditions associated with peristomal care

Contraindications
- Contraindicated in patients with hypersensitivity to acemannan hydrogel or other components of the dressing

Application
- Clean the wound with a suitable cleanser, such as UltraKlenz, Carra-Klenz, or MicroKlenz, by spraying the affected area.
- Gently dry the surrounding skin with soft gauze. No rinsing is required.
- Apply a layer of Ultrex Gel $\frac{1}{8}''$ to $\frac{1}{4}''$ (0.3 to 0.5 cm) thick on areas of ulceration.
- Cover with an appropriate secondary dressing, such as CarraDres, Carra-Film, or CarraSmart Foam.

Removal
- Change dressing according to the wound condition and the amount of exudate, or as directed by the physician.
- Rinse away any remaining gel with gentle irrigation.

Woun'Dres Collagen Hydrogel

Coloplast Corporation

How supplied
Tube: 1 oz, 3 oz; A6248

Action
Woun'Dres Collagen Hydrogel maintains a moist healing environment and gently absorbs exudate. Assists in protecting new granulation tissue, and promotes autolytic debridement.

Indications
To manage pressure ulcers (stages 2, 3, and 4), venous stasis ulcers, superficial wounds, scrapes, first- and second-degree burns, and partial- and full-thickness wounds; may also be used on tunneling wounds, infected and noninfected wounds, wounds with minimal or moderate drainage, wounds with serosanguineous drainage, and red, yellow, or black wounds

Contraindications
■ Contraindicated for third-degree burns

Application
■ Clean the wound thoroughly with wound cleanser or normal saline solution.
■ Apply Woun'Dres Collagen Hydrogel directly into the wound.
■ Cover with a secondary dressing.

Removal
■ Remove the secondary dressing.
■ Flush the wound with a wound cleanser or normal saline solution.

HYDROGELS

XCell Antimicrobial Cellulose Wound Dressings
Xylos Corporation

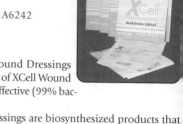

How supplied
$3^1/_2$" × $3^1/_2$", $^3/_4$" × 8"; A6242
$5^1/_2$"× 8"; A6243

Action
XCell Antimicrobial Cellulose Wound Dressings have all of the performance benefits of XCell Wound Dressings, plus a gentle yet highly effective (99% bactericidal) antimicrobial agent.

All XCell Cellulose Wound Dressings are biosynthesized products that actively balance the moisture content within a wound by hydrating and absorbing simultaneously in different parts of the wound. The process of "microenvironment moisture management" enables continuous autolytic debridement and optimizes the process of wound bed preparation.

Indications
To manage infected and noninfected chronic wounds at all stages (venous, pressure, arterial, and diabetic), postoperative wounds, first- and second-degree burns, donor sites, skin grafts, and dermal lesions; actively enables autolytic debridement; may be used for up to 7 days

Contraindications
- Contraindicated for third-degree burns
- Contraindicated on patients with sensitivity to the dressing

Application
- XCell is a primary dressing that may be cut to size, as needed, or inserted into tunnels or sinuses.
- Overlap the wound margins by at least 1" (2.5 cm) on all sides.
- Use appropriate cover dressing in accordance with the amount of exudate and anticipated wear time.

Removal
- There are no special removal requirements. If the dressing becomes dried over the periwound area (which is normal and should be anticipated), it may be rehydrated with water or saline for a few minutes.

XCell Cellulose Wound Dressings

Xylos Corporation

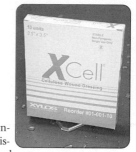

How supplied

$3^{1}/_{2}$" × $3^{1}/_{2}$", $^{3}/_{4}$" × 8"; A6242
$5^{1}/_{2}$" × 8"; A6243

Action

XCell Cellulose Wound Dressings are biosynthesized products that actively balance the moisture content within a wound by hydrating and

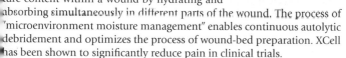

absorbing simultaneously in different parts of the wound. The process of "microenvironment moisture management" enables continuous autolytic debridement and optimizes the process of wound-bed preparation. XCell has been shown to significantly reduce pain in clinical trials.

Indications

To manage all chronic wounds at all stages (venous, pressure, arterial, and diabetic), postoperative wounds, first- and second-degree burns, donor sites, skin grafts, and dermal lesions; actively enables autolytic debridement; may be used for up to 7 days

Contraindications

- Contraindicated for third-degree burns
- Contraindicated on patients who are sensitive to the dressing

Application

- XCell is a primary dressing that may be cut to size, as needed, or inserted into tunnels or sinuses.
- Overlap the wound margins by at least 1" (2.5 cm) on all sides.
- Use appropriate cover dressing in accordance with the amount of exudate and anticipated wear time.

Removal

- There are no special removal requirements. If the dressing becomes dried over the periwound area (which is normal and should be anticipated), it may be rehydrated with water or saline for a few minutes.

Specialty absorptives

ACTION

Specialty absorptives are unitized, multilayered dressings that consist of highly absorptive layers of fibers, such as absorbent cellulose, cotton, or rayon. These dressings may or may not have an adhesive border.

INDICATIONS

Specialty absorptive dressings may be used as primary or secondary dressings to manage light to heavy drainage from partial- and full-thickness wounds, infected and noninfected wounds, and red, yellow, or black wounds.

ADVANTAGES

- Can be used as secondary dressing over most primary dressings
- Are semiadherent or nonadherent
- Are highly absorptive
- Are easy to apply and remove
- May have an adhesive border, making additional tape unnecessary

DISADVANTAGES

- May not be appropriate as a primary dressing for undermining wounds

HCPCS CODE OVERVIEW

The HCPCS codes normally assigned to specialty absorptive wound covers without an adhesive border are:

A6251—pad size < 16 in^2

A6252—pad size > 16 in^2 but < 48 in^2

A6253—pad size > 48 in^2.

The HCPCS codes normally assigned to specialty absorptive wound covers with an adhesive border are:

A6254—pad size < 16 in^2

A6255—pad size > 16 in^2 but ≤ 48 in^2

A6256—pad size > 48 in^2.

Covaderm Adhesive Wound Dressing
DeRoyal

How supplied
Multilayered pad with fabric tape border: 2^1/$_2$" × 2^1/$_2$" with 4" × 4" tape, 2^1/$_2$" × 4" with 4" × 6" tape, 2" × 5^1/$_2$" with 4" × 8" tape, 2" × 7^1/$_2$" with 4" × 10" tape; A6254 2" × 11" with 4" × 14" tape; A6255

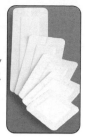

Action
Covaderm Adhesive Wound Dressing is an absorbent island dressing with a protective, air-permeable, adhesive fabric tape border for aseptic, one-step application. Rounded edges conform to jointed, curved, or irregular wound areas.

Indications
For use as a primary or secondary dressing to manage surgical incisions, superficial lacerations, and abrasions; may also be used as an all-purpose dressing

Contraindications
- None provided by the manufacturer

Application
- Peel back the edge of the folded release liner.
- Anchor the exposed edge of the tape to the skin, and then peel off the remaining release paper.
- Smooth all the tape edges onto the skin.

Removal
- Carefully lift the edges of the tape, and peel off the dressing.

SPECIALTY ABSORPTIVES

CURITY Abdominal Pads
Tyco Healthcare/Kendall

How supplied
Sterile pad: 5″ × 9″, 7¹/₂″ × 8″, 8″ × 10″

Nonsterile pad: 5″ × 9″, 7¹/₂″ × 8″, 8″ × 10″, 12″
                     × 16″, 24″ × 8″, 12″ × 8″, 12″
                     × 10″, 24″ × 10″, 10″ × 12″

Nonsterile roll: 8″ × 2 yd

Action
CURITY Abdominal Pads are a secondary dressing that absorb excess wound fluid and protect the wound by cushioning it.

Indications
To prevent skin breakdown and to manage moderately to heavily exuding wounds; may also be used as part of a decreasing system for virtually any wound requiring fluid retention and cushioning

Contraindications
- Contraindicated for tunneling wounds

Application
- Choose a primary dressing based on wound type and apply it.
- Cover the primary dressing with a CURITY Abdominal Pad.
- Secure the abdominal pad with tape, bandage roll, or another appropriate product.

Removal
- Carefully remove the securing product.
- Remove the CURITY Abdominal Pad from the primary dressing.

DuPad Abdominal Pads, Open End
Derma Sciences, Inc.

How supplied

Sterile pad: 5″ × 9″, 8″ × 8″, 8″ × 10″, 8″ × 24″

Nonsterile pad: 5″ × 9″, 8″ × 8″, 8″ × 10″, 8″ × 12″, 10″ × 12″,
8″ × 24″, 10″ × 24″, 12″ × 16″, 8″ × 20 yd

Action
These highly absorbent cotton-filled sterile and nonsterile pads provide protection for heavily exuding wounds.

Indications
For use as a secondary dressing for highly exuding wounds

Contraindications
■ None provided by the manufacturer

Application
■ Clean the wound with PrimaDerm Dermal Cleanser or saline solution. Dry the periwound skin.
■ Apply an appropriate primary dressing.
■ Cover the primary dressing with DuPad Abdominal Pad, and secure with tape, gauze roll, or other appropriate dressing.

Removal
■ Gently remove all layers.

SPECIALTY ABSORPTIVES

DuPad Abdominal Pads, Sealed End
Derma Sciences, Inc.

How supplied
Sterile pad: 5″ × 9″, 8″ × 8″, 8″ × 10″
Nonsterile pad: 5″ × 9″, 8″ × 8″, 8″ × 10″

Action
These highly aborbent cotton-filled pads provide cushioning to protect heavily exuding wounds. Sterile and nonsterile pads are available.

Indications
For use as a secondary dressing for highly exuding wounds

Contraindications
- None provided by the manufacturer

Application
- Clean the wound with PrimaDerm Dermal Cleanser or saline solution. Dry the periwound skin.
- Choose an appropriate primary dressing.
- Cover the dressing with DuPad Abdominal Pad, and secure with tape, gauze roll, or other appropriate dressing.

Removal
- Gently remove all layers.

EXU-DRY
Smith & Nephew, Inc.
Wound Management

How supplied
Specialty dressing: Arm 6″ × 9″, Arm
      9″ × 15″, Arm/Shoulder;
      A6253
      Scalp/Face, Elbow/Knee/Heel, Boot/Foot L; A6252
      Hand, Boot/Foot M/S; A6251
      Neck, Buttocks, Leg, Burn Jacket/Vest; A6253
Slit disk: 3″; A6251
Slit tube: 2″ × 3″, 3″ × 4″; A6251
      4″ × 6″; A6252
Disk: 2″, 3″, 3″ × 4″; A6251
      4″ × 6″; A6252
      6″ × 9″, 9″ × 15″, 15″ × 18″, 15″ × 24″, 20″ × 28″; A6253
Incision dressing: 3″ × 9″; A6252
Nonpermeable pad: 24″ × 36″, 36″ × 72″; A6253
Permeable sheet: 36″ × 72″; A6253
Pediatric specialty dressing: Scalp, Infant/Toddler Vest; A6252
      Hand, Foot; A6251
Arm, Leg, Child Vest: 6″ × 9″, 9″ × 15″; A6253
Pad/sheet: 20″ × 28″ Crib Sheet (permeable), 20″ × 28″ Receiving Blanket, 24″ × 36″ Pad (nonpermeable); A6253

Action
EXU-DRY's highly absorptive properties may reduce the need for frequent dressing changes. The dressings are designed to minimize adherence and improve patient comfort. The antishear layer helps to minimize friction and shear. It may be used wet or dry.

Indications
To manage exudate in partial- and full-thickness wounds, such as burns and donor or skin graft sites

Contraindications
■ None provided by the manufacturer

Application
■ Select a dressing slightly larger than the wound.
■ Place the dressing on the wound with the words "Use other side against wound" face up.
■ Secure the dressing with gauze, tape, or netting.

Removal
■ Remove the gauze, tape, or netting.
■ Lift off the dressing.

MPM Woundgard Bordered Gauze Dressing
MPM Medical, Inc.

How supplied
Nonsterile dressing: 4″ × 4″, 6″ × 6″; A6254
6″ × 8″; A6255
Sterile dressing: 2″ × 2″, 4″ × 4″, 5″ × 5″, 6″ × 6″; A6254

Action
MPM Woundgard specialty absorptive dressing protects wound from the outside environment and helps the body maintain a moist healing environment.

Indications
To manage cuts, burns, abrasions, skin tears, pressure ulcers, and leg ulcers

Contraindications
- None provided by the manufacturer

Application
- Clean the wound of dirt, debris, and necrotic tissue, and make sure the periwound skin is dry.
- Remove the backing from the dressing, and apply the dressing to the wound.

Removal
- Gently peel the dressing away from the wound.

Multipad Non-Adherent Wound Dressing
DeRoyal

How supplied
Pad: 2″ × 2″, 4″ × 4″; A6251
4″ × 8″; A6252
7¹/₂″ × 7¹/₂″

Action
Multipad Non-Adherent Wound Dressing is a thick, multilayered, absorbent wound dressing that won't stick to the wound site or damage fragile granulation tissue. It's composed of a highly absorptive nonwoven pad between two wound contact layers.

Indications
To manage pressure ulcers (stages 2, 3, and 4), partial- and full-thickness wounds, donor sites, tunneling wounds, infected and noninfected wounds, and red, yellow, or black wounds

Contraindications
- None provided by the manufacturer

Application
- Clean the wound, and then position the dressing over it.
- Secure the dressing with tape, roll gauze, or tubular elastic bandages if using it as a primary dressing.
- If using Multipad as a secondary dressing, apply the primary dressing or filler before securing Multipad to the wound.

Removal
- Remove any secondary dressing.
- Gently lift the dressing from the wound.

SPECIALTY ABSORPTIVES

Sensiplex CRL Wound Dressing
Winfield Laboratories, Inc.

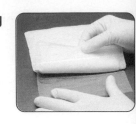

How supplied
Sterile pad: 4″ × 6″; A6252
6″ × 9″, 9″ × 18″, 15″ × 24″,
24″ × 36″, 32″ × 72″; A6253
Vest: Large   33″ × 30″; A6253

Action
Sensiplex CRL Wound Dressing is a one-piece, multilayered, nonadherent, highly absorbent dressing with the patented releasably attached BreakAway wound contact layer that can be used wet or dry. It protects the wound, supports healing, reduces shearing action and friction, and wicks away drainage. It allows observation of the wound surface before removal of the wound contact layer, preventing disruption of the healing wound surface. The air-permeable and absorptive dressing backing is reinforced to provide strength when wet.

Indications
To manage pressure ulcers (stages 2, 3, and 4), partial- and full-thickness wounds, skin graft sites, dermatologic conditions, fungating neoplasms, burns, tunneling wounds, and infected and noninfected wounds; may be used for wounds with serosanguineous or purulent drainage, wounds with heavy drainage, minor lacerations; and also as a wet or dry postoperative dressing

Contraindications
- Contraindicated for preventing skin breakdown
- Contraindicated for areas needing an occlusive dressing
- Contraindicated for third-degree burns

Application
- Use Sensiplex CRL Wound Dressing wet or dry.
- Select a dressing size that covers the wound and periwound area.
- Apply a desired topical agent directly to the wound or dressing.
- If using dressing wet, soak it with normal saline solution or a solution of choice. Squeeze out excess fluid; don't wring.
- Apply dressing with releasably attached wound contact layer toward wound. Secure dressing with stretch netting, roll gauze, or tape.

Removal
- Change the dressing daily or more frequently, if needed.
- Lift the dressing gently off the wound.
- If the wound has dried or is overly bloody, hold the wound contact layer in place, and release the absorbent pad component. If the wound contact layer has points of sticking, clean it with normal saline solution and then remove the wound contact layer.

Sofsorb Wound Dressing

DeRoyal

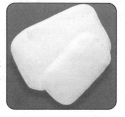

How supplied

Pad: 3″ × 3″; A6251
  4″ × 6″, 4″ × 6″ with drain slit; A6252
  4″ × 9″, 6″ × 9″, 9″ × 15″, 15″ × 18″,
  15″ × 24″; A6253

Action

Sofsorb Wound Dressing is a nonadherent, absorbent, multilayered, one-piece dressing used wet or dry to treat various wounds. The nonwoven layer permits passage of wound drainage into the absorbent pad and prevents it from returning. The center layer absorbs drainage. The cellulose layer wicks drainage horizontally along the pad to increase dressing capacity. The air-permeable backing provides strength and integrity.

Indications

For use as a postoperative dressing and as a primary or secondary dressing to manage burns, minor lacerations, abrasions, and heavily draining skin ulcers; may also be used on pressure ulcers (stages 2, 3, and 4), partial- and full-thickness wounds, tunneling wounds, infected and noninfected wounds, wounds with heavy drainage, wounds with serosanguineous or purulent drainage, and red, yellow, or black wounds

Contraindications

- None provided by the manufacturer

Application

- Apply the dry dressing with the wound contact layer toward the wound surface.
- Alternatively, soak the dressing with normal saline solution or another topical solution. Squeeze out excess fluid, and then apply the dressing with the wound contact layer toward the wound surface.
- Secure with a stretch net dressing, roll gauze, or tape.

Removal

- Moisten with normal saline solution, if necessary.
- Carefully lift the dressing off the wound.

TENDERSORB WET-PRUF
Abdominal Pads
Tyco Healthcare/Kendall

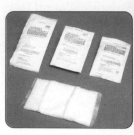

How supplied
Sterile pad: 5″ × 9″; A6252
                    7½″ × 8″, 8″ × 10″; A6253
Nonsterile bulk: 5″ × 9″; A6252
                    7½″ × 8″, 8″ × 10″; A6253

Action
TENDERSORB WET-PRUF Abdominal Pads can be used as secondary dressings to absorb excess wound fluid. They also protect the wound by cushioning it.

Indications
For use as part of a dressing system for virtually any wound requiring fluid retention and cushioning; may also be used to prevent skin breakdown and to manage wounds with moderate to heavy drainage

Contraindications
- Contraindicated for tunneling wounds

Application
- Apply a primary dressing based on wound type.
- Cover the primary dressing with a TENDERSORB WET-PRUF Abdominal Pad.
- Secure the pad with tape, bandage roll, or another appropriate product.

Removal
- Remove the securing tape or bandage roll.
- Remove the TENDERSORB WET-PRUF Abdominal Pad from the primary dressing.

Surgical supplies, miscellaneous

When the Statistical Analysis Durable Medical Equipment Regional Carrier and the four Durable Medical Equipment Regional Carriers (DMERCs) perform a Coding Verification Review and fail to reach a consensus coding decision, they sometimes assign the product or procedure to a general category. Therefore, various dissimilar products and procedures are usually assigned to this category. These products in this category don't have a universal definition, use guidelines, or a rate on the DMERC Fee Schedule. Yet, each product listed under this category has an individual action, indication, contraindication, and application and removal process. It remains the clinician's responsibility to understand each product before using it.

When submitting claims for products or procedures in this category, the provider and supplier must check with the payer for the supporting documentation that's required.

HCPCS CODE OVERVIEW

The HCPCS code normally assigned to miscellaneous surgical supplies is: A4649—surgical supplies, miscellaneous.

BIAFINE
OrthoNeutrogena

How supplied
Tube: 45g, 90g; A6250

Action
BIAFINE is a versatile, oil-in-water topical emulsion that provides hydration and occlusion for wound care. It provides up to a 10-fold increase in macrophage recruitment, autolytic debridement, and a moist healing environment.

Indication
For use in full-thickness wounds, pressure ulcers, dermal ulcers, including lower leg ulcers, dermal donor and graft site management, and radiation dermatitis

Contraindication
- Contraindicated for use on bleeding wounds
- Contraindicated on skin rashes related to food or medicine allergies
- Contraindicated when an allergy to one of the ingredients is known

Application
For full-thickness wounds, dermal donor and graft site management:
- Wash the affected area with saline solution, clean water, or wound cleanser.
- Apply BIAFINE on and around the affected area in layers $1/4''$ to $1/2''$ thick.
- If applying gauze dressing, moisten the dressing lightly before application.
- Reapply BIAFINE as described above every 24 to 48 hours or as directed until the wound or lesion has healed fully.
- For donor site management, apply BIAFINE after the skin removal, and cover with moist dressing. Reapply as directed.
- For dermal graft site management, apply BIAFINE to graft site only after graft has taken sucessfully. BIAFINE can be washed away with saline solution or clean water without damaging the newly formed tissues.

For radiation dermatitis
- Apply a generous amount of BIAFINE three times per day, 7 days per week, to the treated areas, gently massaging the areas until BIAFINE is completely absorbed.
- Continue to apply BIAFINE as described until the skin has fully recovered.
- Don't interrupt applications during the course of radiation therapy, even for 1 day.
- Don't apply BIAFINE 4 hours or less before a radiation session.

Removal
- Remove BIAFINE with normal saline solution or clean water.

Burn Blok After Care Lotion

Medi-Tech International Corp.

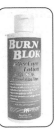

How supplied

Lotion with 80% Aloe Vera: 1 oz, 2 oz, 6 oz

Action

Burn Blok After Care Lotion is an effective treatment for burns, scars, and radiation-induced reactions. Nongreasy and alcohol-free, it provides deep dermal hydration and reduces the severity of radiation-induced skin reaction. It also provides an effective barrier to heat buildup, replenishes lost moisture to the skin, and encourages production of collagen fibration.

Indications

For management of radiation-induced reactions, skin reactions after radiation therapy, first- and second-degree burns, laser resurfacing, and keloid and hypertrophic scars; also for conditioning the skin before radiation therapy

Contraindications

- None provided by the manufacturer

Application

- Begin application immediately after the first radiation session.
- Apply Burn Blok liberally two or three times daily.
- Use Burn Blok daily throughout the entire treatment period.
- Burn Blok can be used either in closed or open treatment.

Removal

- Remember that Burn Blok is water-soluble, so you can rinse it off with water or Medi-Tech Wound Cleanser.

GlucanPro Cream with Oat Beta-Glucan
Brennen Medical, LLC

How supplied
Tube: 25 g (0.9 oz), 85 g (3 oz); A6250

Action
GlucanPro topical burn and wound cream combines oat beta-glucan with a gentle oil-in-water emulsion. GlucanPro Cream may be used in the management of partial-thickness burns; acute and chronic skin injuries; dermatological disorders; and dry, irritated, and itchy skin. GlucanPro Cream may also aid in the autolytic debridement of wounds with scattered areas of necrosis and slough.

Indications
May be used to aid in the management of superficial abrasions, scrapes, cuts, and lacerations; minor burns and scalds; partial- and full-thickness wounds; and irritations of the skin; may also be used under the supervision of a health care professional for pressure ulcers; venous, diabetic, and arterial ulcers; partial-thickness burns, donor graft sites; and surgical wounds

Contraindications
- For external use only
- Not for use on patients with known allergies to plants such as gum oat or any of the ingredients

Application
- Clean the affected area.
- Apply GlucanPro liberally to the affected area one to three times daily.
- If desired, cover with a nonstick bandage.

Removal
- If applicable, remove secondary dressing and discard.
- Gently clean the wound.
- Repeat application of GlucanPro Cream as needed.

MTSPANDAGE (Latex-Free)

MTSPANDAGE PRE-CUTS (Latex-Free)

SPANDAGE (Latex-Free)

SPANDAGE CUSTOM PRE-CUTS (Latex-Free)

Medi-Tech International Corp.

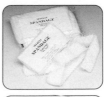

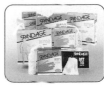

How supplied

MTSPANDAGE (Latex-Free) and SPANDAGE (Latex-Free)
Tube: Uncut

MTSPANDAGE CUSTOM PRE-CUTS (Latex-Free) and SPANDAGE CUSTOM PRE-CUTS (Latex-Free)
Tube: Individual precuts in sizes to fit a wide range of body areas from head to toes; A4649

Action

These secondary dressing retainers hold a dressing in place, eliminating the use of adhesive tape as well as the discomfort of tape removal, tape excoriation problems, tape residue on the skin, and the need for hypoallergenic tapes. They provide freedom of movement and allow aeration to the wound, which promotes healing.

Indications

To hold firmly and comfortably any wet or dry dressing or compress on almost any part of the body

Contraindications

■ None provided by the manufacturer

Application

■ Usually, place both hands into the appropriate size MTSPANDAGE tube and stretch it over the dressing.
■ Withdraw your hands from the tube, allowing MTSPANDAGE to fit the contour of the dressed area.
Head
■ Cut 10″ to 12″ (25.5 to 30.5 cm) of tubing, or use a precut size.
■ Stretch the tube over the head, from the top of the head to under the chin, creating a face mask.
■ Cut the tube away from the face, from the midforehead to under the chin. If the face is to remain covered, don't cut.

SURGICAL SUPPLIES
MISCELLANEOUS

Skull cap
- Cut 12″ to 14″ (30.5 to 35.5 cm) of tubing, or use a precut size.
- Stretch one end of the tube over the cranium to just above the eyebrows.
- Make one full twist of the remaining tube, place both of your hands into the opening, and restretch the remainder down over the cranium.

Finger/Toe (using applicator)
- Push a length of tubing onto applicator equal to twice the applicator's length, and place the applicator over the entire dressed appendage.
- Pull a small amount of tubing off the applicator, hold it with thumb and forefinger at the base of the appendage, and pull the applicator off. Cut tubing at the tip of the appendage.
- Repeat the process if additional pressure is required to secure the dressing, but never apply more than two layers.

Hand
- Cut 14″ (35.5 cm) of tubing, or use a precut size.
- Stretch one end of the tube over the hand.
- Make one full twist in the remaining tube at the fingertip, and restretch the remainder back over the hand as far as the wrist.
- Uninjured fingers may be left free by cutting finger holes.

Shoulder/Axilla/Breast/Mastectomy
- Cut 20″ (51 cm) of tubing, or use a precut size.
- Make a 3″ (7.5 cm) vertical cut in the tube's fold about 6″ (15 cm) from one end. This cut will be a neck hole.
- Insert the affected arm into the long piece of net and bring the net up to the neck.
- Pass the head through the 3″ (7.5 cm) cut so that the net fits like a sling.

Chest/Upper abdomen
- Cut 20″ (51 cm) of tubing, or use a precut size.
- About 3″ (7.5 cm) from the top of the tube, make two identical 3″ vertical cuts in the opposite folds.
- Place both hands into the tube at the end farthest from the 3″ cuts. Then, stretch the tube over the patient's head and raised arms, pulling each arm through one of the 3″ cuts, as if putting on a sweater.
- Draw the stretched tube down over the shoulders to the waist.
- This "sweater" can also serve to secure electrodes for ECG monitoring.

Elbow/Forearm/Leg/Knee
- Cut 8″ (20.5 cm) of tubing, or use a precut size.
- Allow tube to extend about 2″ (5 cm) beyond the dressing at each end.

Genital/Anal/Perineal areas
- Cut 20″ (51 cm) of tubing, or use a precut size.
- Make a 4″ (10 cm) vertical cut directly in the center of the fold.
- With both hands in the top part of the tube, stretch the pantylike tube up the legs and over the hips to the waist, while keeping the lower length of the tube (or tail) hanging in the rear.
- With the tail hanging in the rear and below, pass the legs through the indicated side leg cuts and bring the tail up to the waist, passing over the first layer.

Gluteus/Lower abdomen/Hip/Groin/Buttocks/Thigh
- Cut 14" (35.5 cm) of tubing, or use a precut size.
- At a point 2" (5 cm) from the top of the tube, make a 2" cut through one side of the net.
- For bandaging the right side of the affected areas: With the 2" cut on the left side of the tube, pass the affected right leg through the long part of the tube and the left leg through the 2" cut.
- For bandaging the left side of the affected areas: With the 2" cut on the right side of the tube, draw the legs through the two stretched openings and pull the panty upward to above the waist.

Amputation
- Cut 12" (30.5 cm) of tubing, or use a precut size.
- Apply one end of tube over the stump.
- Make one full twist in the remaining tube at the stump tip, and restretch the remainder back over the stump.

Foot
- Cut 10" (25.5 cm) of tubing, or use a precut size.
- Extend the tube from ankle to toes.

Removal
- If not soiled, MTSPANDAGE may remain in place for 3 days or more. For examination or dressing change, lift or roll it back over the dressed area.
- Lift one end of MTSPANDAGE, raise the lower end of the tube, and remove. Because the dressing retainer molds itself to the contours of the body without adhesion, removing it from hairy skin doesn't cause pain.

Transparent films

ACTION

Transparent films are adhesive, semipermeable, polyurethane membrane dressings that vary in thickness and size. They're waterproof and impermeable to bacteria and contaminants, yet they permit water vapor to cross the barrier. These dressings maintain a moist healing environment, promoting formation of granulation tissue and autolysis of necrotic tissue.

INDICATIONS

Transparent films may be used as a primary or secondary dressing to prevent and manage stage 1 pressure ulcers, partial-thickness wounds with little or no exudate, and wounds with necrotic tissue or slough.

ADVANTAGES

- Retain moisture
- Are impermeable to bacteria and other contaminants
- Facilitate autolytic debridement
- Allow wound observation
- Don't require a secondary dressing

DISADVANTAGES

- May not be recommended for infected wounds
- Not recommended for wounds with moderate to heavy drainage because they don't absorb
- Not recommended for use on fragile skin
- Require a border of intact skin for adhesive edge of dressing
- May be difficult to apply and handle
- May dislodge in high-friction areas

HCPCS CODE OVERVIEW

The HCPCS codes normally assigned to transparent film dressings are:
A6257—pad size < 16 in^2
A6258—pad size > 16 in^2 but ≤ 48 in^2
A6259—pad size > 48 in^2.

BIOCLUSIVE Select Transparent Dressing
Johnson & Johnson
Wound Management
A division of ETHICON, Inc.

How supplied
Film: $1^3/4'' \times 2^3/4''$, $2^3/8'' \times 2^3/4''$,
$3'' \times 4''$; A6257
$4'' \times 5''$; A6258

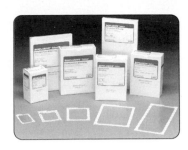

Action
BIOCLUSIVE Select Transparent Dressing is a semiocclusive bacterial and viral barrier that protects skin from exogenous fluid and contaminants. It allows evaporation, promotes gas and water vapor exchange, and creates a moist healing environment.

Indications
To manage access devices, central venous catheters, and peripheral I.V., total parenteral nutrition, central venous pressure, and neonatal I.V. sites; may also be used for care of endoscopy incisions, small surgical incisions, skin biopsy sites, donor sites, and second-degree burns

Contraindications
■ None provided by the manufacturer

Application
■ Peel away the middle section from the frame of the dressing.
■ Place the window frame over the wound area or I.V. site.
■ Gently smooth and secure the dressing to skin.
■ Remove the frame using a circular motion. Perforation will release with gentle pressure.

Removal
■ Gently pick up a corner of the dressing. Stretch the dressing away from the center of the wound, partially lifting it.
■ Peel the dressing back until you feel resistance.
■ Repeatedly stretch and peel the dressing as necessary until it's removed.

TRANSPARENT FILMS

BIOCLUSIVE Transparent Dressing

Johnson & Johnson
Wound Management
A division of ETHICON, Inc.

How supplied

Film: $1^1/_2'' \times 1^1/_2''$, $2'' \times 3''$; A6257
          $4'' \times 5''$, $5'' \times 7''$, $4'' \times 10''$; A6258
          $8'' \times 10''$; A6259

Action

BIOCLUSIVE Transparent Dressing is a semiocclusive bacterial and viral barrier that protects skin from exogenous fluid and contaminants. It allows evaporation, promotes gas and water vapor exchange, and creates a moist healing environment.

Indications

To manage I.V. sites, total parenteral nutrition sites, pressure ulcers (stages 1 and 2), second-degree burns, donor sites, minimally draining or nondraining clean surgical wounds, lacerations, and abrasions, and to prevent skin breakdown; may also be used on partial-thickness wounds, noninfected wounds, and red wounds, and for autolytic debridement

Contraindications

■ Contraindicated for infected wounds

Application

■ Clean the wound with an appropriate topical antiseptic, such as hydrogen peroxide or normal saline solution.
■ Remove oil from the surrounding skin with alcohol or acetone alcohol, and dry the skin thoroughly. To ensure proper adhesion of the dressing, maintain a 1″ (2.5 cm) margin of dry periwound skin.
■ Hold the dressing with the center paper tab faceup, and remove the center backing paper.
■ Grasp the side paper tabs, position the dressing over the wound site, and smooth the center portion into place.
■ Peel away the side backing papers one at a time while smoothing the film onto the skin.
■ Don't require secondary dressings.

Removal

■ Gently pick up a corner of the dressing. Stretch the dressing away from the center of the wound, partially lifting it.
■ Peel the dressing back until you feel resistance.
■ Repeatedly stretch and peel the dressing as necessary until it's removed.

CarraFilm Transparent Film Dressing

Carrington Laboratories, Inc.

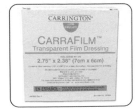

How supplied

Film sheet: $2^3/4'' \times 2^3/8''$; A6257

$4'' \times 5^1/4''$; A6258

Action

CarraFilm Transparent Film Dressing is an adhesive, semipermeable membrane dressing that's sterile and impervious to moisture and bacteria but permeable to moisture vapor and oxygen.

Indications

For use as a protective wound dressing on minor abrasions, closed surgical wounds, superficial pressure ulcers, skin grafts, and donor sites, or as a secondary cover dressing over other types of primary dressings; may also be used on superficial, partial-thickness wounds; wounds with necrosis or slough; wounds with low, medium, or high exudate; and red, yellow, or black wounds

Contraindications

- Contraindicated for infected wounds

Application

- Clean the wound and periwound tissue. Dry the periwound skin.
- Clip or shave excess hair at site, if desired. A skin barrier wipe may be used on intact skin.
- Gently pull the paper tabs away from the center of the dressing to partially expose the dressing.
- Apply the exposed dressing to the wound site without tension, to prevent skin shear. Press and smooth into place.
- Pull the tabs at an angle with even pressure to release them from the dressing.

Removal

- Change the dressing as needed according to the wound condition and amount of exudate or as directed by the physician.
- CarraFilm may remain in place up to 7 days.

CarraSmart Film Transparent Film Dressing

Carrington Laboratories, Inc.

How supplied
Film sheet: 4" × 5"; A6258

Action
CarraSmart Film Transparent Film Dressing has the same properties as CarraFilm, an adhesive semipermeable membrane dressing, but also allows selective drainage evaporation through the film and thus may be used as a primary or secondary dressing over highly exuding wounds. It has an extremely high moisture vapor transport rate (MVTR)—the measure of a surface's "breathability," or its ability to allow evaporation of moisture. MVTR is measured in grams per square meter per day ($g/m^2/day$). Normal skin releases 240 to 1,800 $g/m^2/day$, whereas burn patients lose 3,000 to 5,200 $g/m^2/day$. Wound care products with high MVTR maintain an optimum wound care environment by venting and retaining moisture as needed. On wounds with high exudate levels, these products can reduce the frequency of dressing changes and can prevent maceration under the film.

Indications
For use as a protective wound dressing on minor abrasions, closed surgical wounds, superficial pressure ulcers, skin grafts, and donor sites, and as a secondary cover dressing over other types of primary dressings; may also be used on superficial, partial-thickness wounds; wounds with necrosis or slough; wounds with low, medium, or high exudate; and red, yellow, or black wounds

Contraindications
- Contraindicated for infected wounds

Application
- Clean the wound and periwound tissue. Dry the periwound skin. Clip or shave excess hair at site, if desired. A skin barrier wipe may be used on intact skin.
- Gently pull the paper tabs away from the center of the dressing to partially expose the dressing.
- Apply the exposed dressing to the wound site without tension, to prevent skin shear. Press and smooth it into place.
- Pull the tabs at an angle with even pressure to release them from the dressing.

Removal
- Change the dressing as needed according to the wound condition and amount of exudate or as directed by the physician.
- Dressing may stay in place up to 7 days.

TRANSPARENT FILMS

ClearSite Transparent Membrane Dressing

Conmed Corporation

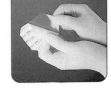

How supplied
Film: 2" × 3"; A6257
4" × 5", 6" × 8"; A6258
2" × 2", 3" × 4", 4" × 4", 4" × 8", 8" × 10"

Action
ClearSite Transparent Membrane Dressing is a latex-free, semipermeable polyurethane adhesive film that provides a moist healing environment and allows transmission of moisture to reduce the risk of maceration.

Indications
To cover and protect wounds and minor skin irritations

Contraindications
- Contraindicated for infected wounds

Application
- Gently clean and dry the wound and surrounding area. Remove excessive hair at site, if necessary.
- Holding the dressing's tabs, remove the printed liner.
- Apply the dressing to the wound.
- Remove the dressing's clear liner, then pull to remove the white tab.

Removal
- Change the dressing according to facility policy.
- While supporting the skin, firmly grasp an edge of the dressing, and pull or stretch it parallel to the skin surface. This will release the adhesive film from the skin.

Comfeel Film
Coloplast Corp.

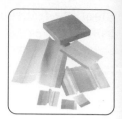

How supplied
Comfeel Film: $2^3/_8'' \times 2^3/_4''$; A6257
                 $4'' \times 4^3/_4''$; A6258
                 $9'' \times 5^1/_2''$, $8'' \times 11^1/_2''$,
                 $11^1/_2'' \times 15^3/_4''$; A6259

Action
Comfeel Film is a sterile, semipermeable film dressing that provides a moist environment and protects the wound from contamination. Excellent moisture vapor transmission rate of 1,700 $g/m^2/24$ hours allows excess moisture to quickly evaporate, minimizing maceration.

Indication
As a primary or secondary dressing to manage dry or minimally exuding acute and chronic wounds, including pressure ulcers, leg ulcers, skin tears, superficial lacerations and abrasions, minor burns, and donor sites; may be used as a dressing for peripheral and central I.V. catheters

Contraindications
- Not for use on third-degree burns
- May be used on infected wounds under the supervision of a health care professional
- Should be removed before radiation treatment (X-ray, ultrasonic treatment, diathermy, microwave)

Application
- Remove film from the pouch.
- Remove the paper liner, center the film over the site, and apply while avoiding tension or wrinkles.
- Completely remove the paper liner to apply the remaining part of dressing. Before removing the supporting film, gently press along colored edge to ensure the film has adhered.
- Remove the protective supporting film by pulling the colored edge gently parallel to the skin. The film is now applied.

Removal
- Gently grasp an edge of the dressing, and pull parallel to the skin to stretch the dressing, which will cause the adhesive to release.
- You may apply a piece of tape to the dressing edge to facilitate lifting the dressing to start removal procedure.
- The film should be removed and a new dressing applied if the film isn't intact or if the seal integrity has been compromised.

DermaView
DermaRite Industries, LLC

How supplied
Film:　　2″ × 3″; A6257
　　　　　　4″ × 5″; A6258

Action
DermaView is a semiocclusive bacterial and viral barrier that protects skin from urine and fecal breakdown. This semipermeable dressing maintains a moist healing environment.

Indications
May be used as a primary or secondary dressing, to secure other dressings, or for infected wounds that need autolytic debridement

Contraindications
- Contraindicated for infected areas
- Contraindicated for patients with deep systemic infections
- Contraindicated for full-thickness wounds involving muscle, tendon, or bone

Application
- Clean the wound area.
- Consulting the dressing instructions, peel off area surface labeled #1.
- Position the dressing over the wound, and press it down gently around the wound's perimeter.
- Pull out tab #2 and discard it. Peel back tab #3.
- Smooth the dressing out firmly from the center toward the edges.

Removal
- Lift and slowly stretch one corner of the dressing in the direction of the hair growth.
- Continue stretching or pulling around the perimeter of the dressing, and then remove remaining film.

TRANSPARENT FILMS

DermaView II
DermaRite Industries, LLC

How supplied
Dressing: 2″ × 3″; A6257
4″ × 5″; A6258

Action
DermaView II is a transparent, semipermeable
dressing with an utlrathin conformable film, coat-
ed with hypoallergenic adhesive and laminated between two protective sil-
icon release papers. A properly applied dressing is impermeable to bacteria and liquids but offers excellent moisture vapor permeability properties.

Indications
May be used as a primary or secondary dressing, to secure other dressings,
or for infected wounds that need autolytic debridement

Contraindications
- Contraindicated as a primary dressing on heavily draining wounds
- Not intended to replace wound closures

Application
- Clean the wound area with DermaKlenz wound cleaner.
- Consulting the dressing instructions, remove the primary adhesive lin-
  er from the film adhesive.
- Place the dressing over the wound site. Use the notch in the frame to
  place over the catheter hub when using for I.V.
- Smooth the dressing in place using firm, but gentle pressure.
- Carefully remove the paper frame from the perimeter of the film dress-
  ing. Secure any loose edges, if necessary.

Removal
- Carefully loosen the perimeter of the film dressing.
- Holding down one edge of the film, gently pull the opposite edge to
  break the adhesive bond.

Mefilm Transparent Film Dressing

Mölnlycke Health Care

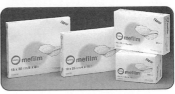

How supplied

Dressing: 2.4" × 2.8"; A6257
          4" × 4.8", 4" × 10";
          A6258
          6" × 8"; A6259

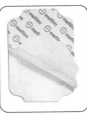

Action

Mefilm is a breathable, transparent self-adhesive film dressing that conforms easily to body contours, helps protect the wound surface, and provides a barrier to leakage and bacterial contamination. Mefilm helps maintain a moist wound environment, and the adhesive is gentle to the skin and wound site.

Indications

Designed for a wide range of clean wounds in the granulation phase, such as superficial burns, I.V. sites, abrasions, lacerations, superficial pressure ulcers, closed surgical wounds, and donor sites with low exudate levels, as well as for prevention of skin breakdown

Contraindications

- Not for use on full-thickness wounds involving muscle, tendon, or bone
- Not for use on third-degree burns

Application

- Clean the wound area. Make sure that the surrounding skin is dry.
- Choose the correct dressing size to overlap dry skin by at least ³/₈" (1 cm).
- For sizes 4" × 10" and 6" × 8" only. Remove center cutout paper and discard.
- Remove the protective backing to expose the adhesive.
- Position the dressing, and smooth it onto the skin.
- Remove the paper frame and the two white paper side tabs.

Removal

- The dressing may be left in place for up to 7 days, depending on the condition of the wound and surrounding skin.

OPSITE
OPSITE FLEXIGRID
OPSITE FLEXIFIX
Smith & Nephew, Inc.
Wound Management

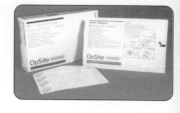

How supplied
OPSITE

Film: $5^1/_2'' \times 4''$, $11'' \times 4''$; A6258
         $5^1/_2'' \times 10''$, $11'' \times 6''$, $11'' \times 11^3/_4''$, $11'' \times 17^3/_4''$, $17^3/_4'' \times 2^5/_8''$;
         A6259

OPSITE FLEXIGRID

Film: $2^3/_8'' \times 2^1/_2''$; A6257
         $4'' \times 4^3/_4''$, $6'' \times 8''$, $4^3/_4'' \times 10''$; A6258

OPSITE FLEXIFIX

Film: $2'' \times 11$ yd, $4'' \times 11$ yd; A6257

Action
OPSITE consists of a polyurethane membrane that creates a moist environment by trapping the wound exudate. It's waterproof and aids in preventing bacterial contamination. OPSITE FLEXIGRID dressings provide a unique wound measurement grid that can be written on to record the change in wound size. OPSITE FLEXIFIX is easily applied to awkward areas of the body and over dressings and tubes. The film is highly conformable and extensible to increase patient comfort.

Indications
To protect skin from friction and for use as secondary dressings to secure foams, alginates, and gauzes while protecting the wound

Contraindications
None provided by the manufacturer

Application
- Remove the backing from the dressing to expose the adhesive surface.
- Place the dressing gently over the wound, allowing the film to cover at least 1″ (2.5 cm) of undamaged skin around the wound.
- If using OPSITE FLEXIGRID, remove the flexible plastic grid.

Removal
- Lift a corner of the dressing, and begin stretching it horizontally along the skin surface, breaking the adhesive bond.
- Continue stretching from the edges toward the center. When two sides of the dressing are partially removed, grasp both sides and stretch horizontally, parallel to the skin, until the entire dressing can be removed.

Polyskin II Transparent Dressing
Tyco Healthcare/Kendall

How supplied
Sterile film sheet: $1^1/2'' \times 1^1/2''$, $2'' \times 2^3/4''$; A6257
                         $4'' \times 4^3/4''$, $4'' \times 8''$, $6'' \times 8''$; A6258
                         $8'' \times 10''$; A6259

Action
Polyskin II Transparent Dressing supports autolytic debridement of wounds with eschar by maintaining a moist healing environment and acting as a barrier against bacteria.

Indications
To manage partial-thickness wounds or dry necrotic wounds that require debridement and to prevent skin breakdown; may be used to dress I.V. sites, donor sites, ulcers, and surgical sites; may also be used to help manage pressure ulcers (stages 1 and 2), noninfected wounds, and wounds with minimal drainage

Contraindications
- Contraindicated for exuding wounds, friable skin around wounds, and wounds with sinus tracts

Application
- Check that the wound has a margin of intact skin to ensure successful application.
- Peel tab #1 from the backing of the dressing to expose the adhesive surface.
- Apply the dressing to the wound, and smooth it into place.
- Remove tab #2.

Removal
- Change the dressing based on the amount of accumulated exudate.
- Lift and slowly pull the dressing in the direction of hair growth.
- Alternatively, affix a small piece of surgical tape to the edge of the dressing, and peel back.

Polyskin MR Moisture Responsive Transparent Dressing
Tyco Healthcare/Kendall

How supplied
Sterile film sheet: 2" × 2³/₄"; A6257
                        4" × 4³/₄"; A6258

Action
POLYSKIN MR Moisture Responsive Transparent Dressing responds to fluid by increasing or decreasing its moisture vapor transfer rate and provides an optimal wound-healing environment.

Indications
To manage pressure ulcers (stages 1, 2, 3, and 4), partial- and full-thickness wounds, infected and uninfected wounds, wounds with light drainage, and red wounds

Contraindications
None provided by the manufacturer

Application
- Check that the wound has a margin of intact skin to ensure successful application.
- Peel tab #1 from the backing of the dressing to expose the adhesive surface.
- Apply the dressing to the wound, and smooth it into place.
- Remove tab #2.

Removal
- Lift one corner of the dressing.
- Pull or stretch the dressing gently in the direction of hair growth.

TRANSPARENT FILMS

Suresite Transparent Film

Medline Industries, Inc.

How supplied

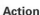

Film: 1.52″ × 1.52″ 1*2*3 style, 2″ × 3″, 2³/₄″ × 2³/₈″ window style, 2³/₄″ × 2³/₈″ 1*2*3 style; A6257
4″ × 4.5″, 4″ × 4.5″ matrix style, 4″ × 4.5″ window style, 4″ × 4.5″ 1*2*3 style, 6″ × 8″ matrix style, 6″ × 8″ 1*2*3 style, 4″ × 10″ 1*2*3 style; A6258
8″ × 12″ 1*2*3 style, A6259

Action

Suresite is a sterile, hypoallergenic film dressing that acts as a barrier to bacteria and water while creating a moist healing environment. It's permeable to oxygen and vapor.

Indications

To manage peripheral and central I.V. catheter sites and minor abrasions and skin tears, and to help prevent skin breakdown; may also be used for pressure ulcers (stages 1 and 2), partial-thickness wounds, noninfected wounds, and wounds with minimal drainage

Contraindications

- Contraindicated for use as a primary dressing on moderately to heavily draining wounds

Application

- Clean the wound with normal saline solution or another appropriate cleanser, such as Skintegrity Wound Cleanser. Dry the surrounding area. Allow any skin preparation to dry completely.
- Remove the backing paper from the dressing, exposing the adhesive.
- Gently place the dressing over the wound and apply it, leaving at least 1¹/₄″ to 1¹/₂″ (3 to 4 cm) of healthy periwound skin.
- Remove the flexible plastic grid, paper window frame, or top paper carrier, if applicable.

Removal

- Suresite can be worn during showering to protect the wound or the I.V. hub. If exudate accumulates under the dressing, change the dressing immediately.
- Lift a corner of the dressing, and begin stretching it horizontally along the skin surface. When two sides are partially removed, grasp both sides, and stretch parallel to the skin.

3M Tegaderm HP Transparent Dressing

3M Tegaderm Transparent Dressing
3M Health Care

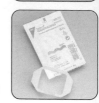

How supplied
3M Tegaderm HP Transparent Dressing

Film sheet:	2³/₄″ × 2³/₄″; A6257
	4″ × 4³/₄″; A6258
Film sheet (sacral):	4¹/₂″ × 4³/₄″; A6258
Oval:	2¹/₈″ × 2¹/₂″; A6257
	4″ × 4¹/₂″, 5¹/₂″ × 6¹/₂″; A6258

3M Tegaderm Transparent Dressing

Film sheet (picture frame):	1³/₄″ × 1³/₄″, 2³/₈″ × 2³/₄″; A6257
	4″ × 4³/₄″; A6258
Film sheet (original frame):	2³/₈″ × 2³/₄″; A6257
	4″ × 4³/₄″, 4″ × 10″, 6″ × 8″; A6258
	8″ × 12″; A6259
Film sheet (oval frame):	4″ × 4¹/₂″; A6258
Film sheet (I.V. frame):	2³/₄″ × 3¹/₄″, 3¹/₂″ × 4¹/₄″; A6257
Film sheet (first aid style):	2³/₈″ × 2³/₄″; A6257
	4″ × 5¹/₂″; A6258

Action
3M Tegaderm Transparent Dressing consists of a thin film backing with a hypoallergenic adhesive. The dressing is breathable, allowing good oxygen and moisture vapor exchange. It's waterproof and impermeable to liquids, bacteria, and viruses. An intact dressing protects the site from outside contamination.

Indications
To cover and protect catheter sites and wounds, to maintain a moist environment for wound healing or to facilitate autolytic debridement, as a secondary dressing, as a protective cover over at-risk skin, to secure devices to the skin, to cover first- and second-degree burns, and as a protective eye covering

Contraindications
- Contraindicated for infected wounds and infected catheter sites
- Not intended to replace sutures or other primary wound closure methods

Application
- Peel the liner from the dressing, exposing the adhesive surface.

3M Tegaderm HP Dressing

■ Center the dressing over the catheter site or wound.

3M Tegaderm HP Dressing with Secure Strip

■ Position the dressing so the notch fits over the catheter hub and the insertion site is centered in the transparent film.
■ Slowly remove the frame while smoothing down the dressing edges.
■ Then, smooth the dressing from the center toward the edges, using firm pressure to enhance adhesion.

Removal

■ Gently grasp an edge, and slowly peel the dressing from the skin in the direction of hair growth. Avoid skin trauma by peeling the dressing back, rather than pulling it up from the skin.
■ Alternatively, for removal from I.V. sites or other devices, grasp one edge of the dressing, and gently pull it straight out to stretch it and release the adhesion. A medical solvent can also facilitate removal.
■ Take care not to dislodge catheters or other devices or to disrupt the wound surface while removing the dressing. Support the skin and the catheter while removing the dressing.
■ If the dressing adheres to the wound surface where epithelialization has taken place, gently soak it off.

Transeal Transparent Wound Dressing
DeRoyal

How supplied
Film: 1³/₄″ × 1³/₄″, 2 ¹/₂″ × 2³/₄″; A6257
             4″ × 4³/₄″, 4″ × 10″, 6″ × 8″; A6258
             8″ × 12″; A6259

Action
Transeal is a transparent, breathable polyurethane wound dressing coated with an acrylic, pressure-sensitive adhesive that acts as a second skin. Transeal has the highest vapor transmission rate available, yet it's impermeable to external contaminants, such as water, dirt, debris, and bacteria.

Indications
To prevent skin breakdown and to manage pressure ulcers (stages 1, 2, 3, and 4), partial- and full-thickness wounds, tunneling wounds, donor sites, I.V. sites, first- and second-degree burns, acute wounds, infected and non-infected wounds, draining wounds, and red, yellow, or black wounds; may be used as a primary or secondary dressing depending on wound type

Contraindications
- Contraindicated as a primary dressing for heavily draining wounds

Application
- Clean and thoroughly dry the wound and surrounding skin.
- Peel off the backing layer of the dressing to expose the adhesive side of the dressing.
- Position the dressing over the wound, and press it gently into place.
- Peel off the clear carrier film to leave the dressing in place.

Removal
- Remove the dressing by gently peeling away in the direction of hair growth.

TRANSPARENT FILMS

Wound fillers

Action
Wound fillers are available as pastes, granules, powders, beads, and gels that provide a moist healing environment, absorb exudate, and help debride the wound bed by softening the necrotic tissue.

Indications
Wound fillers may be used as primary dressings to manage partial- and full-thickness wounds, minimally to moderately exuding wounds, infected and noninfected wounds, and wounds requiring packing to fill dead space

Advantages
- May be absorbent
- Promote autolytic debridement
- Are easy to apply and remove
- May be used with other products
- Fill dead space

Disadvantages
- Most not recommended for use in wounds with little or no exudate
- Require secondary dressing

HCPCS code overview
The HCPCS codes normally assigned to wound fillers not elsewhere classified are.
A6261—paste, per fluid ounce
A6262—dry form, per gram.

Catrix 5 Rejuvenation Cream
Lescarden, Inc.

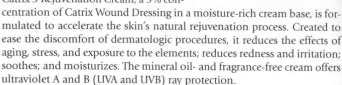

How supplied
Tube: 1.25 oz

Action
Catrix 5 Rejuvenation Cream, a 5% concentration of Catrix Wound Dressing in a moisture-rich cream base, is formulated to accelerate the skin's natural rejuvenation process. Created to ease the discomfort of dermatologic procedures, it reduces the effects of aging, stress, and exposure to the elements; reduces redness and irritation; soothes; and moisturizes. The mineral oil- and fragrance-free cream offers ultraviolet A and B (UVA and UVB) ray protection.

Indications
To counteract the irritating adverse effects often associated with topical retinoids, chemical acid peels, AHAs, and fluouroplex; used primarily in cosmetic dermatology and plastic surgery patients

Contraindications
- For external use only
- Not for contact with eyes

Application
- Smooth the cream onto clean skin morning and night.
- If also using a dermatologic therapy, first clean the skin, and then apply the therapy as instructed by the physician, followed by Catrix 5 Rejuvenation Cream.
- For 1 week before a dermatologic procedure, apply Catrix 5 Rejuvenation Cream daily, and then follow the directions above.
- Catrix 5 Rejuvenation Cream may be used in place of Catrix 10 Ointment starting 7 to 10 days after a dermatologic procedure, such as laser resurfacing. Apply according to directions above.
- Continued daily use after healing will keep the skin healthy and supple.

Removal
- Continue to use product under the direction of the physician.

Catrix 10 Ointment

Lescarden, Inc.

How supplied

Tube: 0.15 oz, 2 oz

Action

Catrix 10 Ointment by Catrix Skincare is a clinically tested postprocedural application that helps relieve discomfort and restores skin to its naturally healthy condition after laser resurfacing, chemical peels, and microdermabrasion. Catrix 10 promotes the development of epithelial cells and expedites the healing process. It reduces redness, soothes itchiness, controls oozing and crusting, and limits tautness. The nonirritating nonsteroidal formula is an effective therapy for wounds, surgical incisions, and skin problems from incontinence, abrasions, and psoriasis.

Indications

To manage wounds including laser resurfacing, microdermabrasion, and surgical incisions; used primarily in cosmetic dermatology and plastic surgery patients; also useful for mild psoriasis

Contraindications

- For external use only
- Not for contact with eyes

Application

- After procedure, apply a liberal layer of Catrix 10 Ointment every 2 to 5 hours or as often as needed to keep the treated area moist.
- Apply enough to fully coat and occlude the treated area.
- Continue using for 7 days or as directed by the physician.

Removal

- In the unlikely event of crust formation, gently soak off ointment using water or another solution, as directed.
- Reapply the ointment.

Catrix Wound Dressing
Lescarden, Inc.

How supplied
Topical powder: 1-g packet; A6262

Action
Topically applied powder made from
bovine tracheal cartilage containing micronized collagen, and mucopoly-saccharides is clinically proven to accelerate the healing of cutaneous wounds. The dressing maintains a moist healing environment, promotes angiogenesis, promotes the proliferation and migration of fibroblasts, stimulates the growth of keratinocytes, and creates a protective barrier against bacterial infections and other agents.

Indications
To manage pressure ulcers (stages 1, 2, 3, and 4), stasis ulcers, first- and second-degree burns, diabetic ulcers, foot ulcers, postsurgical incisions, radiation dermatitis, cuts and abrasions, partial-thickness wounds, and skin conditions associated with peristomal care; also used to absorb wound exudate

Contraindications
■ Contraindicated in patients with an adverse reaction to bovine products

Application
■ Debride and clean the wound. Treat with medication, if needed.
■ Apply Catrix Wound Dressing to the wound in an even manner to a thickness of no more than $^1/_{16}$".
■ In hard-to-reach wounds, mix Catrix Wound Dressing with 2 to 5 ml glyceride or 4 to 10 ml saline solution to form a paste that can be applied directly to the wound, completely covering it.
■ If needed, apply a nonocclusive dressing, such as Telfa.
■ Apply one or two times a day, as needed.

Removal
■ Reapply as ordered.

New Product

DiaB F.D.G. Freeze Dried Gel Wound Dressing with Acemannan Hydrogel

Carrington Laboratories, Inc.

How supplied
Wafer:　　4″ diameter

Action
DiaB F.D.G. is a freeze-dried gel that absorbs excess fluid. When rehydrated, it becomes a gel, forming a protective layer over diabetic ulcers. Sterile and preservative free, it contains acemannan hydrogel.

Indications
For diabetic foot and leg ulcers with moderate drainage

Contraindications
- Contraindicated on patients who are sensitive to acemannan hydrogel or any other component of the dressing

Application
- Flush the wound with a suitable cleanser such as DiaB Klenz.
- Peel open the package, and remove DiaB F.D.G. following sterile protocol.
- Apply to the wound bed by folding into the wound or tearing to pack in undermined areas.
- Cover with a secondary dressing such as CarraSmart Foam or CarraSmart Film.
- If the wound is dry, wet F.D.G. with a small amount of DiaB Klenz and place resulting semi-gel in wound and cover.

Removal
- Flush wound with a suitable wound cleanser such as DiaB Klenz.

WOUND FILLERS

FlexiGel Strands Absorbent Wound Dressing

Smith & Nephew
Wound Management, Inc.

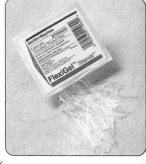

How supplied
Packet: 6 g; A6262

Action
FlexiGel Strands Absorbent Wound Dressing is a sterile, single-use bundle of absorbent matrix for use in moist wound dressing applications. The synthetic matrix absorbs excess exudate fluid, swells to conform to the wound contours, and entraps slough and necrotic debris within its strands to assist in debridement. FlexiGel Strands is flexible, pliable, and nonadherent to aid in comfort.

Indications
For use as an external wound dressing, for the management of exudate from chronic wounds such as ulcers (venous, arterial, diabetic); pressure sores; donor sites; surgical incisions and excisions; lacerations; and burns (first and second degree)

Contraindications
- Not for use if wound gets larger or shows signs of irritation (reddening, inflammation), maceration (over-hydration of skin), hypergraulation (excess tissue), or sensitivity (allergic reactions); in this event, a health care professional should be contacted
- Contraindicated if package is open or damaged before use
- For single-use only; shouldn't be reused (FlexiGel Strands should be removed during the dressing change and at the end of treatment)
- Contraindicated on third-degree burns

Application
- Cleanse wound.
- Apply a skin preparation to the periwound skin.
- Apply FlexiGel Strands.
- Apply a secondary dressing such as CovRSite or roll gauze (for venous leg ulcers, apply a compression wrap).
- Dressing may be cut at the middle connecting band to accommodate wounds of various volume. FlexiGel Strands expands as it absorbs. Apply to fill half of the wound cavity. Don't pack.

Removal
- Change once a day or when secondary dressing reveals wound drainage.

Gold Dust
Southwest Technologies, Inc.

How supplied
Packet: 3 g

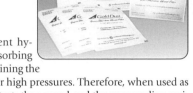

Action
Gold Dust is a highly absorbent hydrophillic polymer capable of absorbing 100 times its own weight and retaining the exudate in the matrix, even under high pressures. Therefore, when used as a wound dressing, Gold Dust protects the wound and the surrounding peri-wound area from maceration and degradation. Once the granules interact with wound exudate, the powder turns into a gel.

Indications
To manage heavy drainage

Contraindications
■ Not for use on wounds without drainage

Application
■ Wet the tissue with a small amount of water or saline solution, or add a thin layer of high-water-content amorphous hydrogel. It's recommended that Gold Dust be covered with a nonadherent dressing, such as Elastro-Gel wound dressing.
■ In some cases, Gold Dust must be removed, especially for patients with low tolerance for pain.
■ Gold Dust may be used as dry granules on highly exuding wounds, but the wounds must be monitored for the potential of overdrying of the tissue.
■ When managing moderate- to low-exuding wounds, premoisten Gold Dust granules to form a gel, to avoid overdrying the tissue.
■ Because of the high absorption capacity of the product, even Gold Dust as a premoistened gel can cause a burning or stinging sensation for the patient.

Removal
■ Product doesn't have to be changed daily.
■ Gold Dust may be flushed using saline solution or an irrigation system.

IODOFLEX
0.9% Cadexomer Iodine Pad

Smith & Nephew
Wound Management, Inc.

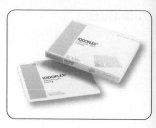

How supplied

Sterile pad: 5 g ($1^{1}/_{2}''$ × $2^{3}/_{8}''$), 10 g
                  ($2^{3}/_{8}''$ × $3''$); A6262

Action

IODOFLEX is an antimicrobial pad with the benefits of 0.9% Cadexomer
Iodine. Its unique smart-release formulation provides a slow, sustained release of iodine while absorbing slough, debris, and exudate from the wound
bed. IODO delivers sustained, broad-spectrum antimicrobial activity for
up to 72 hours. The pliable dressing allows easy shaping to fit wound contours.

Indications

For use in cleaning wet ulcers and wounds such as venous stasis ulcers,
pressure sores, and infected traumatic and surgical wounds

Contraindications

- Contraindicated in patients with a sensitivity to iodine
- Contraindicated in patients with Hashimoto's thyroiditis, Graves' disease, or nontoxic nodular goiter; only for cautious use in patients with
  a history of thyroid disorder, who are more susceptible to a change in
  thyroid metabolism with long-term use
- Contraindicated in pregnant or breast-feeding patients
- Contraindicated for internal use and use in eyes

Application

- Clean the wound and surrounding area with either a gentle stream of
  sterile water or saline. Gently blot any excess fluid, leaving the wound
  surface slightly moist.
- With gloved hand, remove carrier gauze on one or both sides of the
  IODOFLEX Pad. Place the pad in contact with the wound surface.
- Cover the wound with dry sterile gauze or dressing of choice. Apply compression bandaging where appropriate.

Removal

- Change IODOFLEX three times a week or when all the IODOFLEX has
  changed from brown to a yellow/gray.
- If necessary, soak the gauze for a few minutes, then remove.
- Remove IODOFLEX with sterile water or saline.
- Gently blot any excess fluid, leaving the wound surface slightly moist,
  before reapplying IODOFLEX. The number of applications should be
  reduced as the exudate diminishes.

IODOSORB

0.9% Cadexomer Iodine Gel

Smith & Nephew
Wound Management, Inc.

How supplied
Sterile tube: 40 g; A6261

Action
IODOSORB is an antimicrobial gel with the benefits of 0.9% Cadexomer Iodine. Its unique smart-release formulation provides a slow, sustained release of iodine while absorbing slough, debris, and exudate from the wound bed. IODOSORB delivers sustained, broad-spectrum antimicrobial activity for up to 72 hours.

Indications
For use in cleaning wet ulcers and wounds such as venous stasis ulcers, pressure sores, and infected traumatic and surgical wounds

Contraindications
- Contraindicated in patients with a sensitivity to iodine
- Contraindicated in patients with Hashimoto's thyroiditis, Graves' disease, or nontoxic nodular goiter; only for cautious use in patients with a history of thyroid disorder, who are more susceptible to a change in thyroid metabolism with long-term use
- Contraindicated in pregnant or breast-feeding patients
- Contraindicated for internal use and use in eyes

Application
- Clean the wound and surrounding area with either a gentle stream of sterile water or saline. Don't dry surface.
- Apply ¹⁄₈" to ¹⁄₄" thickness (0.3 to 0.5 cm) IODOSORB Gel onto dry gauze, sufficient to cover all parts of the wound. Larger amounts are unnecessary though not problematic.
- With gloved hands, position the prepared gauze onto the wound.
- A single application shouldn't exceed 1.8 oz (50 g) gel, and the total amount used in 1 week shouldn't exceed 5.3 oz (150 g).

Removal
- Change IODOSORB three times a week or when all the IODOSORB has changed from brown to a yellow/gray.
- Remove IODOSORB with either a gentle stream of sterile water or saline, using a sterile wet swab if necessary.
- Gently blot any excess fluid, leaving the wound surface slightly moist, before reapplying IODOSORB.

Multidex Maltodextrin Wound Dressing Gel or Powder
DeRoyal

How supplied
Powder: 6-g tube, 12-g tube, 25-g tube, 45-g tube; A6262
Gel: ¼ fl oz tube, ½ fl oz tube, 3 fl oz tube

Action
Multidex Maltodextrin Wound Dressing establishes and maintains a moist environment for tissue granulation by mixing with wound exudate, thus controlling dehydration, drainage, and odor.

Indications
To be used as a primary or secondary dressing to manage pressure ulcers (stages 2, 3, and 4), venous stasis ulcers, diabetic ulcers, neuropathic ulcers, and poorly healing wounds; may also be used on tunneling wounds, partial- and full-thickness wounds, infected and noninfected wounds, wounds with heavy or purulent drainage, and red, yellow, or black wounds

Contraindications
- None provided by the manufacturer

Application
- Irrigate the wound with normal saline solution.
- Apply the dressing over the entire wound to a minimum thickness of 1⅛" to 1¼" (0.3 to 0.5 cm). For deep wounds, fill to the skin surface.
- Cover with a nonadherent dressing.

Removal
- Remove the secondary dressing.
- Irrigate the wound with normal saline solution. Any remaining dressing may be left in the wound.

New Product

RadiaFDG Freeze Dried Gel Wound Dressing with Acemannan Hydrogel

Carrington Laboratories, Inc.

How supplied
Wafer: 4″ diameter

Action
RadiaFDG Freeze Dried Gel absorbs excess fluid. When rehydrated, it becomes a gel, forming a protective layer over affected skin. Sterile and preservative free, it contains acemannan hydrogel and facilitates the natural healing process.

Indications
For radiation dermatitis with moderate exudate and moist desquamation

Contraindications
- Contraindicated on patients with a sensitivity to acemannan hydrogel or any other component of the dressing

Application
- Flush wound with a suitable cleanser such as RadiaKlenz.
- Peel open package, and remove RadiaFDG in an aseptic manner.
- Apply to wound bed by folding into wound or tearing to pack undermined areas.
- Cover with a secondary dressing such as RadiaDres Gel Sheet, CarraSmart Foam, or CarraSmart Film.

Removal
- Flush wound with a suitable cleanser such as RadiaKlenz.

Other products

This category comprises a wide variety of products used to facilitate skin and wound management. Each entry details the product's:

- action
- indications
- contraindications
- application
- removal.

Please refer to each product listing for further information about these products.

In this section, the manufacturer has either received a HCPCS code or hasn't yet received or applied for a code. It's the clinician's responsibility to verify coding of each product with the product's manufacturer.

Biobrane and Biobrane-L Temporary Wound Dressings
Mylan Bertek Pharmaceuticals Inc.

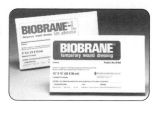

How supplied
Biobrane
Dressing: 5″ × 5″, 5″ × 15″, 10″ × 15″, 15″ × 20″

Biobrane-L
Dressing: 5″ × 5″, 5″ × 15″, 10″ × 15″

Action
Biobrane is a biocomposite dressing made from an ultrathin, semipermeable silicone membrane bonded to a flexible knitted trifilament nylon fabric; Biobrane-L utilizes a monofilament nylon. A nontoxic mixture of highly purified peptides derived from porcine dermal collagen has been bonded to the nylon/silicone membrane to provide a highly flexible and conformable composite dressing with adherence properties and a hydrophilic, biocompatible surface. The semipermeable silicone membrane controls water vapor loss at rates comparable to normal skin and provides a flexible adherent covering for the wound surface. It conforms to surface irregularities, allowing joint movement and early ambulation, and minimizes the proliferation of bacteria on the wound surface by minimizing dead space.

Indications
For clean partial-thickness burn wounds and donor sites (Biobrane); for meshed autografts (Biobrane-L)

Contraindications
- Not for use if a patient shows evidence of an allergic reaction (remove the dressing, and discontinue its use)

Application
- Application should be made to freshly debrided or excised wounds. The debridement or excision must be done thoroughly to remove all coagulum or eschar. Biobrane or Biobrane-L won't adhere to dead tissue, and any remaining necrotic tissue may cause infection.
- Establish hemostasis before applying the dressing.
- Apply Biobrane or Biobrane-L dull side down, wrinkle-free against the wound surface with slight tension.
- Secure the dressing in place. Under slight tension, immobilize the dressing using staples, tape, sutures, or skin closure strips. Wrap the area with a dry gauze dressing or another stenting device to hold the dressing firmly in contact with the wound surface for 24 to 36 hours.

OTHER PRODUCTS

Patient teaching

- 24 hours postapplication
  - Don't remove the outer dressing. Don't get the dressing wet.
  - Don't move the covered area more than necessary.
- 24 to 36 hours postapplication
  - Remove the outer dressing down to Biobrane/Biobrane-L, and observe the following:
  - If Biobrane or Biobrane-L is adherent and no fluid has accumulated, rewrap with gauze for protection.
  - If Biobrane or Biobrane-L is loose, but the underlying tissue is still viable, aspirate or roll out any nonpurulent fluid collection, rewrap with a gauze dressing, and observe in 24 hours for adherence.
  - If Biobrane or Biobrane-L is loose and there is purulent drainage underneath, remove the purulent nonadherent areas, and use conventional topical antimicrobial therapy to reduce bacterial contamination to safe levels.
- 48 to 72 hours postapplication
  - Remove the outer dressing down to Biobrane or Biobrane-L, and check for adherence. If adherent, the outer dressing need not be reapplied. If nonadherent, treat as referenced above.
  - Observe the covered wound daily for bubbles and purulence, and treat as referenced above. Biobrane or Biobrane-L should be removed from wound areas showing signs of infection.
  - Remove staples, tape, sutures, or skin-closure strips 3 to 4 days after application or when adherence is achieved.
  - Once Biobrane or Biobrane-L is adherent, bathing according to standard burn unit protocols and motion of the burned area can be initiated.

Removal

- Remove Biobrane or Biobrane-L when the tissue underneath is healed, typically 7 to 14 days. The dressing should be dry and loose in spots, and the patient may report itching.
- If edges are loose, they can be trimmed away until the entire wound has healed.
- Remove by starting at one corner and pulling gently.
- Biobrane or Biobrane-L will peel off healed tissue relatively easily. The application of a petroleum-based ointment or soaking prior to removal facilitates the removal process.

Caution: If bleeding occurs, or if patient complains of excessive pain, stop removal of the dressing, and wait 1 to 2 additional days. Forced removal may result in wound reinjury. Also, if Biobrane or Biobrane-L becomes adherent to a partial-thickness wound that has progressed to a full-thickness wound, it should be removed in the operating room.

Carrington Oral Wound Rinse
Carrington Laboratories, Inc.

How supplied
Powder: 9.4 g

Action
Carrington Oral Wound Rinse is a mild, pleasant tasting, slightly viscous liquid when reconstituted. It's provided in a powdered form and mixed with water before use. Carrington Oral Wound Rinse relieves the pain of oral lesions by adhering to injured tissue of the oral mucosa, cooling the wound surface, and due to high moisture content, protecting exposed nerve surfaces while allowing the injury to heal.

Indications
For all types of oral wounds (mouth sores and injuries), aphthous ulcers, canker sores, and traumatic ulcers such as those caused by ill-fitting braces or dentures

Contraindications
- None provided by the manufacturer

Application
- Fill the bottle with water to the first arrow, then shake vigorously until all particles go into suspension. Fill the bottle with water to the second arrow and shake again to mix.
- Swish or gargle 1 tablespoon of Carrington Oral Wound Rinse liquid suspension in the mouth for at least 1 minute or as long as possible. Increased contact time enhances effectiveness. Carrington Oral Wound Rinse is safe if swallowed.
- Swish or gargle four times a day or more often, if needed. Again, Carrington Oral Wound Rinse is safe if swallowed
- Avoid eating or drinking for 1 hour after use, allowing Carrington Oral Wound Rinse to remain in contact with irritated tissue for as long as possible.

Removal
- Not applicable.

OTHER PRODUCTS

CHONDROPROTEC
The Hymed Group Corporation

How supplied
Vial: 5 ml/500 mg
            10 ml/1,000 mg

Action
CHONDROPROTEC, a polysulfated glycosaminoglycan, is a
unique topical wound management dressing. CHONDROPROTEC creates
a moist healing environment, protects new granulation tissue, conforms
to any wound site, is easy to apply and redress, and promotes natural autolysis by rehydrating and softening necrotic tissue and eschar, thereby encouraging autolytic debridement.

Indications
To manage pressure ulcers (stages 1, 2, 3, and 4), venous stasis ulcers, first-
and second-degree burns, secreting and bleeding dermal lesions, trauma
injuries, partial- and full-thickness wounds, surgical incisions, and donor
sites

Contraindications
- Not indicated for use as a long-term or permanent dressing.

Application
- If the wound is contaminated or infected, debride it before using CHON-
  DROPROTEC.
- Irrigate wound with normal saline solution.
- Either pour contents of vial or dispense from syringe to withdraw solu-
  tion and cover wound site.
- Cover with a nonadherant dressing such as polyurethane film (PUF) or
  Telfa. *Note:* Subsequent applications of CHONDROPROTEC can be ad-
  ministered through the dressing to not disturb the wound bed.

Removal
- Reapply CHONDROPROTEC daily, and redress the wound site every 5
  to 7 days or as needed.

E-Z Derm Biosynthetic Porcine Wound Dressing

Brennen Medical, LLC

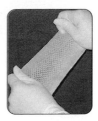

How supplied

Patch, non-perforated: 2″ × 2″, 3″ × 4″
Patch, perforated/meshed: 2″ × 2″, 3″ × 4″

Action

E-Z Derm protects partial-thickness wound beds from bacteria during proliferation and migration of the epithelial cells from the wound margins or
skin appendages.

Indications

For temporary protective coverage of partial-thickness wounds, such as
burns, ulcers, donor sites, and nail avulsion, and as an autograft test graft
for full-thickness wounds

Contraindications

- Contraindicated on patients with multiple or serum allergies
- Contraindicated over large areas of adherent eschar
- Not for use on deep, split-thickness, skin donor sites

Application

- Apply E-Z Derm to partial-thickness wounds as soon as possible after
  the injury occurs. Delay allows for wound bed drying or crusting, which
  retards epithelial regeneration.
- Thoroughly clean the wound and remove all debris and necrotic tissue.
  Even small amounts of resident bacteria or excessive fluid loss may pre-
  vent E-Z Derm from adhering.
- Sterilely remove E-Z Derm from its package. Apply either side of the E-Z
  Derm to the wound.
- Wrap with light gauze or tubular net dressing.
- Monitor for 24 hours, then inspect every 12 to 24 hours to detect any
  purulent accumulations under the skin. If a rash unrelated to other therapy or systemic antibiotic therapy occurs, discontinue use of E-Z Derm.
- If E-Z Derm doesn't adhere, thoroughly clean the wound and reapply
  new E-Z Derm. If E-Z Derm hasn't begun to adhere after 48 hours or
  four to five changes, take wound cultures to monitor wound status. Use
  an appropriate antibiotic to eradicate any gram-negative bacteria. Failure to adhere usually indicates original misdiagnosis of wound depth
  or bacterial proliferation.

Removal

- As epithelium regenerates, E-Z Derm sloughs from the injured area.
- Areas of dry, nonadherent E-Z Derm indicate subsurface healing and
  should be trimmed away.

OTHER PRODUCTS

Flexi-Seal Fecal Management System*
ConvaTec

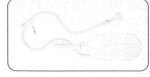

How supplied
Flexi-Seal FMS Kit: 1 kit or box
Flexi-Seal FMS Replacement Collection Bags: 10/box

Action
The Flexi-Seal Fecal Management System contains 1 soft silicone catheter tube assembly, 1 syringe, and 3 collection bags. The soft silicone catheter is inserted into the rectum for fecal management to contain and divert fecal waste to protect the patient's skin and keep the bedding clean. There is a low-pressure retention balloon at one end and a connector for attaching the collection bag at the other end.

Indications
For the fecal management of patients with little or no bowel control and liquid or semiliquid stool

Contraindications
- Not intended for use
  - for more than 29 consecutive days
  - for pediatric patients.
- Not for use on individuals who
  - have suspected or confirmed rectal mucosal impairment (that is, severe proctitis, ischemic proctitis, mucosal ulcerations)
  - have had rectal surgery within the past year
  - have any rectal or anal injury
  - have hemorrhoids of significant size and/or symptoms
  - have a rectal or anal stricture or stenosis
  - have a suspected or confirmed rectal or anal tumor
  - have any in-dwelling rectal or anal device (for example, thermometer) or delivery mechanism (for example, suppositories or enemas) in place
  - are sensitive to or who have had an allergic reaction to any components within the kit.

Application
Preparation of device
- In addition to the device kit, gloves and lubricant will be required.
- Using the syringe provided, remove any residual air that may be in the balloon by attaching the syringe to the inflation port and withdrawing the plunger. Ensure that the syringe is empty by expelling any air. Then fill this empty syringe with 45 ml tap water or saline. Don't overfill beyond 45 ml.

- Attach the syringe to the inflation port (marked 45 ml).
- Securely snap the collection bag to the connector at the end of the catheter.

Preparation of patient
- Position the patient in left side-lying position; if unable to tolerate, position the patient so access to the rectum is possible.
- Perform a digital rectal exam to evaluate suitability for insertion of device.

Insertion of device
- Remove any indwelling or anal device prior to insertion of the Flexi-Seal FMS device.
- Unfold the length of the catheter to lay it flat on the bed, extending the collection bag toward the foot of the bed. Insert a lubricated, gloved index finger into the retention balloon cuff finger pocket for digital guidance during device insertion. The finger pocket is located above the position indicator line. Coat the balloon end of the catheter with lubricating jelly. Grasp the catheter and gently insert the balloon end through the anal sphincter until the balloon is beyond the external orifice and well inside the rectal vault. The finger may be removed or remain in place in the rectum during balloon inflation.
- Inflate the balloon with 45 ml of water or saline by slowly depressing the syringe plunger. Under no circumstances should the balloon be inflated with more than 45 ml. The oval inflation indication chamber on the inflation port will expand as fluid is injected. This normal expansion should subside once the plunger stops. If the inflation indication chamber remains excessively expanded after the plunger stops, the balloon is not properly inflating. This is likely the result of improper balloon positioning in the rectal vault. In this case, use the syringe to withdraw the fluid from the balloon, reposition the balloon in the rectal vault and reinflate the balloon.
- Remove the syringe from the inflation port, and gently pull on the soft silicone catheter to check that the balloon is securely in the rectum and that it's positioned against the rectal floor.
- Position the length of the flexible silicone catheter along patient's leg avoiding kinks and obstructions. Take note of the position indicator line relative to the patient's anus. Regularly observe changes in the location of the position indicator line as a means to determine movement of the retention balloon in the patient's rectum. This may indicate the need for the balloon or device to be repositioned.
- Hang the bag by the strap on the bedside at a position lower than that of the patient.

Irrigation of the device
- The silicone catheter can be rinsed by filling the syringe with tap water at room temperature and attaching the syringe to the irrigation port (marked IRRIG.) and depressing the plunger. Make sure that the syringe

OTHER PRODUCTS

isn't inadvertently attached to the balloon inflation port (marked 45 ml). Repeat the irrigation procedure as often as necessary to maintain proper functioning of the device. Flushing the device as described above is an optional procedure for use only when needed to maintain the unobstructed flow of stool into the collection bag. If repeated flushing with water does not return the flow of stool through the catheter, the device should be inspected to ascertain that there is no external obstruction (pressure from a body part, piece of equipment, or resolution of diarrhea). If no source of obstruction of the device is detected, use of the device should be discontinued.

Maintenance of device

- Change the collection bag as needed. Snap the cap onto each used bag and discard according to institutional protocol for disposal of medical waste. Observe the device frequently for obstructions from kinks, solid fecal particles, or external pressure.

Removal

- To remove the catheter from the rectum, the retention balloon must first be deflated. Attach the syringe to the inflation port, and slowly withdraw all water from the retention balloon. Disconnect the syringe and discard.
- Grasp the catheter as close to the patient as possible, and slowly slide it out of the anus.
- Dispose of the device in accordance with institutional protocol for disposal of medical waste.

*See package insert for complete instructions for use.

OTHER PRODUCTS

Hyalofill-F Biopolymeric Wound Dressing*

ConvaTec

How supplied

Dressing: 2″ × 2″, 4″ × 4″; A6196
Ribbon: 0.5 g

Action

Hyalofill-F Biopolymeric Wound Dressing is an absorbent and conformable, fibrous fleece composed of Hyaff, an ester of hyaluronic acid. As it absorbs wound exudate, it forms a soft, cohesive gel that provides a moist wound environment, aiding autolytic debridement and allowing nontraumatic removal without damaging newly formed tissue.

Indications

To manage leg ulcers, pressure ulcers (stages 1, 2, 3, and 4), diabetic ulcers, surgical wounds, second-degree burns, and wounds prone to bleeding, such as mechanically or surgically debrided wounds, donor sites, and traumatic wounds. May also be used on abrasions, lacerations, and minor cuts

Contraindications

- Contraindicated in patients with hypersensitivity to this product or to avian proteins

Application

- Clean the wound, rinse well, and dry the surrounding skin.
- Place the Hyalofill Biopolymeric Wound Dressing onto the surface of the lesion.
- Cover with a sterile secondary dressing.

Removal

- Dressings applied to heavily exuding or sloughy wounds may need daily replacement initially, then every 2 to 3 days as exudate decreases
- Thoroughly irrigating the wound with sterile saline solution or using forceps or gloved fingers may aid removal.

*See package insert for complete instructions for use.

OTHER PRODUCTS

HYCOAT
The Hymed Group

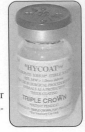

How supplied
Vial: 2 ml/20 mg, 6 ml/30 mg, 10 ml/50 mg

Action
HYCOAT is a sterile solution of sodium hyaluronate for use in chronic and acute wounds and as a protective tissue coating.

Indications
For use on pressure ulcers (stages 1, 2, 3, and 4), acute wounds, first- and second-degree burns, surgical wounds, venous stasis wounds, autograft procedures

Contraindication
- Not for use as a permanent or long-term dressing

Application
- Wounds that are contaminated and/or infected should be debrided before using the HYCOAT product.
- Cleanse wound/surgical site with saline.
- Open vial or use syringe to withdraw the solution.
- Either pour directly from vial or dispense from syringe onto affected area.
- Cover treated area with a nonadherent dressing.

Removal
- Change dressing as needed, repeating application of HYCOAT.

InterDry Ag
Coloplast Corp.

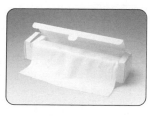

How supplied
Box/Roll: 10″ × 12″ impregnated textile

Action

InterDry Ag is a nonsterile skin protectant composed of polyurethane-coated polyester textile impregnated with an antimicrobial silver complex as the active component. It's a single-patient-use product that is custom cut from a multiuse package. The textile provides moisture transportation to keep skin dry, while the antimicrobial in the textile reduces odor. The textile's low friction surface aids lubrication, thereby reducing skin-to-skin friction. The product provides a protective environment for the skin and an effective protection against microbial contamination in the device. The device is an effective antimicrobial barrier against gram-positive and gram-negative bacteria and fungi, including methicillin-resistant *Staphylococcus aureus* (MRSA), methicillin-resistant *S. epidermidis* (MRSE), vancomycin-resistant *Enterococcus faecalis* (VRE), *Klebsiella pneumoniae*, *Pseudomonas aeruginosa*, *Aspergillus niger*, and *Candida albicans*.

Indications

For management of skin folds and other skin-to-skin contact areas; to provide an antimicrobial barrier to microbial colonization in the dressing; for use with compression bandaging (may be placed over wound dressings)

Contraindication

- Not for use on patients with a sensitivity to silver. In case of suspected allergic reaction, contact Coloplast for further information.
- Not for use during radiation treatment or examinations that include X-rays, ultrasonic treatment, diathermy, microwaves, or MRI
- Not for use on highly exudating wounds

Application

- The use of InterDry Ag during pregnancy and lactation and on children hasn't been demonstrated.
- Measure and cut the appropriate length of textile allowing for 5 cm (2″) of textile exposure to the air on each side of the skin fold.
- Place one edge of the textile in the base of the skin fold. Gently smooth the rest of the cloth over the skin keeping the textile flat, covering any wound dressings.
- Gently place skin fold together, with 5 cm (2″) of textile exposed to air at each cut end.
- Separate the skin fold to assess the skin and placement of the textile daily or as indicated by normal practice.

OTHER PRODUCTS

- For use on an extremity, loosely wrap the textile around the area of skin to be protected. Secure with tape or other suitable device.

Removal

- InterDry Ag may be left in place for up to 5 days, depending on the amount of moisture, the general skin condition and the use of wound dressings.
- When removing the textile from a skin fold, gently separate the skin fold, and lift away the textile.

Mepiform Soft Silicone Gel Sheeting
Mölnlycke Health Care

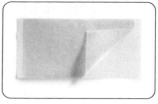

How supplied
Dressing: 2″ × 3″, 4″ × 7″, 1.6″ × 12″

Action
Mepiform is a self-adherent soft silicone gel sheeting for scar management featuring Safetac technology that's breathable, comfortable, and waterproof. Mepiform is thin, flexible, and discreet and can be worn during all daily activities.

Indications
For the management of old and new hypertrophic and keloid scars; can be used on closed wounds where it may prevent the formation of hypertrophic and keloid scars; may be used prophylactically for 2 to 6 months, depending on the condition of the scar

Contraindications
- None provided by the manufacturer

Application
- Clean the scar tissue or closed wound with mild soap and water. Rinse and pat dry. Make sure the scar and surrounding skin are dry.
- If necessary, cut the dressing to the appropriate shape.
- Remove the release film, and apply the dressing to the scar without stretching the dressing.
- Avoid the use of creams or ointments under Mepiform.

Removal
- Optimally, Mepiform should be worn 24 hours/day. It's recommended that Mepiform be removed once a day for showering or bathing and reapplied.
- Change the dressing when it begins to lose its adherent properties. Dressing wear time varies by person.

OTHER PRODUCTS

NovaGel Silicone Gel Sheeting
Brennen Medical, LLC

How supplied
Sheet: 5" × 6" A6025

Action
NovaGel Silicone Gel Sheeting is a soft, slightly adhesive
scar dressing intended to reduce the height and coloring of the scar. It's
made from medical-grade silicone and reinforced with a polyester mesh
placed within the silicone sheet.

Indications
For use as a scar management dressing on old and new hypertropic (raised)
or keloid scars

Contraindications
- Contraindicated in patients with mitigating medical conditions (such
  as open wounds), dermatologic conditions (such as rashes), or disorders that may cause the skin to break out during use of NovaGel
- Contraindicated for open wounds

Application
- Wash scar site, then dry with a clean, dry towel.
- Remove NovaGel from the tray. The nylon net overlay may remain on
  the top side of NovaGel to help prevent adherence to clothes.
- If needed, trim NovaGel to a size and shape slightly larger than the scar
  to be covered. Multiple sheets may be used, side by side, to cover a large
  scar. Place NovaGel on the scar.
- Secure with an appropriate tape or support bandage covering to ensure
  that the NovaGel doesn't slide off the scar site.

Removal
- NovaGel may be worn for up to 24 hours per day (a minimum of 12
  hours per day is recommended). After 24 hours, remove, clean, and reapply NovaGel.
- After removing NovaGel, wash scar site and NovaGel gently with mild
  soap and warm water. Dry scar site and NovaGel, then reapply NovaGel.
  (Remove the nylon net overlay when cleaning the NovaGel. Replace nylon net overlay before reapplying the NovaGel.)
- Each NovaGel sheet can be used for 10 to 14 days. NovaGel may lose its
  adhesive qualities or become imbedded with surface dirt over time. If
  this occurs, discard the used NovaGel and apply a fresh sheet.
- If rash and pruritus occur beneath NovaGel (usually from poor hygiene
  at the scar site), limit application of the NovaGel to 12-hour periods,
  then remove for 12 hours. If symptoms persist, discontinue use of Nova-
  Gel.

OTHER PRODUCTS

OASIS Wound Matrix
Healthpoint, Ltd.

How supplied
Fenestrated: 3 × 3.5 cm (10 sheets), 3 × 7 cm
(10 sheets), 7 × 10 cm (5 sheets),
7 × 20 cm (5 sheets)
Meshed: 7 × 10 cm (5 sheets), 7 × 20 cm (5 sheets)
Burn Matrix: 7 × 20 cm bilaminate mesh (5 sheets)
CPT codes: 15430 and 15431
J code: J7341

Action
OASIS works by providing a natural, extracellular matrix with a three-dimensional structure that acts as a scaffold for host-tissue remodeling.

Indications
For the management of partial- and full-thickness skin loss injury, such as pressure and chronic vascular ulcers, diabetic ulcers, second-degree burns, abrasions, and autograft donor sites

Contraindications
- Not for use on patients with sensitivity to porcine material

Application
- Gently clean the wound.
- Cut the dry OASIS sheet to size, and apply the sheet on the wound surface.
- Rehydrate using sterile saline or lactated Ringer's solution, and anchor with choice of fixative.

Removal
- OASIS remodels like tissue and, therefore, isn't removed from the wound. Additional OASIS is added as needed.

New Product

Oleeva Clear
Bio Med Sciences, Inc.

How supplied
Dressing: 1.5″ × 5″, 5″ × 5″, 5″ × 10″, 8″ × 12″; A6025

Action
Oleeva Clear is used topically to reduce or prevent hypertrophic scars and keloids.

Indications
Used topically to reduce or prevent hypertrophic scars and keloids resulting from traumatic or surgical injury

Contraindications
- Not for use on open wounds
- Not for use with creams or lotions
- Not for use on patients with sensitivity to silicone

Application
- Remove the product from its package. If necessary, use scissors to trim the product so it extends beyond the area of the scar.
- Peel away the paper protective liner and save it for later use.
- Place the product sticky side down, directly on the scarred area.
- Keep the product in place from 12 to 23 hours per day.
- At least once a day, wash the scarred area and both sides of the product with mild soap and water. Rinse the product thoroughly to remove all traces of soap.
- Allow the product to air-dry, or pat it dry with a lint-free towel before reapplying.
- Between uses, product may be stored on the protective paper liner.

Removal
- Remove daily, wash with mild soap and water, allow product to dry, and reapply.

OTHER PRODUCTS

New Product

Oleeva Fabric

Bio Med Sciences, Inc.

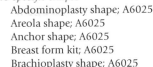

How supplied

Dressing: 1.5" × 5", 5" × 5", 5" × 10", 8" × 12"; A6025

Procedure-specific shapes

> Abdominoplasty shape; A6025
> Areola shape; A6025
> Anchor shape; A6025
> Breast form kit; A6025
> Brachioplasty shape; A6025
> C Section shape, A6025
> Umbilicoplasty shape; A6025
> Vertical mastopexy; A6025

OTHER PRODUCTS

Action

Oleeva Fabric is used topically to reduce or prevent hypertrophic scars and keloids.

Indications

Used topically to reduce or prevent hypertrophic scars and keloids resulting from traumatic or surgical injury

Contraindications

- Not for use on open wounds
- Contraindicated with creams or lotions
- Contraindicated on patients with sensitivity to silicone

Application

- Remove the product from its package. If necessary, use scissors to trim the product so it extends beyond the area of the scar.
- Peel away the paper protective liner, and save it for later use.
- Place the product sticky side down, directly on the scarred area.
- Keep the product in place from 12 to 23 hours per day.
- At least once a day, wash the scarred area and both sides of the product with mild soap and water. Rinse the product thoroughly to remove all traces of soap.
- Allow the product to air-dry, or pat it dry with a lint-free towel before reapplying.
- Between uses, product may be stored on the protective paper liner.

Removal

- Remove daily, wash with mild soap and water, allow product to dry, and reapply.

Provant Wound Therapy System

Regenesis Biomedical, Inc.

How supplied

Durable Medical Equipment product (portable system carrying case, treatment applicator pad, and disposable infection-control covers): E0769

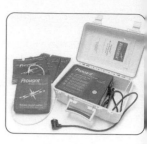

Action

The Provant Wound Therapy System, based on Cell Proliferation Induction (CPI) technology, is a medical device that induces proliferation of fibroblasts and epithelial cells. Fibroblasts initiate wound healing and trigger the biochemical cascade that leads to granulation in the wound bed. Epithelial cells complete the healing and closure process. This device also stimulates secretion of multiple growth factors within the first treatment through a calcium-dependent cellular mechanism. Recent studies show that Provant induced the expression of hundreds of genes controlling all phases of wound healing, including inflammatory, granulation, epithelialization, and remodeling. The CPI treatment signal penetrates 7 to 8 cm through dressings and damaged tissue layers to initiate these critical events.

Provant is a lightweight and portable medical device about the size and shape of a briefcase. Provant is so simple to use that a patient or caregiver can perform the treatment without the aid of a skilled practitioner.

Indications

To treat symptoms of the inflammatory phase of wound healing in soft tissues, thus inducing subsequent granulation, epithelialization, and angiogenesis throughout multiple phases of the wound-healing process; may be used on patients soon after surgery or on patients with chronic and recalcitrant wounds after surgical debridement; intended for use in conjunction with all other wound therapies

Contraindications

- Contraindicated for treatment of bone or deep internal organs and for use over joints of patients with immature bone development
- Contraindicated on pregnant patients
- Contraindicated on patients who have metallic implants in the area of application or who have cardiac pacemakers

Application

- Connect the system's base unit to a power outlet.
- Place a single-use, disposable, infection control cover over the treatment applicator pad before each use.
- The system delivers a manufacturer-preset therapeutic dose to the treatment area through the applicator pad. The recommended Provant ther-

apy schedule is 30 minutes in the morning and again in the evening until the desired effect is achieved. No adjustments by patient or caregiver are necessary or possible.

- Provant treatment dosing penetrates directly through wound dressings, casts, Unna boots, and clothes. No removal of dressings is required. When treatment is complete, Provant turns off automatically.
- In hospitals and long-term care facilities, a wound care nurse or a physical therapist typically administers the therapy. In outpatient settings, the primary care provider typically prescribes the therapy for administration by the patient, family member, or other caregiver twice daily at home between regular office visits for supervision of wound protocols.

Removal

- Discard the infection control cover after each 30 minute treatment.

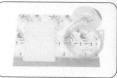

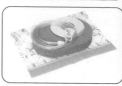

New Product

V.A.C. Dressings*
KCI

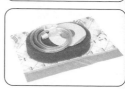

How supplied
Foam: Variety

Action
V.A.C. GranuFoam Dressing is a black, polyurethane foam dressing with a reticulated, open
cell design that provides uniform distribution
of pressure at the wound site. The 400- to 600-
micron pore size induces promotion of granulation tissue formation and new cell growth.
Hydrophobic (moisture repelling) foam effectively removes fluid and infectious materials,
allowing wound healing progression.

The V.A.C. GranuFoam Silver Dressing is the
above-mentioned open-celled, reticulated poly-
urethane foam that has been microbonded with metallic silver via a proprie-
tary metallization process. During V.A.C. Therapy, exposure of the dressing
to wound fluid results in oxidation of metallic silver to ionic silver, allowing the continuous, sustained release of silver ions for antimicrobial activity
against microorganisms that come in contact with the ions.

V.A.C. WhiteFoam Dressing is a polyvinyl alcohol foam with a dense,
open pore design and a high tensile strength, ideal for use in tunnels and
undermining. It's hydrophilic (or moisture retaining) and premoistened
with sterile water. It's generally recommended for use in wounds where the
growth of granulation tissue into the foam needs to be controlled or when
the patient cannot tolerate V.A.C. GranuFoam because of discomfort.

Indications
For use with the V.A.C. family of negative-pressure wound therapy systems
to help promote wound healing in chronic, acute, traumatic, sub-acute and
dehisced wounds, partial-thickness burns, pressure and diabetic ulcers,
flaps, and grafts

Contraindications
- Not intended to come into direct contact with exposed blood vessels,
  organs, or nerves
- Contraindicated on patients with malignancy in the wound, untreated
  osteomyelitis, nonenteric and unexplored fistulas, necrotic tissue with
  eschar present, sensitivity to silver (V.A.C. GranuFoam Silver Dressing
  only)

OTHER PRODUCTS

Application

- Always use V.A.C. Dressings from sterile packages that have not been opened or damaged.
- Don't place any foam dressing into blind or unexplored tunnels. The V.A.C. WhiteFoam Dressing may be more appropriate for use with explored tunnels.
- Don't force foam dressings into any area of the wound, as this may damage tissue, alter delivery of negative pressure, or hinder exudate removal.
- Always count the total number of pieces of foam used in the dressing, and document that number on the drape and in the patient's chart. Also document the dressing change date on the drape.
- Consult a physician, and review all V.A.C. Therapy Instructions for Use and the V.A.C. Therapy Clinical Guidelines Reference Manual before use.

Removal

- Routine dressing changes are recommended every 48 hours unless the patient status requires earlier removal.
- Dressing changes for infected wounds should occur every 12 to 24 hours.
- Always replace all disposable components with new sterile dressing components.

*See package insert for complete instructions for use and safety information.

OTHER PRODUCTS

V.A.C. Therapy*

KCl

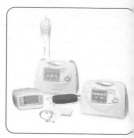

How supplied

*V.A.C. ATS unit, V.A.C. Freedom unit, V.A.C.
          Instill unit;* E2402
V.A.C. Dressing kit (small, medium, large);
          A6550
Other V.A.C. Dressing kit components; A6550
V.A.C. Canister with or without Isolyser; A6551

Action

V.A.C. Therapy is the controlled application of subatmospheric pressure to
a wound using a therapy unit to intermittently or continuously convey negative pressure to a specialized wound dressing to help promote wound
healing. The wound dressing is a resilient, open-cell foam surface dressing
(such as GranuFoam and Vers-Foam) that assists tissue granulation and is
sealed with an adhesive drape that contains the subatmospheric pressure
at the wound site. Special T.R.A.C. technology** enhances patient safety
by regulating pressure at the wound site. Additionally, the V.A.C. Therapy
System helps direct drainage to a specially designed canister that reduces
the risk of exposure to exudate fluids and infectious materials.

Indications

Used to help promote wound healing, through means including removal
of infectious material or other fluids, under the influence of continuous
and/or intermittent negative pressure, particularly for chronic, acute, traumatic, subacute, and dehisced wounds, partial-thickness burns, ulcers (such
as diabetic or pressure), flaps, and grafts

Contraindications

- Not intended to come into direct contact with exposed blood vessels,
  organs, or nerves
- Not for use if there is a malignancy in the wound
- Not for use with untreated osteomyelitis
- Not for use with nonenteric and unexplored fistulas
- Not for use with necrotic tissue with eschar (may be used after de-
  bridement of necrotic tissue and complete removal of eschar)
- Not for use on patients with a sensitivity to silver (V.A.C. GranuFoam
  Silver Dressing only)

Application

- V.A.C. Dressings should be changed routinely every 48 hours for noninfected wounds, or every 12 to 24 hours for infected wounds.
- If negative pressure is off for more than 2 hours in a 24-hour period, remove V.A.C. Dressing. When V.A.C. Therapy is restarted, irrigate the

wound per physician or institution protocol, and apply new V.A.C. Dressing from an unopened sterile package.

- Always use a V.A.C. Dressing from an unopened sterile package. V.A.C. Dressing components are disposable and are for single use only. They aren't to be reused.
- Remove and discard previous dressing per institution protocol.
- Debride all necrotic, nonviable tissue, including bone, eschar, or hardened slough, as prescribed by the physician.
- Perform thorough wound and periwound area cleaning per physician order or institution protocol prior to each dressing application.
- Ensure adequate hemostasis has been achieved.
- Protect vessels, organs, and nerves by covering them with natural tissues or several layers of fine-meshed, nonadherent dressing that form a complete barrier between the structures and the foam dressing.
- Consult a physician if bone fragments and/or sharp edges are present in the wound area, as these must be eliminated prior to dressing application.
- Clean and dry periwound tissue. Use of a skin preparation product to protect periwound tissue may also improve adhesion and assist with the integrity of the dressing seal.
- Assess wound dimensions and pathology, including the presence of undermining or tunnels.
- Use V.A.C. WhiteFoam Dressing with explored tunnels. Don't place any foam dressing into blind/unexplored tunnels.
- Cut foam dressing to dimensions that will allow the foam to be placed gently into the wound, but not overlap onto intact skin.
- Don't cut the foam over the wound, as fragments may fall into the wound.
- Gently place foam into wound cavity, ensuring contact with all wound surfaces.
- Don't force foam dressing into any area of the wound.
- Ensure foam-to-foam contact for even distribution of negative pressure.
- Always note the total number of pieces of foam used in the dressing, and document on the drape and in the patient's chart.
- Superficial or retention sutures should be covered with a single layer of nonadherent dressing prior to drape placement.
- Trim and place the V.A.C. Drape to cover the foam dressing and an additional 3- to 5-cm border of intact periwound tissue.
- V.A.C. Drape may be cut into multiple pieces for easier handling.
- Don't cut off the T.R.A.C. Pad or insert the tubing into the foam dressing. This may occlude the tubing and cause the therapy unit to alarm.
- Choose T.R.A.C. Pad application site. Give particular consideration to fluid flow, tubing positioning to allow for optimal drainage, and avoiding placement over bony prominences or within creases in the tissue.
- Pinch the drape, and cut a 2-cm hole through the drape. The hole should be large enough to allow for removal of fluid and/or exudate. It's not necessary to cut into the foam.

- Apply T.R.A.C. Pad.
- Remove V.A.C. Canister from sterile packaging and insert into the V.A.C Therapy Unit until it locks into place.
- Connect T.R.A.C. Pad tubing to canister tubing, and ensure that the clamp on each tube is open. Position clamps away from patient.
- Turn on power to the V.A.C. Therapy Unit, and select the prescribed therapy setting. Refer to the V.A.C. Therapy Clinical Guidelines for specific recommendations.
- Initiate V.A.C. Therapy. Assess dressing to ensure seal integrity. The dressing should be collapsed.
- V.A.C. GranuFoam and V.A.C. GranuFoam Silver Dressings should have a wrinkled appearance. There should be no hissing sounds.
- If there is any evidence of nonintegrity, check T.R.A.C. Pad and drape seals, tubing connections, and canister insertion, and ensure that clamps are open. Secure excess tubing to prevent interference with patient mobility.
- If a leak source is identified, patch with additional drape to ensure seal integrity.
- Multiple layers of the V.A.C. Drape may decrease the moisture vapor transmission rate, which may increase the risk of maceration, especially in small wounds, lower extremities, or load-bearing areas.

Removal

- Change the V.A.C. dressing every 48 hours or, if infection is present, every 12 to 24 hours.
- To remove the dressing, raise the tubing connectors above the level of the therapy unit.
- Tighten the clamp on the dressing tubing.
- Separate the canister tubing and dressing tubing by disconnecting the connector.
- Allow the therapy unit to pull the exudate in the canister tubing into the canister. Then, tighten the clamp on the canister tubing.
- Press the THERAPY ON/OFF button to deactivate the pump.
- Gently stretch the drape horizontally, and slowly pull up from the skin. Don't peel.
- Gently remove the foam from the wound.

Note: If the dressing adheres to the wound base, consider applying a single layer of nonadherent, porous material between the dressing and the wound when reapplying the dressing. The nonadherent material must have wide-enough pores to allow unrestricted passage of air and fluid. Because tissue growth into the V.A.C. dressing may cause adherence, also consider V.A.C. WhiteFoam or more frequent dressing changes.

- Count the number of foam pieces removed; correlate the count with the number of foam pieces previously placed.
- Thoroughly inspect wound to ensure that all pieces of dressing components have been removed.

- If previous dressings were difficult to remove, make sure the dressing tubing is unclamped, then introduce 10 to 30 cc of normal saline solution into the tubing to soak underneath the foam. Wait 15 to 30 minutes, then gently remove the dressing.
- If the patient experiences pain during a dressing change, the physician may order 1% lidocaine solution to be introduced down the tubing. After instilling the lidocaine, clamp the tube, and wait 15 to 20 minutes before gently removing the dressing.
- Discard disposables per facility protocol.

*See manufacturer's Instructions For Use: Safety Information and Dressing Application Instructions for complete information.
**Excludes V.A.C. Classic System.

OTHER PRODUCTS

OTHER PRODUCTS

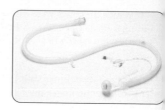

New Product

Zassi Bowel Management System

Hollister Incorporated

How supplied

Catheter kit: 4 cm, 6 cm
Collection bag with drain: 3 L
Single use collection bag: 2 L
Irrigation bag

Action

The Zassi Bowel Management System silicone catheter contains one retention cuff and one intralumenal balloon. The retention cuff is for rectal retention and sealing. The intralumenal balloon aids insertion of the catheter through the anus and occludes the inside of the catheter lumen during bowel irrigation or medication administration to retain the irrigant or medication in the colon-rectum. Adjacent to the retention cuff is a soft collapsible transsphincteric zone 4 or 6 cm long. A sheet clip located on the drain tube can be used to secure the catheter drain tube to the sheet. A flush/sampling port, located on the drain tube, provides access for catheter flushing (rinsing) and stool sampling.

Indications

To minimize external contact of feces with patient skin, to facilitate the collection of fecal matter for patients requiring stool management, to provide access for colonic irrigation and giving enema or medication

Contraindications

- Not for use in patients allergic to the materials used in this device
- Not for use if the patient's distal rectum can't accommodate the inflated volume of the retention cuff or if the distal rectum-anal canal is severely strictured
- Not for use in patients with impacted stool
- Not for use in patients with a recent (less than 6 weeks old) rectal anastomosis or anal or sphincter reconstruction
- Not for use in patients with compromised rectal wall integrity

Application

- Before using Zassi Bowel Management System, read the entire Zassi Bowel Management System Instructions for Use package insert supplied with the product. Read all other package inserts and labels supplied with the product and accessories.

Removal

- Federal law restricts this device for sale by or on the order of a physician.

Drugs

OVERVIEW

In this section, you'll find a list of products that are considered drugs because their administration provokes a series of physiochemical events within the body. The drugs listed in this section each have unique actions, indications, and contraindications specific to the individual product. This information can also be found on the product's package insert. The clinician holds responsibility for understanding how each of these products affects the cascade of wound-healing events.

Products listed in this section are reimbursed as prescription drugs. The clinician must contact the appropriate payor regarding specific payment information for a given drug.

ACCUZYME Papain-Urea
Healthpoint, Ltd.

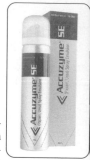

How supplied
Ointment:	6 g, 30 g
Spray:	33 ml
Spray emulsion (SE):	34 ml

Action
ACCUZYME is a debriding product that contains papain, the proteolytic enzyme from the fruit of carica papaya. Papain is a potent digestant of nonviable protein matter but is harmless to viable tissue. In ACCUZYME, papain is combined with urea, a denaturant of proteins, to bring about two supplemental chemical actions: to expose by solvent action the activators of papain, and to denature the nonviable protein matter in lesions and thereby render it more susceptible to enzymatic digestion. The combination of papain and urea results in twice as much digestive activity as papain alone.

Indications
For debridement of necrotic tissue and liquefaction of slough in acute and chronic lesions, such as pressure ulcers, varicose and diabetic ulcers, burns, postoperative wounds, pilonidal cyst wounds, carbuncles, and miscellaneous traumatic or infected wounds

Contraindications
- Contraindicated on patients who are sensitive to papain or any other component of this preparation

Application
- Clean wound with ALLCLENZ Wound Cleanser or saline solution. Avoid using hydrogen peroxide solution because it may inactivate the papain. Apply ACCUZYME ointment directly to wound, ¼" thick. For ACCUZYME spray, hold bottle 1" to 2" from wound, and apply single, even layer to completely cover wound. For ACCUZYME SE, hold bottle 2" to 4" from wound, and apply single layer to cover wound.
- Cover with dressing, and secure into place. Apply once or twice daily. Irrigate the wound at each redressing to remove any accumulation of liquefied necrotic material. *Note:* Papain may also be inactivated by the salts of heavy metals, such as lead, silver, and mercury. Contact with medications containing these metals should be avoided.

Removal
- Clean the wound with AllClenz Wound Cleanser or saline. Avoid using hydrogen peroxide solution because it may inactivate the papain.

BensalHP
AciesHealth, Inc.

How supplied
Topical ointment (tube): 15 g, 30 g

Action
BensalHP topical ointment contains 60 mg benzoic acid and 30 mg salicylic acid per gram in a base containing polyethylene glycol 400, polyethylene glycol 3350, and 30 mg per gram of oak bark extract (QRB-7). BensalHP reduces methicillin-resistant *Staphylococcus aureus* (MRSA) protected by biofilms in wounds using porcine models. BensalHP also stimulates reepithelialization of second-degree burns.

Indications
To treat the inflammation and irritation associated with many common forms of dermatitis, including certain eczematoid conditions; complications associated with pyodermas; insect bites; burns; and fungi

Contraindications
- Contraindicated on patients who are hypersensitive to topical polyethylene glycols

Application
- Hands should be washed thoroughly.
- Don't let the tip of the tube come into contact with the area to be treated.
- If applying with a cotton-tipped applicator, use once and discard.
- BensalHP Ointment should be applied twice per day for best results.
- Gently rinse the area to be treated with saline or water, and then pat dry. BensalHP Ointment can be applied directly to the wound or placed on dry gauze and then placed on the wound.
- Spread a generous quantity of BensalHP Ointment evenly over the desired area to yield a continuous layer about ⅛″ thick.
- The treated area may feel warm or burn for 3 to 5 minutes after application. If irritation occurs or symptoms persist after 10 days, discontinue use, and consult the physician.
- Try to keep the area being treated clean and exposed to air when possible. Apply an appropriate dressing to shield the area from clothes or exposure to water or dirt.
- BensalHP is designed to provide moisture to the wound.
- Wet-packs or wet-to-dry dressings aren't recommended because they dilute the ointment and decrease its effectiveness.
- If the wound doesn't improve in 7 days, consult a physician for further evaluation. If there is no response to the ointment, then the wound should be re-evaluated for other factors inhibiting the healing process.

Removal
- No information given by manufacturer

DRUGS

Cloderm Cream (clocortolone pivalate, 0.1%)
Healthpoint, Ltd.

How supplied
Cream: 15 g, 45 g, 90 g

Action
The mechanism of anti-inflammatory activity of topical steroids, such as Cloderm Cream, is unclear.

Indications
To relieve inflammation and pruritus caused by corticosteroid dermatoses, especially stasis and contact dermatitis; may be used under compression dressings

Contraindications
- Contraindicated in patients with sensitivity to any components of the preparation

Application
- Apply sparingly to affected area three times daily.
- Rub in gently.

Removal
- Gently cleanse the wound per facility protocol.
- Reapply per physician order.

Collagenase Santyl Ointment
Healthpoint, Ltd.

How supplied
Ointment: 15 g, 30 g

Action
Collagenase Santyl Ointment is a sterile enzymatic debriding ointment which contains 250 collagenase units per gram of white petrolatum USP. The enzyme collagenase is derived from the fermentation by *Clostridium histolyticum*. It possesses the unique ability to digest collagen in necrotic tissue.

Because collagen accounts for 75% of the dry weight of skin tissue, the ability of collagenase to digest collagen in the physiological pH and temperature range makes it particularly effective in the removal of detritus. Collagenase thus contributes to the formation of granulation tissue and subsequent epithelialization of dermal ulcers and severely burned areas. Collagen in healthy tissue or in newly formed granulation tissue isn't attacked. No information is available on collagenase absorption through skin or its concentration in body fluids associated with therapeutic or toxic effects, degree of binding to plasma proteins, degree of uptake by a particular organ or in the fetus, and passage across the blood-brain barrier.

Indications
For debriding chronic dermal ulcers and severely burned areas

Contraindications
- Contraindicated on patients who have local or systemic hypersensitivity to collagenase

Application
- Before application, wound should be cleansed of debris and digested material by gently rubbing with a gauze pad saturated with normal saline solution, or with the desired cleansing agent compatible with Collagenase Santyl Ointment, followed by a normal saline solution rinse.
- Whenever infection is present, it is desirable to use an appropriate topical antibiotic powder. The antibiotic should be applied to the wound prior to the application of Collagenase Santyl Ointment. Should the infection not respond, therapy with Collagenase Santyl Ointment should be discontinued until remission of the infection.
- Collagenase Santyl Ointment may be applied directly to the wound or to a sterile gauze pad, which is then applied to the wound and properly secured.

Removal
- Use of Collagenase Santyl Ointment should be terminated when debridement of necrotic tissue is complete and granulation tissue is well established.

DRUGS

Ethezyme

Ethezyme 830

Ethex Corporation

How supplied
Tube: 1 oz (30 g)

Action
Each gram of Ethezyme enzymatic debriding ointment contains Papain, USP, (1.1×10^6 USP units of activity) and 100 mg Urea, USP. Each gram of Ethezyme 830 enzymatic debriding ointment contains Papain, USP (8.3×10^5 USP units of activity) and 100 mg Urea, USP. Papain is a potent digestant of nonviable protein matter but is harmless to viable tissue. It's active over a wide pH range, from 3 to 12. Despite its recognized value as a digestive agent, papain is relatively ineffective when used alone as a debriding agent, primarily because it requires activators for its digestive function. Urea is combined with papain to provide two supplementary chemical actions to produce twice as much digestion as papain alone.

Indications
For debridement of necrotic tissue and liquefaction of pus in acute and chronic lesions, such as pressure, varicose, and diabetic ulcers; burns; postoperative wounds; pilonidal cyst wounds; carbuncles; and miscellaneous traumatic or infected wounds

Contraindications
- Contraindicated on patients who have shown sensitivity to papain or any other component of this preparation
- Not for contact with medications containing salts of heavy metals, such as lead, silver, and mercury

Application
- Apply either Ethezyme or Ethezyme 830 debriding ointment directly to lesion, and cover with appropriate dressing. Daily or twice-daily changes of dressings are preferred.
- At each redressing, the lesion should be irrigated with isotonic saline solution, or other mild cleansing solution (except hydrogen peroxide solution, which may inactivate the papain) to remove any accumulation of liquefied necrotic material.

Removal
- Gently cleanse the wound per facility protocol.
- Reapply per physician order.

Gladase Papain-Urea Debriding Ointment
Smith & Nephew, Inc.
Wound Management

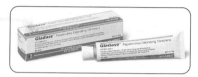

How supplied
Tube: 30 g

Action
Papain is a potent digestant of nonviable protein matter but is harmless to viable tissue. It's active over a pH range of 3 to 12. Papain is relatively ineffective when used alone as a debriding agent and requires the presence of activators to stimulate its digestive potency. In Gladase Papain-Urea Debriding Ointment, papain is combined with urea, a denaturant of proteins, to bring about two supplemental chemical actions: to expose by solvent action the activators of papain, and to denature the nonviable protein matter in lesions and thereby render it more susceptible to enzymatic digestion. The combination of papain and urea result in twice as much digestive activity as papain alone.

Indications
For debridement of necrotic tissue and liquifaction of slough in acute and chronic lesions such as pressure ulcers, varicose and diabetic ulcers, burns, postoperative wounds, pilonidal cyst wounds, carbuncles, and miscellaneous traumatic or infected wounds

Contraindications
- Contraindicated in patients who have a sensitivity to papain or any other component of this preparation
- Not for contact with salts of heavy metals such as lead, silver, and mercury
- Not for contact with hydrogen peroxide solution

Application
- Clean the wound with a wound cleanser or saline solution.
- Irrigate the wound at each redressing to remove any accumulation of liquefied necrotic material.
- Apply Gladase Papain-Urea Debriding Ointment directly to the wound.
- Cover with an appropriate dressing and secure in place.

Removal
- Irrigate the wound at each redressing to remove any accumulation of liquefied necrotic material.
- Reapply product once or twice daily as preferred.

DRUGS

Granulex

Mylan Bertek Pharmaceuticals, Inc.

How supplied

Aerosol can: 2 oz, 4 oz

Action

Granulex is a topical aerosol wound spray that relieves
pain and promotes healing; debrides eschar and necrotic tissue physiologically; stimulates vascular bed; improves epithelization by reducing premature epithe-
lial desiccation and cornification; and reduces odor from malodorous
necrotic wounds.

Indications

To aid in the management of varicose and decubital ulcers, dehiscent
wounds, and sunburn; to promote wound healing and debride eschar

Contraindications

- Not for use on fresh arterial clots

Application

- Gently clean the affected area.
- Shake can well before spraying.
- For stage 1 pressure ulcers, spray lightly into a gloved hand, and very
  gently apply to the area.
- For stages 2 through 4 pressure ulcers, hold can upright and about 12"
  from the area to be treated. Press valve and coat wound rapidly.
- Leave wound unbandaged, or apply a wet dressing.
- Apply twice daily or as often as necessary.

Removal

- Gently wash the affected area with water.

PANAFIL Papain, Urea, Chlorophyllin Copper Complex Sodium
Healthpoint, Ltd.

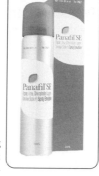

How supplied
Ointment:	6 g, 30 g
Spray:	33 ml
Spray emulsion (SE):	34 ml

Action
PANAFIL is a healing, debriding, and deodorizing product that contains papain, the proteolytic enzyme derived from the papaya fruit. Papain is a potent digestant of nonviable protein matter but is harmless to viable tissue. It's active over a pH range from 3 to 12. Papain is relatively ineffective when used alone as a debriding agent, so it's combined with urea to produce twice as much digestion as papain alone. Chlorophyllin copper complex sodium adds healing action to the cleansing action of the papain-urea combination. Chlorophyllin copper complex sodium promotes healthy granulations, controls local inflammation, and reduces wound odors.

Indications
To facilitate enzymatic debridement of necrotic tissue and liquefaction of fibrinous, purulent debris to cleanse and promote normal healing of varicose, diabetic, and pressure ulcers; burns; postoperative wounds; pilonidal cyst wounds; carbuncles; and miscellaneous traumatic or infected wounds

Contraindications
- Contraindicated for use on patients with sensitivity to papain or any other component of this preparation
- Not for contact with heavy metals, such as lead, silver, and mercury

Application
- Clean the wound with AllClenz Wound Cleanser or saline solution. Avoid using hydrogen peroxide solution because it may inactivate the papain. Apply ¼" thickness of PANAFIL to the wound. For PANAFIL spray, hold bottle 1" to 2" from wound, and apply a single, even layer to completely cover the wound. For PANAFIL SE, hold spray bottle 2" to 4" from wound, and apply a single layer to cover wound bed.
- Once or twice daily, cover with appropriate dressing and secure into place. Irrigate the wound at each redressing to remove any accumulation of liquefied necrotic material.

Removal
- Clean wound with AllClenz Wound Cleanser or saline solution. Avoid using hydrogen peroxide solution because it may inactivate the papain.

PRUDOXIN Doxepin Hydrochloride Cream, 5%
Healthpoint, Ltd.

How supplied
Cream: 45 g

Action
PRUDOXIN's exact mechanism of action is unknown. A histamine blocker, it appears to compete at histamine-1 and histamine-2 receptor sites and inhibit their biological activation.

Indications
For short-term management (up to 8 days) of moderate pruritus in adult patients with atopic dermatitis or lichen simplex chronicus

Contraindications
- Contraindicated on patients with untreated narrow-angle glaucoma
- Contraindicated on patients with a tendency to urine retention

Application
- Apply a thin film of the cream to affected areas three or four times per day.
- Allow at least 3 to 4 hours between applications.

Removal
- The dosage should be repeated as required.

REGRANEX (becaplermin) Gel 0.01%

Johnson & Johnson
Wound Management
A division of ETHICON, Inc.

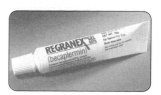

How supplied
Tube: 15 g

Action
Regranex Gel is the only FDA–approved growth factor that activates cells to form new granulation tissue and blood vessels, closing diabetic foot ulcers fast (average healing time 12.3 weeks).

Indications
For the treatment of lower-extremity diabetic neuropathic ulcers that extend into the subcutaneous tissue or beyond and have an adequate blood supply

Contraindications
- Not for treatment of ischemic diabetic ulcers, pressure ulcers, venous stasis ulcers, or diabetic neuropathic ulcers that don't extend through the dermis into subcutaneous tissue (stage 1 or 2, International Association of Enterostomal Therapy staging classification)
- Contraindicated on patients with hypersensitivity to any of the product's components (such as parabens)
- Contraindicated on patients with neoplasms at the site of application
- Not for use on wounds that close by primary intention because it's a nonsterile, low-bioburden, preserved product

Application
- Debride the wound. (Sharp debridement is recommended.)
- Apply the gel once daily in a carefully measured quantity. The daily dose should be recalculated weekly or biweekly by the physician.
- Squeeze the calculated length of gel onto a clean, firm, nonabsorbent surface, such as waxed paper. Don't allow the tip of the tube to touch the wound or any other surface.
- Using a clean cotton swab, tongue blade, or similar tool, spread the measured gel evenly over the wound in a continuous layer ¼" (0.2 cm) thick.
- Cover with a saline-moistened gauze dressing.

Removal
- After about 12 hours, gently rinse the ulcer with normal saline solution or water to remove residual gel.
- Cover with saline-moistened gauze; don't reapply the gel.

DRUGS

Xenaderm Ointment

Balsam Peru, Castor Oil USP/NF, Trypsin USP

Healthpoint, Ltd.

How supplied
Tube: 30 g, 60 g

Action
Balsam Peru is an effective capillary bed stimulant used to increase blood supply to the wound site. Castor oil is used to improve epithelialization by reducing premature epithelial desiccation and cornification. Also, it can act as a protective covering and aids in the reduction of pain. Trypsin is intended for debridement of eschar and other necrotic tissue. It appears that, in many instances, removal of wound debris strengthens humoral defense mechanisms sufficiently to retard proliferation of local pathogens.

Indications
To promote healing and the treatment of pressure ulcers, varicose ulcers, and dehiscent wounds

Contraindications
■ Contraindicated in patients with sensitivity to any of the product's components

Application
■ Apply a thin film of Xenaderm twice daily or as often as necessary. The wound may be left unbandaged or appropriate dressing may be applied.

Removal
■ To remove, wash gently with appropriate cleanser.

PART THREE

ADDITIONAL DRESSINGS AND PRODUCTS

OVERVIEW

Part 3 provides a comprehensive listing of additional products: abdominal dressing holders and binders, tapes and closures, wound pouches, wound cleansers, gauzes, elastic bandages, and compression bandage systems.

Because of the high volume of general products that are manufactured, the section groups similar products into tables. The table headings closely follow the categories outlined by the Medicare Part B Surgical Dressing Policy. Each table may include more than one category. In that case, as appropriate, each representative category and its respective Health Care Financing Administration Common Procedure Coding System (HCPCS) code are identified above the table.

Inclusion in these tables doesn't mean that the manufacturers have applied for or received the HCPCS code identified above the tables. The provider and supplier are responsible for verifying the correct HCPCS codes before submitting claims to any payer.

To ensure uniform Medicare claim coding by all suppliers of wound care dressings, the Statistical Analysis Durable Medical Equipment Regional Carrier (SADMERC) performs a Coding Verification Review. If manufacturers wish to have a HCPCS code assigned to their products, they must formally apply to the SADMERC.

SADMERC and the four Durable Medical Equipment Regional Carriers (DMERCs) review the applications to determine the correct HCPCS codes for Medicare billing. These reviews result in a consensus coding decision. The assignment of an HCPCS code to a product should not be construed as an approval or endorsement of the product by SADMERC or Medicare and doesn't imply or guarantee reimbursement or coverage.

Many other payers also require the assigned HCPCS codes on their claim forms.

Abdominal dressing holders or binders

Abdominal dressing holders or binders are hypoallergenic adhesive straps used in place of standard surgical tapes to avoid removing and reapplying tape during dressing changes.

The HCPCS code normally assigned to abdominal dressing holders or binders is A4462.

Product name
Medfix Montgomery Straps

Manufacturer/Distributor
Medline Industries, Inc.

Compression bandage systems

Compression therapy products are used to manage edema and promote the return of venous blood flow to the heart. Conventional management with zinc oxide–impregnated bandaging systems, such as an Unna boot, provides inelastic compression. Multilayered, sustained, graduated, high-compression bandages aid in the management of wounds caused by venous insufficiency.

Each component used in the compression therapy system is billed using a specific code for the component, if available. The HCPCS codes normally assigned to compression bandage systems are:

Light compression bandage
A6448: Width < 3″ per yard
A6449: Width ≥ 3″ and < 5″ per yard
A6450: Width ≥ 5″ per yard

Moderate-high compression bandage
A6451: Moderate compression bandage, load resistance of 1.25 to 1.34 foot pounds at 50% maximum stretch, width > 3″ and < 5″ per yard
A6452: High compression bandage, load resistance ≥ 1.35 foot pounds at 50% maximum stretch, width ≥ 3″ and < 5″ per yard

Self-adherent bandage
A6453: Width < 3″ per yard
A6454: Width ≥ 3″ and < 5″ per yard
A6455: Width ≥ 5″ per yard

Conforming bandage
A6442: Width < 3″ per yard
A6443: Width ≥ 3″ and < 5″ per yard
A6444: Width > 5″ per yard
A6445: Width < 3″ per yard
A6446: Width ≥ 3″ and < 5″ per yard
A6447: Width ≥ 5″ per yard

Padding bandage
A6441: Width $\geq$ 3″ and < 5″ per yard

Zinc paste-impregnated bandage
A6456: Width $\geq$ 3″ and < 5″ per yard

Product name	Manufacturer/ Distributor	Type of compression	Subcategory
AltoPress	Derma Sciences, Inc.	Elastic	Single-layer compression system
DeWrap	DeRoyal	Elastic	Multi-layer compression system
Duboot Two-Layer Paste Bandage System	Derma Sciences, Inc.	Elastic/ Inelastic	Cohesive wrap/Unna boot
Dufore Four-Layer Compression Bandaging System	Derma Sciences, Inc.	Elastic	Multi-layer compression system
DYNA-FLEX Multi-Layer Compression System	Johnson & Johnson Wound Management A division of ETHICON, Inc.	Elastic	Multi-layer compression system
FourFlex 4-Layer Bandage System	Medline Industries, Inc.	Elastic	Multi-layer compression system
Profore Four Layer Bandaging System	Smith & Nephew, Inc. Wound Management	Elastic	Multi-layer compression system
Profore Latex Free Four Layer Bandage System	Smith & Nephew, Inc. Wound Management	Elastic	Multi-layer compression system
Profore Lite Multi-Layer Compression Bandage System	Smith & Nephew, Inc. Wound Management	Elastic	Multi-layer compression system
Profore LF Multi-Layer High Compression Bandage System	Smith & Nephew, Inc. Wound Management	Elastic	Multi-layer compression system
Profore Lite Multi-Layer Reduced Compression Bandage System	Smith & Nephew, Inc. Wound Management	Elastic	Multi-layer compression system
Profore Multi-Layer High Compression Bandage System	Smith & Nephew, Inc. Wound Management	Elastic	Multi-layer compression system
ProGuide Multi-Layer High Compression Bandage System	Smith & Nephew, Inc. Wound Management	Inelastic	Unna boot/paste bandage

*Denotes new product

Product name	Manufacturer/Distributor	Type of compression	Subcategory
Tenderwrap Unna Boot Bandage	Tyco/Kendall Healthcare	Elastic	Multi-layer compression system
*ThreeFlex Three-Layer Compression Bandaging System	Medline Industries, Inc.	Elastic	Multi-layer compression system
Tresflex Three-Layer Compression Bandaging System	Derma Sciences, Inc.	Inelastic	Paste bandage
Unna Boot	DeRoyal	Elastic	Unna boot
UNNA FLEX Plus Venous Ulcer	ConvaTec	Elastic	Unna boot
UNNA-FLEX Plus Venous Ulcer Convenience Pack	ConvaTec	Inelastic	Unna boot/paste bandage
UnnaPress Paste Bandage	Derma Sciences, Inc.	Inelastic	Unna boot/paste bandage

Conforming bandages

The HCPCS codes normally assigned to conforming bandages are:

Conforming bandage, nonsterile
A6442: Width < 3" per yard
A6443: Width ≥ 3" and < 5" per yard
A6444: Width ≥ 5" per yard

Conforming bandage, sterile
A6445: Width < 3" per yard
A6446: Width ≥ 3" and < 5" per yard
A6447: Width ≥ 5" per yard

Packing strips, nonimpregnated
A6407: Up to 2" wide, per linear yard

Product name	Manufacturer/Distributor
Bulkee II	Medline Industries, Inc.
Bulkee Lite 100% Nonsterile Cotton Bandage	Medline Industries, Inc.
Bulkee Lite 100% Sterile Cotton Bandage	Medline Industries, Inc.
Cotton Plain Packing	Derma Sciences, Inc.
CURITY Packing Strips	Tyco Healthcare/Kendall
Duform Synthetic Conforming Bandage	Derma Sciences, Inc.

*Denotes new product

Product name	Manufacturer/Distributor
FLUFTEX Rolls	DeRoyal
KERLIX LITE	Tyco Healthcare/Kendall
Kerlix Rolls	Tyco Healthcare/Kendall
Medline Plain Packing Strips	Medline Industries, Inc.
Pak-Its Gauze Packing Strips – Plain	Derma Sciences, Inc.
Packing Strips	Medline Industries, Inc.
Packing Strips with Iodoform	Medline Industries, Inc.

Elastic bandage rolls

The HCPCS codes normally assigned elastic bandage rolls are:

Light compression bandage
A6448: Width < 3″ per yard
A6449: Width ≥ 3″ and < 5″ per yard
A6450: Width ≥ 5″ per yard

Moderate-high compression bandage
A6451: Moderate compression bandage, load resistance of 1.25 to 1.34 foot pounds at 50% maximum stretch, width ≥ 3″ and < 5″ per yard
A6452: High compression bandage, load resistance greater than or equal to 1.35 foot pounds at 50% maximum stretch, width ≥ 3″ and < 5″ per yard

Self-adherent bandage
A6453: Width < 3″ per yard
A6454: Width ≥ 3″ and < 5″ per yard
A6455: Width ≥ 5″ per yard
A6457: Tubular dressing with or without elastic, any width, per linear yard

Product name	Manufacturer/Distributor
3M Coban Self-Adherent Wrap	3M Health Care
Compriband	Derma Sciences, Inc.
CURITY Elastic Bandage	Tyco Healthcare/Kendall
Duban Cohesive Elastic Bandage	Derma Sciences, Inc.
Duflex Synthetic Conforming Bandage	Derma Sciences, Inc.
DuGrip Tubular Bandage	Derma Sciences, Inc.
Dsor Elastic Bandage – with Clips	Derma Sciences, Inc.
Elastive Adhesive Bandage - Nonlatex	Derma Sciences, Inc.
FLEX-WRAP Self-Adherent Wrap	Tyco Healthcare/Kendall
Matrix Latex Free Elastic Bandage with Double Velcro	Medline Industries, Inc.
MediGrip Tubular Elastic Bandage	Medline Industries, Inc.

Product name	Manufacturer/Distributor
SetoPress High Compression Banadage	ConvaTec
Soft Wrap Elastic Bandage	Medline Industries, Inc.
SurePress High Compression Bandage	ConvaTec
Swift Wrap Elastic Bandage with Single Velcro	Medline Industries, Inc.
TENSOR Elastic Bandage	Tyco Healthcare/Kendall
Tubigrip Shaped Support Bandage	ConvaTec
Tubifast Cut Dressing Retention Bandage	ConvaTec

Gauze, impregnated with other than water, normal saline, or hydrogel, without adhesive border

Impregnated gauze dressings are woven or nonwoven materials in which substances such as iodinated agents, petrolatum, zinc compounds, crystalline sodium chloride, chlorbexadine gluconate, bismuth tribromophenate, aqueous saline, or other agents have been incorporated into the dressing material by the manufacturer.

The HCPCS codes normally assigned to gauze, impregnated with other than water, normal saline, or hydrogel, without adhesive border are:

A6222: Pad size ≤ 16 in^2
A6223: Pad size > 16 in^2 but < 48 in^2
A6224: Pad size > 48 in^2

Product name	Manufacturer/Distributor
ADAPTIC Non-Adhering Dressing	Johnson & Johnson Wound Management, a division of ETHICON, Inc.
ADAPTIC X Xeroform Gauze Non Adherent Dressing	Johnson & Johnson Wound Management, a division of ETHICON, Inc.
Bulkee II 4" × 4" 12 ply sponges	Medline Industries, Inc.
Bulkee II Super Fluff Sponges	Medline Industries, Inc.
CURASALT Sodium Chloride Dressing	Tyco Healthcare/Kendall
Curity AMD–Antimicrobial Dressings	Tyco Healthcare/Kendall
Curity Oil Emulsion Dressing	Tyco Healthcare/Kendall
CUTICERIN Low Adherent Dressing	Smith & Nephew, Inc. Wound Management
DERMAGRAN (Zinc-Saline) Wet Dressing	Derma Sciences, Inc.
Kerlix AMD–Antimicrobial Dressing	Tyco Healthcare/Kendall
Kerlix/Curity Saline Dressing	Tyco Healthcare/Kendall

*Denotes new product

Product name	Manufacturer/Distributor
Medline Oil Emulsion	Medline Industries, Inc.
Medline Petrolatum Gauze	Medline Industries, Inc.
Medline Xeroform Gauze	Medline Industries, Inc.
Medi-Tech Hydrophilic Gauze	Medi-Tech International Corporation
Mesalt	Mölnlycke Health Care
Mesalt Ribbon	Mölnlycke Health Care
*Oil Emulsion	DeRoyal
Pak-Its Gauze Packing Strips – Iodoform	Derma Sciences, Inc.
Vaseline Petrolatum Gauze	Tyco Healthcare/Kendall
Xeroflo Gauze Dressing	Tyco Healthcare/Kendall
Xeroform Petrolatum Gauze	Tyco Healthcare/Kendall
*Xerofoam	DeRoyal

Gauze, impregnated with water or normal saline, without adhesive border

The HCPCS codes normally assigned to gauze, impregnated with water or normal saline, without an adhesive border are:
A6228: Pad size $\leq$ 16 in^2
A6229: Pad size > 16 in^2 but $\leq$ 48 in^2
A6230: Pad size > 48 in^2

Product name	Manufacturer/Distributor
CURITY Saline Dressing	Tyco Healthcare/Kendall
Dumex Wet Dressings	Derma Sciences, Inc.
MPM Gauze Impregnated Saline Dressing	MPM Medical, Inc.
Pak-Its Saline Impregnated Gauze	Derma Sciences, Inc.

Gauze, nonimpregnated, with adhesive border

The HCPCS codes normally assigned to gauze, nonimpregnated, with an adhesive border are:
A6219: Pad size $\leq$ 16 in^2
A6220: Pad size > 16 in^2 but $\leq$ 48 in^2
A6221: Pad size > 48 in^2

Product name	Manufacturer/Distributor
Bordered Gauze Dressing	Carrington Laboratories
CovRSite	Smith & Nephew, Inc. Wound Management

*Denotes new product

Product name	**Manufacturer/Distributor**
ConvaTec	Smith & Nephew, Inc. Wound Management
DermaRite Bordered Gauze	DermaRite Industries
Gentell Bordered Gauze	Gentell, Inc.
Medline Bordered Gauze	Medline Industries, Inc.
Mepore Absorbent Island Dressing	Mölnlycke Health Care
*Mepore Pro	Mölnlycke Health Care

Gauze, nonimpregnated, without adhesive border

The HCPCS codes normally assigned to gauze, nonimpregnated, without an adhesive border are:

Gauze, nonimpregnated, sterile
A6402: Pad size $\leq$ 16 in^2
A6403: Pad size > 16 in^2 but $\leq$ 48 in^2
A6404: Pad size > 48 in^2

Gauze, nonimpregnated, nonsterile
A6216: Pad size $\leq$ 16 in^2
A6217: Pad size > 16 in^2 but $\leq$ 48 in^2
A6218: Pad size > 48 in^2

Product name	**Manufacturer/Distributor**
Avant Gauze—Nonsterile	Medline Industries, Inc.
Avant Gauze Drain Sponge	Medline Industries, Inc.
Bulkee Super Fluff Sponges	Medline Industries, Inc.
Curity Cover Sponges	Tyco Healthcare/Kendall
Curity Gauze Pads	Tyco Healthcare/Kendall
Curity Gauze Sponges	Tyco Healthcare/Kendall
Ducare Gauze Dressings/Sponges	Derma Sciences, Inc.
Dulix 6-ply Fluff Sponge	Derma Sciences, Inc.
Dusoft Non-Woven Dressings/Sponges	Derma Sciences, Inc.
EXCILON Drain Sponge	Tyco Healthcare/Kendall
FLUFTEX Sponges	DeRoyal
Kerlix 4x4 Sponges	Tyco Healthcare/Kendall
Kerlix Packing Sponges	Tyco Healthcare/Kendall
Mediline Borderless Composite Dressing	Medline Industries, Inc.
Medline Gauze Pads—Bulk, Nonsterile	Medline Industries, Inc.

---

*Denotes new product

Product name	Manufacturer/Distributor
*Medline Gauze Pads–Sterile	Medline Industries, Inc.
PrimaPad Nonadherent Absorbent Pad	Derma Sciences, Inc.
Sof-Form	Medline Industries, Inc.

Tapes

Securing a wound cover is an essential step in the management process. One way to secure a wound cover is with the use of tapes. Each product is manufactured using various materials, widths, adhesives, and hypoallergenic properties.

The HCPCS codes normally assigned tapes and closures are:
A4450: Nonwaterproof, per 18 in^2
A4452: Waterproof, per 18 in^2

Product name	Manufacturer/Distributor
3M Blenderm Surgical Tape	3M Health Care
3M Cloth Adhesive Tape	3M Health Care
3M Durapore Surgical Tape	3M Health Care
3M Medipore H Soft Cloth Surgical Tape	3M Health Care
3M Medipore Pre-Cut Dressing Covers	3M Health Care
3M Medipore Soft Cloth Surgical Tape	3M Health Care
3M Microfoam Surgical Tape	3M Health Care
3M Microfoam Surgical Tape Patch	3M Health Care
3M Micropore Surgical Tape	3M Health Care
3M Transpore White Dressing Tape	3M Health Care
3M Transpore Surgical Tape	3M Health Care
CONFORM Elastic Tape	Tyco Healthcare/Kendall
CURASILK	Tyco Healthcare/Kendall
CURITY Clear	Tyco Healthcare/Kendall
CURITY Standard Porous	Tyco Healthcare/Kendall
Episeal	DeRoyal
Hypafix Dressing Retention Rolls	Smith & Nephew, Inc. Wound Management
Medfix Dressing Retention Waterproof Tape	Medline Industries, Inc.
Medfix Cloth Tape	Medline Industries, Inc.
Medfix EZ Dressing Retention Tape	Medline Industries, Inc.
Medfix Ortho-Porous Sports Tape	Medline Industries, Inc.
Medfix Paper Tape	Medline Industries, Inc.

---

*Denotes new product

---

i refers to an illustration; t refers to a table; **boldface** indicates color pages.
